Innovative Production Strategies for High-Quality, Traditional Pig Products

Innovative Production Strategies for High-Quality, Traditional Pig Products

Editors

Giovanna Martelli
Eleonora Nannoni

MDPI • Basel • Beijing • Wuhan • Barcelona • Belgrade • Manchester • Tokyo • Cluj • Tianjin

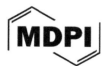

Editors
Giovanna Martelli
Department of Veterinary
Medical Sciences (DIMEVET)
University of Bologna
Ozzano Emilia (BO)
Italy

Eleonora Nannoni
Department of Veterinary
Medical Sciences (DIMEVET)
University of Bologna
Ozzano Emilia (BO)
Italy

Editorial Office
MDPI
St. Alban-Anlage 66
4052 Basel, Switzerland

This is a reprint of articles from the Special Issue published online in the open access journal *Animals* (ISSN 2076-2615) (available at: www.mdpi.com/journal/animals/special_issues/Innovative_production_strategies_high-quality_traditional_pig_products).

For citation purposes, cite each article independently as indicated on the article page online and as indicated below:

LastName, A.A.; LastName, B.B.; LastName, C.C. Article Title. *Journal Name* **Year**, *Volume Number*, Page Range.

ISBN 978-3-0365-1400-0 (Hbk)
ISBN 978-3-0365-1399-7 (PDF)

Contents

Preface to "Innovative Production Strategies for High-Quality, Traditional Pig Products"

In a number of European countries (e.g., Spain, Italy, France, Portugal, Slovenia, Croatia, Poland), a portion of the pig sector is aimed at the production of traditional and certified products (e.g., PDO—Protected Designation of Origin, PGI—Protected Geographical Indication). Dry-cured ham is probably the most famous traditional pork product; however, typical pork products are produced in (and exported to) many countries worldwide. The meat used for producing these high-quality delicacies needs to be suitable for seasoning and dry-curing, and these characteristics are the result of complex interactions between the animal (breed, genotype, rearing condition, feeding regime, age and weight at slaughter, etc.) and the environment, without disregarding the importance of ethical attributes such as animal welfare and the environmental impact.

This Special Issue focuses on all the innovative production strategies for pigs intended for high-quality, typical productions (in terms of higher sustainability of the whole production chain, improvement of animal welfare, innovative feeding and farming techniques, reduction in environmental impact, improvement in meat and fat quality, etc.), with emphasis on PDOs, PGIs, and other recognized production schemes, and it is aimed at providing new insights for a wide range of stakeholders from different countries.

Giovanna Martelli, Eleonora Nannoni
Editors

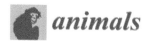

Article

High Altitude Adaptability and Meat Quality in Tibetan Pigs: A Reference for Local Pork Processing and Genetic Improvement

Mailin Gan [1,2,†], Linyuan Shen [1,2,†], Yuan Fan [1,2], Zhixian Guo [1,2], Bin Liu [1,2], Lei Chen [1,2], Guoqing Tang [1,2], Yanzhi Jiang [1,2], Xuewei Li [1,2], Shunhua Zhang [1,2], Lin Bai [1,2,*] and Li Zhu [1,2,*]

[1] College of Animal Science and Technology, Sichuan Agricultural University, Chengdu 611130, Sichuan, China; gml1660600546@163.com (M.G.); shenlinyuan0815@163.com (L.S.); fanyuan0701@163.com (Y.Z.); guozhixian521@outlook.com (Z.G.); 13018240830@163.com (B.L.); chenlei815918@163.com (L.C.); tyq003@163.com (G.T.); jiangyz04@163.com (Y.J.); xuewei.li@sicau.edu.cn (X.L.); zhangsh1919@163.com (S.Z.)

[2] Farm Animal Genetic Resources Exploration and Innovation Key Laboratory of Sichuan Province, Sichuan Agricultural University, Chengdu 611130, Sichuan, China

* Correspondence: blin16@126.com (L.B.); zhuli7508@163.com (L.Z.); Tel.: +86-28-8629-1133 (L.B. & L.Z.)

† These authors contributed equally to this work.

Received: 2 October 2019; Accepted: 20 November 2019; Published: 3 December 2019

Simple Summary: The increase in altitude will bring about a complex change in a series of elements of nature, which will have a profound impact on human production and life. Studying domestic animals in the native environment is an effective way to explore the impact of high altitude on human life, and at the same time is conducive to the development of local animal husbandry. Here, we found that the hypoxic adaptation of Tibetan pigs may be related to higher levels of *VEGFA*, *HIF1* and myoglobin expression. The higher aerobic oxidative capacity of Tibetan pigs is beneficial to improve energy utilization, and the higher UFA content of Tibetan pigs is beneficial to cold resistance. In addition, Tibetan pigs have higher levels of BCAA and *Myh2* expression, which serve to relieve muscle fatigue and improve endurance. In addition, it was observed that there are obvious differences in carcass and meat quality traits of different altitudes pigs. Taken together, our findings illustrate the adaptability of Tibetan pigs to high altitude from various perspectives and compare carcass and meat quality traits of three pig breeds.

Abstract: The carcass and meat quality traits of pig breeds living at three different altitudes (Yorkshire pigs, YP: 500 m; Qingyu Pigs, QYP: 1500 m; Tibetan pigs, TP: 2500 m) were compared. It was observed that there are obvious differences in pig breeds with respect to performance parameters. Specifically, YP had the best carcass traits, showing high slaughter rates and leanest meat. Conversely, QYP had the highest back fat thickness and intramuscular fat (IMF) content. For the high-altitude breed TP, the animals exhibited low L* and high a* values. The genotypes contributing to the observed phenotypes were supported by a PCR analysis. The glycolytic genes expression (HK, PFK, PK) were highest in YP, whereas expression of genes related to adipogenesis (C/EBPα, FABP4, SCD1) were highest in QYP. As expected, genes associated with angiogenesis and hypoxia (*HIF1a*, *VEGFA*) were expressed at the highest levels in TP. The composition and proportion of amino and fatty acids in pig muscles at the three altitudes examined also varied substantially. Among the breeds, TP had the highest proportion of umami amino acids, whereas QYP had the highest proportion of sweet amino acids. However, TP also exhibited the highest proportion of essential fatty acids and the lowest proportion of n6:n3. This study explains the high-altitude adaptive evolution and the formation of meat quality differences in different altitude pigs from various angles and provides a reference for local pork food processing and genetic improvement of local pigs.

Keywords: altitude; carcass quality; meat quality; amino acid; fatty acid

1. Introduction

In many countries and regions, the various cultures have a tradition of eating pork as a central part of their diet. According to Food and Agriculture Organization of the United Nations (FAO, http://www.fao.org/faostat/zh/#data/QL), global pork production and consumption have long exceeded 30% of the total meat production and consumption. The development of pig production and related industries has greatly improved the quality of life of people worldwide [1]. Pig carcass and meat quality traits are the most economically important features for breeders, food developers, and consumers. Traditionally, pig breeders have pursued high growth rates and lean meat. Consequently, these traits have resulted in less desirable pork. However, consumers have recently begun to pursue meat of higher quality and flavor [2]. Heirloom and local pig breeds provide these rich traits for the development of pork [3,4].

Yorkshire pigs (YP) are one of the main varieties of the modern pig industry, with high growth rates and lean meat percentage, which is representative of the advanced breeding levels. Qingyu Pigs (QYP) are typical fat-type Chinese local pig breeds that is widely distributed throughout the mountain areas around the Sichuan Basin [5]. Tibetan pigs (TP) are typical high-altitude pig breeds that live on the Qinghai-Tibet Plateau, and are important to the lives of about 11 million people residing on the plateau. The extremely high-altitude adaptability of Tibetan pigs is not observable in other pig breeds [6]. In-depth research on Tibetan pigs also helps us understand the hypoxic adaptation of plateau species [7].

The development of novel pig breeds through selective breeding is a long and complex process, which is often determined by both the local environment and people's eating habits [8]. In-depth studies of pork quality not only provide a reference for improved breeding and food development of pigs, but can also provide insights into the local history and social culture. Protecting local germplasm resources is of great significance for the maintenance and promotion local food culture.

In the current study, the carcass traits, meat quality, amino acid, and fatty acid composition of pig breeds were examined. Additionally, the expression of genes involved in muscle development, fat deposition, and glycolysis were examined as well. All of these traits were examined in the context of the environmental and social factors that influence pork quality differences, and sought to understand food development strategies based on meat quality indicators. The results of this research can serve as a reference for local specialty food development and local pig genetic improvement.

2. Materials and Methods

All experimental protocols and procedures conducted are in accordance with the requirements of the Sichuan Agricultural University Ethics Committee.

2.1. Animals and Treatments

A total of 80 pigs were used in this study: 39 Yorkshire pigs (YP), including 20 males and 19 females, slaughtered at 180 days of age; 17 Qingyu pigs (QYP), including 8 males and 9 females (QYP1—5 pigs slaughtered at 180 days of age; QYP2—12 pigs, slaughtered at 300 days of age); 24 Tibetan pigs (TP), including 12 males and 12 females, slaughtered at 300 days of age. Altitude distribution of three pig breeds was shown in Figure 1. All male pigs were castrated. Ingredients of the basal experiment diets is shown in Table S1. After fasting with ad libitum access to water for 24 h, pigs were electrically stunned and exsanguinated. Approximately 10 g of a tissue core was collected from the last rib of the longissimus dorsi muscle, immediately placed in liquid nitrogen, and transferred to −80 °C for subsequent amino and fatty acid analysis, and qRT-PCR.

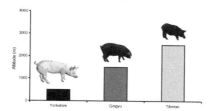

Figure 1. Altitude distribution of three pig breeds.

2.2. Measurement of Carcass Characteristics

Carcass weight was recorded after evisceration. Dressing percentage was calculated from the individual live weight and carcass weight measures (pig's head, internal organs, hooves and tail were removed from the carcasses) [4]. Accurately strip the muscles and bones of the pig carcass (the difference between the sum of each part and the weight before splitting was less than 1%). The carcass lean, fat, and bone percentages were calculated. Back fat depth (average of the seventh and last ribs, and the thickest part of the shoulder) were also assessed. Marbling score was performed using the standard 5 scoring scale system [4].

2.3. Measurement of Physical Correlates of Meat Quality

Muscle pH values of the longissimus dorsi muscle were measured at 45 min and 24 h postmortem using a portable pH meter (model 720A; Orion Research Inc., Boston, MA, USA). Meat color, including lightness (L*), redness (a*), and yellowness (b*) were assessed at 45 min and 24 h postmortem on the longissimus dorsi muscle using a Minolta CR-300 colorimeter (Minolta Camera, Osaka, Japan). Warner–Bratzler shear force (WBS) was determined using a texture analyzer (TA.XT. Plus, Stable Micro Systems, Godalming, UK) equipped with a Warner–Bratzler shearing device. After being stored at 4 °C for 72 h, a cuboid muscle of longissimus dorsi muscle was cooked in a circulating water bath held at 80 °C until the core temperature reached 70 °C, then cooled to room temperature. Hot dog shearing procedure was used in the test. Drip loss, shear force, and cooking loss of the longissimus dorsi muscle samples were measured as previously described [9,10].

2.4. Muscle Chemical Composition

Muscle chemical composition determination was performed as previously defined [10,11]. The crude protein was determined using the Kjeldahl method, and intramuscular fat content was determined by the Soxhlet extraction. Ash refers to the residue remaining after incineration of all organic materials in a high temperature furnace at 600 °C.

2.5. Quantitative Real-Time PCR

The frozen longissimus dorsi muscle was ground to a powder using liquid nitrogen, and total RNA was extracted from 40 mg of tissue homogenate using the triazole reagent (TaKaRa, Dalian Plateau, China). First strand cDNA was synthesized using the PrimeScript First Strand cDNA Synthesis Kit (TaKaRa). Quantitative real-time PCR (qRT-PCR) was performed using the SYBR Premix Ex Taq kit (TaKaRa) on a CFX96 real-time PCR detection system (Bio-Rad, Richmond, CA, USA). To calculate relative mRNA expression, the $2-\Delta\Delta Ct$ method [12] was used with β-actin as the internal reference. The primer sequences used for qRT-PCR are listed in Table S2.

2.6. Analysis of Free Amino Acids (FAA) and Fatty Acid

Prior to FAA analysis, 80 mg of tissue was homogenized, and 1000 uL pre-treatment solution (acetonitrile: water 1:1) was added. The suspensions were then shaken for 60 min. Next, the samples were centrifuged at 13,200 rpm/min for 10 min, and the supernatants were collected. The supernatant fluids were used to determine FAA composition using liquid chromatography-mass spectrometry (Liquid phase: LC-20AD, Shimadzu, Japan; Mass Spectrometry: 5500 Q TRAP LC-MS/MS, AB SCIEX, USA). Pretreatment of fatty acid samples was accomplished by homogenizing 100 mg of tissue. Next, 2 mL of n-hexane was added, and shaken at 50 °C for 30 min, at which point 3 mL of KOH methanol solution (0.4 mol/L) was added. The samples were then shaken for 30 min at 50 °C. Next, 1 mL of water and 2 mL of n-hexane were added, and the samples mixed. The mixture was then allowed to stand for stratification. The upper layer was collected, and fatty acids were detected using gas chromatography-mass spectrometry (GC-MS 7890B-5977A, Agilent, USA).

2.7. Statistical Analysis

All data were reported as mean ± standard deviation (SD). The differences between two groups were analyzed by Student's *t*-test. Groups of three or more were analyzed by one-way ANOVA. Statistical analyses were conducted using SPSS 20.0 software (IBM, Almond, NY, USA). Differences were considered significant when $p < 0.05$.

3. Results

3.1. Carcass Traits

The carcass traits of the three pig breeds all showed significant differences (Table 1). The lean carcass percentage and loin eye area of YP were significantly higher ($p < 0.05$) than both QYP and TP. Furthermore, the carcass fat percentage, back fat thickness, and marbling scores of YP were significantly lower ($p < 0.05$) than was observed in the other breeds. The carcass weight and length of TP were significantly lower ($p < 0.05$) than both QYP and YP. The designations of QYP1 and QYP2 refer to Qingyu pigs of 180 days old and 300 days old, respectively. The carcass fat percentage, backfat thickness, and marbling scores of QYP1 and QYP2 were all significantly higher ($p < 0.05$) than YP and TP. Notably, the body weight, carcass length and backfat thickness of QYP2 were all significantly higher ($p < 0.05$) than QYP1. However, none of the other parameters assessed exhibited any significant differences between the two ages.

Table 1. Pig carcass traits.

Carcass Traits	YP (*n* = 39)	QYP1 (*n* = 5)	QYP2 (*n* = 12)	TP (*n* = 24)	Significance
Carcass weight, kg	84.60 ± 9.39 [a]	44.64 ± 3.99 [b]	70.32 ± 16.96 [a]	28.88 ± 4.04 [c]	<0.001
Carcass length, cm	81.09 ± 2.27 [a]	64.4 ± 2.97 [b]	73.83 ± 11.74 [a]	57.4 ± 2.71 [c]	<0.001
Dressing, %	74.87 ± 3.05 [a]	66.85 ± 5.03 [b]	71.61 ± 7.8 [ab]	69.69 ± 2.23 [b]	0.002
Bone rate, %	13.1 ± 2.07 [a]	9.26 ± 1.78 [b]	11.41 ± 3.57 [ab]	10.84 ± 1.62 [b]	0.037
Carcass lean, %	64.11 ± 5.59 [a]	43.32 ± 2.94 [bc]	40.68 ± 5.12 [b]	47.87 ± 3.63 [c]	<0.001
Carcass fat, %	22.79 ± 4.80 [a]	47.34 ± 3.96 [b]	47.79 ± 8.41 [b]	41.16 ± 3.64 [c]	<0.001
Back fat thickness, cm	1.89 ± 0.48 [a]	3.33 ± 0.54 [b]	4.14 ± 1.14 [c]	2.59 ± 0.5 [d]	<0.001
Loin eye area, cm^2	49.39 ± 8.27 [a]	17.84 ± 3.67 [bc]	20.85 ± 3.42 [c]	14.08 ± 3.48 [b]	<0.001
Marbling scores	1.05 ± 0.5 [a]	2.63 ± 0.48 [b]	3.13 ± 0.53 [bc]	2.46 ± 0.45 [b]	<0.001

Different letters indicate significant difference ($p < 0.05$).

3.2. Meat Quality and Muscle Chemical Composition

The characteristics affecting meat quality are presented in Table 2. Among the three pig breeds, the L*45 min value, b*45 min value, L*24 h value, b*24 h value, and drip loss of the YP were significantly higher ($p < 0.05$) than those of QYP and TP. However, the pH 45 min value, pH 24 h value and a*45 min value were significantly lower ($p < 0.05$) than the QYP and TP breeds. The L*45 min and a*45 min values of TP were significantly lower ($p < 0.05$) than QYP and YP. The b*45 min value and ash content of the two stages of QYP were significantly lower ($p < 0.05$) than YP and TP.

3.3. Expression of Genes in Longissimus Dorsi Muscle

In order to better understand the differences in the meat quality of the three pig breeds, the expression of genes associated with pig carcass traits, meat quality, and high altitude adaptation were analyzed. The expression levels of *MyoD* and *MyoG* in YP were significantly higher ($p < 0.05$) than those of QYP and TP, while the expression of *MSTN* in TP was significantly higher ($p < 0.05$) than that of QYP and YP (Figure 2A). The expression levels and content ratios of *Myh4* and *Myh7* in the longissimus dorsi muscle of YP were significantly higher ($p < 0.05$) than those of the other two breeds, and the expression and proportion of *MYh2* in TP were significantly higher ($p < 0.05$) than those in YP and QYP (Figure 2B,C). The expression of *HK*, *PFK*, and *PK* in TP were significantly higher ($p < 0.05$) than QYP and TP (Figure 2D). The expression of *VEGFA*, *HIF1*, and Mb in TP were significantly higher ($p < 0.05$) than was observed in QYP and YP (Figure 2E). The expression of *C/EBPα*, *FABP4*, and *SCD1* in YP were significantly lower than QYP and TP (Figure 2F).

Table 2. Meat quality and chemical composition of the longissimus dorsi muscle.

Meat Quality	YP ($n = 32$)	QYP1 ($n = 5$)	QYP2 ($n = 12$)	TP ($n = 12$)	Significance
PH 45 min	6.28 ± 0.17 [a]	6.8 ± 0.31 [b]	6.6 ± 0.3 [bc]	6.51 ± 0.15 [c]	<0.001
PH 24 h	5.7 ± 0.29 [a]	6.11 ± 0.17 [b]	5.92 ± 0.33 [b]	6 ± 0.11 [b]	0.002
L*45 min	46.99 ± 1.98 [a]	43.65 ± 3.25 [b]	41.03 ± 2.76 [b]	38.84 ± 2.7 [c]	<0.001
a*45 min	5.93 ± 1.15 [a]	8.42 ± 2.08 [b]	10.59 ± 2.99 [b]	12.57 ± 2.27 [c]	<0.001
b*45 min	6.75 ± 0.73 [a]	0.6 ± 0.42 [b]	1.7 ± 1.57 [c]	3.14 ± 0.64 [d]	<0.001
L*24 h	52.63 ± 3.31 [a]	47.71 ± 4.61 [b]	45.77 ± 2.46 [b]	44.89 ± 4 [b]	<0.001
a*24	9.82 ± 1.94 [a]	8.83 ± 1.97 [a]	11.05 ± 2.96 [ab]	12.14 ± 2.73 [b]	0.026
b*24 h	7.83 ± 0.91 [a]	3.49 ± 1.21 [b]	4.97 ± 2.03 [b]	5.11 ± 2.57 [b]	<0.001
Drip loss, %	3.75 ± 1.81 [a]	1.91 ± 0.48 [b]	2.12 ± 0.59 [b]	2.37 ± 0.35 [b]	0.013
Cooking loss, %	34.40 ± 1.82	33.96 ± 2.29	36.94 ± 8.23	33.26 ± 4.08	0.341
Shear force, kg	9.9 ± 3.49	6.05 ± 2.68	6.44 ± 2	4.7 ± 1.86	0.694
Crude protein, %	21.58 ± 3.77 [ab]	24.22 ± 0.52 [a]	21.89 ± 0.96 [ab]	20.27 ± 2.36 [b]	0.077
Intramuscular fat, %	1.43 ± 0.55 [a]	2.48 ± 0.3 [b]	4.62 ± 1.85 [c]	1.88 ± 0.33 [ab]	<0.001
Ash, %	2.19 ± 0.5 [a]	1.35 ± 0.07 [b]	1.15 ± 0.06 [b]	2.73 ± 1.47 [a]	<0.001

Different letters indicate significant difference ($p < 0.05$).

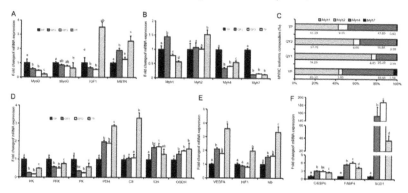

Figure 2. Gene expression in longissimus dorsi muscle. (**A**) The expression of genes involved in muscle development in longissimus dorsi muscle. Myogenic differentiation 1 (*MyoD*), myogenin (*MyoG*), Myocyte enhancer factor 2c (*Mef2c*), Myostatin (*MSTN*). (**B,C**) The expression and abundance of different subtypes of Myosin heavy chain (*MyHC*). (**D**) The expression of genes involved in muscle glycolysis and aerobic oxidation. Hexokinase (*HK*), phosphofructokinase (*PFK*), pyruvate kinase (*PK*), pyruvate dehydrogenase (*PDH*), citrate synthase (*CS*), isocitrate dehydrogenase (*IDH*), oxoglutarate dehydrogenase (*OGDH*). (**E**) The expression of vascular endothelial growth factor-A (*VEGFA*), hypoxia inducible factor-1 (*HIF1*), and myoglobin (*Mb*). (**F**) The expression of CCAAT/enhancer binding protein (*C/EBPα*), adipocyte fattyacid-binding protein (*FABP4*), and stearyl coenzyme A dehydrogenase-1 (*SCD1*), $n = 3$–6. All results are presented as means ± SEM. Different letters indicate significant difference ($p < 0.05$).

3.4. Free Amino Acid Content

In view of small differences between meat quality traits and genes expression between QYP1 and QYP2 and the differences among other pig breeds, Qingyu pigs were represented in the follow-up study by QYP2 (pigs with usual slaughter age). As can be seen in Table 3, with the exception of Phe, Asn, Gly, and Asp, the amino acids in the longissimus dorsi muscle of the three breeds examined were significantly different ($p < 0.05$). The Lys and His content of YP was observed to be significantly higher ($p < 0.05$) than in QYP and TP. Furthermore, Gln of QYP was significantly higher ($p < 0.05$) than YP and TP, whereas ILe, Leu, Val, Trp, Met, Ser, Tyr, and Glu in TP were significantly higher ($p < 0.05$) than the other two breeds.

Table 3. Free amino acid concentration of longissimus dorsi muscle (%).

AA	YP (*n* = 6)	QYP (*n* = 6)	TP (*n* = 6)	*p* Value
Ile	2.09 ± 0.33 [a]	2.16 ± 0.29 [a]	3.69 ± 0.31 [b]	<0.001
Leu	2.76 ± 0.23 [a]	3.47 ± 0.48 [b]	4.01 ± 0.52 [c]	0.001
Lys	5.95 ± 0.5 [a]	3.6 ± 0.53 [b]	3.8 ± 0.48 [b]	<0.001
Thr	2.93 ± 0.26 [a]	3.53 ± 0.4 [b]	3.76 ± 0.32 [b]	0.002
Val	2.62 ± 0.32 [a]	3.49 ± 0.36 [b]	4.18 ± 0.39 [c]	<0.001
Trp	0.93 ± 0.09 [a]	0.25 ± 0.04 [b]	1.05 ± 0.10 [c]	<0.001
Met	1.33 ± 0.11 [a]	0.97 ± 0.38 [b]	3 ± 0.28 [c]	<0.001
Phe	2.18 ± 0.44 [a]	2.61 ± 0.52 [ab]	2.77 ± 0.21 [b]	0.063
Arg	4.02 ± 0.55 [a]	2.92 ± 0.49 [b]	3.89 ± 0.57 [a]	0.005
His	15.31 ± 1.29 [a]	2.69 ± 0.26 [b]	8.36 ± 1.1 [c]	<0.001
Asn	1.86 ± 0.17	1.8 ± 0.35	2.03 ± 0.11	0.246
Ser	2.58 ± 0.2 [a]	3.19 ± 0.54 [b]	3.93 ± 0.46 [c]	<0.001
Gly	7.36 ± 1.53	7.61 ± 1.09	8.01 ± 1.56	0.727
Ala	20.22 ± 2.25 [ab]	21.73 ± 2.11 [a]	17.82 ± 2.5 [b]	0.031
Tyr	2.73 ± 0.11 [a]	1.79 ± 0.26 [b]	4.83 ± 0.34 [c]	<0.001
Gln	17.52 ± 2.61 [a]	30.9 ± 4.33 [b]	14.12 ± 0.97 [a]	<0.001
Glu	3.96 ± 1.44 [a]	4.21 ± 0.39 [a]	7.44 ± 0.86 [b]	<0.001
Asp	0.65 ± 0.15 [ab]	0.86 ± 0.82 [a]	0.19 ± 0.09 [b]	0.079
Pro	3.00 ± 0.13 [a]	2.21 ± 0.32 [b]	3.13 ± 0.31 [a]	<0.001

Different letters indicate significant difference ($p < 0.05$).

Further analysis indicated that the proportion of umami amino acids in TP was 7.67%, which was significantly higher ($p < 0.05$) than was observed in both YP and QYP (Figure 3A). The sweet amino acid concentration of QYP was as high as 72.61%, and 77.01% for essential amino acids (EAA), which were significantly higher ($p < 0.05$) than YP and TP (Figure 3A,B).

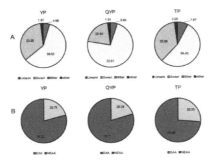

Figure 3. Analysis of amino acid composition in the longissimus dorsi muscle. (**A**) Amino acid ratios of longissimus dorsi muscle with different flavors in different pig breeds. (**B**) Proportion of essential amino acids (EAA) and non-essential amino acids (NEAA) in longissimus dorsi muscle of different pig breeds. All results are presented as means ± SEM. *n* = 6. Umami AA: Glu, Asp; Sweet AA: Gly, Ala, Ser, Thr, Pro, Gln, Lys; Bitter AA: Tyr, Arg, His, Val, Met, Ile, Leu, Trp, Phe.

3.5. Fatty Acid Levels

In the three pig breeds examined, a total of 22 fatty acids were measured. Only C10:0 and C14:0 were observed at similar levels among all three breeds. Among the 20 fatty acids, YP and TP contained the highest proportions of C18:1n9, reaching 49.80% and 54.81%, respectively. The QYP contained the highest proportion of C16:0, reaching 22.90%. In addition, C15:0, C16:0, C17:0, C17:1, C18:2n6, C18:3n3, C20:4n6, C20:5n3, C22:0, and C24:0 in QYP pigs were observed to be significantly higher ($p < 0.05$) than YP and TP. Conversely, TP exhibited the highest levels of C16:1, C18:1n9, C20:0, C20:1, C20:3n3, and C22:1n9 ($p < 0.05$) (Table 4).

Table 4. Fatty acid composition (%) of longissimus dorsi muscle.

FAA	YP (n = 6)	QYP (n = 6)	TP (n = 6)	p Value
C10:0	0.07 ± 0.01	0.06 ± 0.05	0.06 ± 0.01	0.689
C12:0	0.07 ± 0.01 [a]	0.01 ± 0.02 [b]	0.05 ± 0.01 [a]	<0.001
C14:0	1.33 ± 0.13	1.31 ± 0.18	1.34 ± 0.14	0.964
C15:0	0.03 ± 0.01 [a]	0.10 ± 0.01 [b]	0.03 ± 0.02 [a]	<0.001
C16:0	13.95 ± 0.77 [a]	22.90 ± 0.69 [b]	15.60 ± 0.86 [c]	<0.001
C16:1	3.13 ± 0.48 [a]	3.40 ± 0.41 [a]	5.60 ± 1.04 [b]	<0.001
C17:0	0.17 ± 0.04 [a]	0.35 ± 0.02 [b]	0.15 ± 0.05 [a]	<0.001
C17:1	——	0.28 ± 0.01 [a]	0.17 ± 0.04 [b]	<0.001
C18:0	16.37 ± 1.72 [a]	15.81 ± 0.47 [a]	11.77 ± 0.53 [b]	<0.001
C18:1n9	49.80 ± 3.02 [a]	22.79 ± 1.8 [b]	54.81 ± 3.34 [c]	<0.001
C18:2n6	9.91 ± 2.53 [a]	21.46 ± 2.04 [b]	6.48 ± 1.65 [c]	<0.001
C18:3n3	0.56 ± 0.14 [a]	0.60 ± 0.09 [a]	0.33 ± 0.07 [b]	<0.001
C20:0	0.24 ± 0.09 [a]	0.17 ± 0.02 [a]	0.32 ± 0.05 [b]	0.002
C20:1	1.09 ± 0.25 [a]	0.55 ± 0.1 [b]	1.41 ± 0.12 [c]	<0.001
C20:2	0.58 ± 0.12 [a]	0.52 ± 0.08 [a]	0.4 ± 0.07 [b]	0.016
C20:3n3	0.06 ± 0.01 [a]	0.06 ± 0.01 [a]	0.24 ± 0.12 [b]	0.001
C20:4n6	2.56 ± 1.21 [a]	9.13 ± 1.03 [b]	1.08 ± 0.61 [c]	<0.001
C20:5n3	0.04 ± 0.02 [a]	0.23 ± 0.04 [b]	0.03 ± 0.02 [a]	<0.001
C22:0	0.02 ± 0.01 [a]	0.04 ± 0.00 [b]	0.02 ± 0.00 [a]	<0.001
C22:1n9	0.02 ± 0.01 [a]	0.03 ± 0.00 [a]	0.09 ± 0.02 [b]	<0.001
C23:0	——	0.04 ± 0.01	——	——
C24:0	0.02 ± 0.01 [a]	0.05 ± 0 [b]	0.02 ± 0.01 [a]	<0.001

Different letters indicate significant difference ($p < 0.05$).

Next, analysis of the ratios of polyunsaturated fatty acid (PUFA) and PUFA/SFA (saturated fatty acid) indicated significantly higher levels in QYP than in both YP and TP ($p < 0.05$). In contrast, TP were observed to have the highest levels of monounsaturated fatty acids (MUFA) of TP ($p < 0.05$). It is worth noting that the n6/n3 ratio of QYP was observed to be significantly higher ($p < 0.05$) than that of YP and TP (Figure 4).

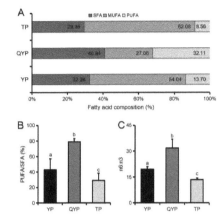

Figure 4. Analysis of fatty acid composition and characteristics in the longissimus dorsi muscle. (**A**) Composition of saturated fatty acids (SFA), monounsaturated fatty acids (MUFA), and polyunsaturated fatty acids (PUFA) in longissimus dorsi muscle of different pig breeds. (**B**) Percentage of PUFA/SFA in longissimus dorsi muscle of different pig breeds. (**C**) Ratio of n6:n3 of longissimus dorsi muscle in different pig breeds. All results are presented as means ± SEM. $n = 6$. Different letters indicate significant difference ($p < 0.05$).

4. Discussion

The differences in body composition among the different breeds were largely expected due to the breed itself and the different rearing conditions. The three pig breeds from low, intermediate, and high altitudes interestingly exhibited not only different body types, but different breeding intensities as well [13]. A workhorse of the pork industry, YP undergoes high-intensity modern breeding, whereas QYP is subjected to medium-intensity traditional breeding, and TP is bred at a low-intensity and is raised in a semi-wild state. The processing of pork for three pig breeds examined here differ substantially. For example, YP is more suitable for the production of bacon, whereas QYP is considered to be a general-purpose meat pig, and TP is predominantly made into jerky. Correspondingly, the three pig breeds correspond to vastly different human social cultures. QYP is adapted to traditional farming culture, and TP are suitable for pasturing [14]. Therefore, the selected breeds are representative of the extremes and intermediate methods and social/environmental climates in which Chinese pigs are produced.

4.1. Plateau Adaptability of Tibetan Pigs

The Tibetan plateau is a harsh, hypoxic environment. It has been reported that *HIF1* is a core regulator of hypoxia-responsive genes involved in the repair of cells in low-oxygen environments [15]. Vascular endothelial growth factor is a key factor in neovascularization, the expression of which is regulated by *HIF1* [16]. Previous studies have found that the heart, liver and kidney of TP all expressed higher levels of *VEGFA* than YP [17]. In the present study, a similar pattern of *VEGFA* and *HIF1* expression was observed in the longissimus dorsi muscle. In addition, the muscle redness of Tibetan pigs was the highest among the pig breeds examined, and the muscle L* value was the lowest. Approximately 80–90% of muscle color is attributable to myoglobin (*Mb*) [18]. This protein has a higher affinity for oxygen than hemoglobin, and was present in the highest concentrations in TP, which would explain the enhanced red coloration of TP meat. In summary, the Tibetan pig muscle exhibited the lowest L* value and the highest a* value, compared with YP and QYP.

Another feature of the plateau environment is the scarcity of food. As a result, it is crucial that Tibetan pigs are more efficient in their energy usage and have exceptional endurance. In order to adapt to different environments, the composition and function of muscle tissue will adjust accordingly. Based on myosin composition, the skeletal muscle fibers can be divided into Myh1, Myh2, Myh4, and Myh7 [19]. Muscles consisting predominantly of Myh2 are classified as fast oxidized muscle fibers, which is in between the oxidized muscle fiber (Myh7) and the glycolytic muscle fiber (Myh4). Therefore, Myh2 can provide energy to the body under both aerobic and anaerobic conditions [18]. Several previously published studies have demonstrated that in order to adapt to the special physiology of excavation activities under hypoxic conditions, the skeletal muscle composition of mole rats has undergone compensatory changes. The cervical trapezius, gastrocnemius, and quadriceps muscles are mainly myosin heavy chain 2a (Myh2) muscle fibers [20]. Similarly, it was observed here that the longissimus dorsi muscle of TP contained significantly higher levels of *Myh2* than YP and QYP.

Glycolysis occurs during the first stage of aerobic oxidation of carbohydrates to provide a rapid energy supply. However, the efficiency of this process is low [11,21]. The expression of glycolytic-related genes in the muscle of Tibetan pigs was at an intermediate level between YP and QYP. The expression of *CS* and *OGDH*, which are located downstream of the aerobic oxidation of carbohydrates were higher than was observed in both YP and QYP. This is logical, as it provides a quick supply energy to respond to dangerous natural environments.

Branches chain amino acids, or BCAAs (leucine, isoleucine, and valine), are essential amino acids [22]. Not only do they serve as raw materials for protein synthesis, but they also promote growth through the promotion of insulin and growth hormone secretion, and enhance metabolism [23]. These three amino acids can slow muscle fatigue, speed up recovery, reduce muscle protein catabolism during exercise, and help the body absorb protein, so they are often used as a muscle protectant [24]. Interestingly, they were observed at significantly higher levels in TP muscle than YP and QYP. Tryptophan has the effect of promoting differentiation of bone marrow T lymphocyte precursors into mature T lymphocytes [25,26]. Therefore, a lack of tryptophan can lead to a decrease in cell mediated immune responses. Here, it was observed that muscle tryptophan of was significantly higher in TP than both YP and QYP.

A cold environment is also a survival challenge for Tibetan pigs. It was observed that this breed has higher levels of unsaturated fatty acids (UFAs). Studies have shown that UFAs are the main factors affecting the fluidity of cell membranes, and are involved in resistance to cold damage in animals [27], plants [28], and microorganisms [29]. As a free-range grazing breed, Tibetan pigs have the opportunity to eat more wild plants, which have higher concentrations of UFAs [30]. High levels of UFAs are likely part of the cold resistance mechanism for Tibetan pigs.

4.2. Carcass Traits and Meat Quality Differences between Yorkshire, Penzhou Mountain, and Tibetan Pigs

Carcass traits are important indicators in the evaluation of meat performance in pigs. Carcass weight, dressing percentage, and carcass lean percentage are the main indicators of concern [31]. Here, the dressing percentage, carcass lean rate, and loin eye area of YP are much higher than those of QYP and TP. It has been reported that *MyoD*, *MyoG*, and *Mef2c* can promote myogenic differentiation, and play a positive role in the development of porcine skeletal muscle [32,33]. The expression of *MyoD* and *MyoG* in YP are significantly higher than was observed in QYP and TP. Myostatin (MSTN) is a negative regulator of skeletal muscle growth [34], which was found to be the highest in Tibetan pig muscles in the present study. The longissimus dorsi muscle fiber type differs between wild and commercial pig breeds [35]. It has been reported that *Myh4* is associated with lean muscle mass and growth rate [36], and that the proportion of *Myh4* expression in the longissimus dorsi muscle of YP was the highest. These results suggest that QYP and TP have great potential for genetic improvement in carcass traits. In addition, Tibetan pigs are small in size, which make them an attractive animal model system for the study of human diseases [37].

Pork pH is closely related to the products of glycolysis in muscle tissue [9,21,38]. The medium level of muscle glycolysis allows the pH of Tibetan pigs to average between that of YP and QYP, while the relatively high levels of tricarboxylic acid cycle-related genes are expressed. Meat color is an important sensory indicator for the evaluation of pork [39,40]. Pork from TP and QYP have higher a* and lower b* values, which implies that Chinese pork sales are based on cultural and visual perceptions of meat freshness. Local pigs show better meat color (higher a* value) and pH value, and further utilize the meat processing technology such as chilled meat processing to better demonstrate the meat quality potential of local pigs.

The muscle amino acid composition of the three pig breeds varied significantly. In the context of the flavors they impart, amino acids are classified into umami amino acids, sweet amino acids, and bitter amino acids [41,42]. Among the breeds examined here, TP had the highest umami amino acid content, and QYP had the highest sweet amino acid content. These may be the reason why QYP and TP meat quality are preferred in many aspects over YP. Furthermore, TP has higher levels of EAAs. Because of the harsh environment and remote location, modern dietary supplements, and ready access to a variety of foods on the Tibetan plateau can be scarce. Therefore, Tibetan pork is an effective way to supplement EAAs in the plateau. The high content of BCAA in Tibetan pork is not only conducive to the survival of Tibetan pigs, but also to the health of people who feed on them [43]. In addition, the high levels of bitter amino acids in Tibetan pork make cooking and seasoning of the meat, such as barbecue, a preferred method of processing and preparation. Although, with the development of food science and technology, amino acid enzymatic technology can expand the choices available for the processing of pork [44]. However, considering local food culture and characteristics, further research on pork jerky may be more conducive to the development of the plateau economy.

Traditional Chinese dishes are full of color, fragrance, and taste, of which local pork has been a preferred protein source in traditional Chinese dishes. Most Chinese local pigs are high-fat breeds. Due to their strong fat deposition capacity and higher saturated fatty acids (SFAs), a diet high in these meats has been demonstrated to affect cholesterol metabolism [45]. Despite the high SFA content of QYP pork, the local climate is warm with abundant green vegetables for consumption throughout the year, which can enhance the health of the people. In contrast, the people of the plateau have a single source of food, with a healthier ratio of PUFA/SFA [46]. Polyunsaturated fatty acids possess many physiological functions, such as maintaining biofilm structures, treating cardiovascular diseases, anti-inflammation, and promotion of brain development [47]. This reflects the harmonious evolution of human and pigs. The content of intramuscular fat (IMF) is closely related to meat tenderness, pH value, marbling, muscle flavor, and other meat quality traits [48,49]. Of the breeds examined here, QYP has the highest IMF as well as *C/EBPα* [50], *FABP4* [51], and *SCD1* [52] expression. All of these genes are related to fat synthesis and were highly expressed in QYP relative to the other breeds examined here. It is worth noting that *SCD1* is a key regulatory gene that catalyzes the synthesis of PUFA [53]. The data presented here suggests that QYP pork is richer and more comprehensive in fatty acids, while the fatty acid composition of TP pork is more favorable to human health.

5. Conclusions

A comparative analysis of three pig breeds showed that the plateau adaptability of Tibetan pigs is likely related to genetics, environment, and production methods. The hypoxic adaptation of Tibetan pigs may be related to higher levels of *VEGFA*, *HIF1*, and myoglobin expression. The higher aerobic oxidative capacity of Tibetan pigs is beneficial to improve energy utilization, and the higher UFA content of Tibetan pigs is beneficial to cold resistance. In addition, Tibetan pigs have higher levels of BCAA and *Myh2* expression, which serve to relieve muscle fatigue and improve endurance. Tibetan pigs have undergone numerous evolutionary changes to enhance their survivability in the harsh environment. Not only have these changes enhanced the survival of Tibetan pigs, but they have also altered meat and carcass quality traits, as well as the health of local people who eat their meat. Further analysis of carcass traits and meat quality indicators showed that YP had excellent carcass traits (higher dressing percentage, carcass lean, and loin eye area), while QYP and TP had better meat quality (higher PH, a* value and intramuscular fat). From the human health and food production perspectives, QYP pork has richer and more comprehensive fatty acid content. In contrast, TP pork exhibits contains higher levels of EAAs and a more favorable fatty acid composition for health. However, it should be noted that excessive fat intake is harmful to human health. There is great potential for cross breeding and further food development of three pig breeds examined here.

Supplementary Materials: The following are available online at http://www.mdpi.com/2076-2615/9/12/1080/s1, Table S1: Ingredients of the basal experiment diets; Table S2: The primer sequences used for qRT-PCR.

Author Contributions: Conceptualization, M.G. and L.Z.; Data curation, L.S. and Y.F.; Funding acquisition, G.T. and Y.J.; Methodology, Z.G. and B.L.; Project administration, X.L. and L.B.; Supervision, L.C. and L.B.; Validation, M.G. and S.Z.; Writing—original draft, M.G.; Writing—review and editing, L.S. and L.Z.

Funding: The study was supported by the Chinese National Sci & Tech Support Program (no. 2015BAD03B01-11), the National Natural Science Foundation of China (no. 31530073), the Sichuan Sci & Tech Support Program (nos. 2016NYZ0050 and SCCXTD-008), the earmarked fund for China Agriculture Research System (no. CARS-36-05B).

Conflicts of Interest: The authors declare they have no conflicts of interest.

References

1. Keenan, D.F. Pork meat quality, production and processing on. *Encycl. Food Health* **2016**, 419–431. [CrossRef]
2. Chen, G.; Cheng, X.; Shi, G.; Zou, C.; Chen, L.; Li, J.; Li, M.; Fang, C.; Li, C. Transcriptome analysis reveals the effect of long intergenic noncoding rnas on pig muscle growth and fat deposition. *Biomed. Res. Int.* **2019**, *2019*, 2951427. [CrossRef]
3. Lebret, B.; Ecolan, P.; Bonhomme, N.; Méteau, K.; Prunier, A. Influence of production system in local and conventional pig breeds on stress indicators at slaughter, muscle and meat traits and pork eating quality. *Animal* **2015**, *9*, 1404–1413. [CrossRef]
4. Luo, J.; Shen, L.; Tan, Z.; Cheng, X.; Yang, D.; Fan, Y.; Yang, Q.; Ma, J.; Tang, Q.; Jiang, A.A.; et al. Comparison reproductive, growth performance, carcass and meat quality of liangshan pig crossbred with duroc and berkshire genotypes and heterosis prediction. *Livest. Sci.* **2018**, *212*, 61–68. [CrossRef]
5. Megens, H.J.; Crooijmans, R.P.M.A.; Cristobal, M.S.; Hui, X.; Li, N.; Groenen, M.A.M. Biodiversity of pig breeds from china and europe estimated from pooled DNA samples: Differences in microsatellite variation between two areas of domestication. *Genet. Sel. Evol.* **2008**, *40*, 103–128.
6. Li, M.; Tian, S.; Jin, L.; Zhou, G.; Li, Y.; Zhang, Y.; Wang, T.; Yeung, C.K.; Chen, L.; Ma, J.; et al. Genomic analyses identify distinct patterns of selection in domesticated pigs and tibetan wild boars. *Nat. Genet.* **2013**, *45*, 1431–1438.
7. Kong, X.; Dong, X.; Yang, S.; Qian, J.; Yang, J.; Jiang, Q.; Li, X.; Wang, B.; Yan, D.; Lu, S.; et al. Natural selection on tmprss6 associated with the blunted erythropoiesis and improved blood viscosity in tibetan pigs. *Comp. Biochem. Physiol. Part B Biochem. Mol. Boil.* **2019**, *233*, 11–22. [CrossRef]
8. Peng, J.H.; Sun, D.; Nevo, E. Domestication evolution, genetics and genomics in wheat. *Mol. Breed.* **2011**, *28*, 281–301. [CrossRef]
9. Luo, J.; Shen, L.Y.; Lei, H.G.; Zhu, K.P.; Jiang, Y.Z.; Bai, L.; Li, M.Z.; Tang, G.Q.; Li, X.W.; Zhang, S.H. Correlation between three glycometabolic-related hormones and muscle glycolysis as well as meat quality in three pig breeds. *J. Sci. Food Agric.* **2016**, *97*, 2706–2713. [CrossRef]
10. Cheng, C.; Liu, Z.; Zhou, Y.; Wei, H.; Zhang, X.; Xia, M.; Deng, Z.; Zou, Y.; Jiang, S.; Peng, J. Effect of oregano essential oil supplementation to a reduced-protein, amino acid-supplemented diet on meat quality, fatty acid composition, and oxidative stability of longissimus thoracis muscle in growing-finishing pigs. *Meat Sci.* **2017**, *133*, 103–109. [CrossRef]
11. Shen, L.; Lei, H.; Zhang, S.; Li, X.; Li, M.; Jiang, X.; Zhu, K.; Zhu, L. The comparison of energy metabolism and meat quality among three pig breeds. *Anim. Sci. J.* **2014**, *85*, 770–779. [CrossRef]
12. Livak, K.J.; Schmittgen, T.D. Analysis of relative gene expression data using real-time quantitative pcr and the 2(-delta delta c(t)) method. *Methods* **2001**, *25*, 402–408. [CrossRef]
13. Wu, Q.; Hao, Y.; Fang, X.; Cheng, Y.; Dong, L.; Wei, W.; Gang, W.; Fu, H.; Liu, S.; Hao, L. The association of haplotypes in igfbp-3 gene promoter region and tissue expressions in three pig breeds. *Anim. Cells. Syst.* **2016**, *20*, 1–10. [CrossRef]
14. Yang, W.; Meng, F.; Peng, J.; Han, P.; Fang, F.; Ma, L.; Cao, B. Isolation and identification of a cellulolytic bacterium from the tibetan pig's intestine and investigation of its cellulase production. *Electron. J. Biotechnol.* **2014**, *17*, 262–267. [CrossRef]

15. Cai, X.H.; Huang, Y.T.; Zhang, Z.P.; Wang, Y.L. Hypoxia inducible factor-1 (hif-1) and its research advance in aquatic animals. *J. Agric. Biotechnol.* **2014**, *22*, 119–132.

16. Hyun Ah, K.; Soyeon, L.; Hyung-Ho, M.; Sung Wan, K.; Ki-Chul, H.; Minhyung, L.; Hwa, K.S.; Donghoon, C. Hypoxia-inducible vascular endothelial growth factor gene therapy using the oxygen-dependent degradation domain in myocardial ischemia. *Pharm. Res.* **2010**, *27*, 2075–2084.

17. Zhang, B.; Qiangba, Y.; Shang, P.; Lu, Y.; Yang, Y.; Wang, Z.; Zhang, H. Gene expression of vascular endothelial growth factor a and hypoxic adaptation in tibetan pig. *J. Anim. Sci. Biotechnol.* **2016**, *4*, 474–481. [CrossRef]

18. Mancini, R.A.; Hunt, M.C. Current research in meat color. *Meat Sci.* **2005**, *71*, 100–121. [CrossRef]

19. Schiaffino, S.; Reggiani, C. Fiber types in mammalian skeletal muscles. *Physiol. Rev.* **2011**, *91*, 1447–1531. [CrossRef]

20. Avivi, A.; Band, M.; Joel, A.; Shenzer, P.; Coleman, R. Adaptive features of skeletal muscles of mole rats (spalax ehrenbergi) to intensive activity under subterranean hypoxic conditions. *Acta Histochem.* **2009**, *111*, 415–419. [CrossRef]

21. Shen, Q.W.; Means, W.J.; Thompson, S.A.; Underwood, K.R.; Zhu, M.J.; Mccormick, R.J.; Ford, S.P.; Du, M. Pre-slaughter transport, amp-activated protein kinase, glycolysis, and quality of pork loin. *Meat Sci.* **2006**, *74*, 388–395. [CrossRef]

22. Wang, F.-H.; Liu, J.; Deng, Q.-J.; Qi, Y.; Wang, M.; Wang, Y.; Zhang, X.-G.; Zhao, D. Association between plasma essential amino acids and atherogenic lipid profile in a chinese population: A cross-sectional study. *Atherosclerosis* **2019**, *286*, 7–13. [CrossRef]

23. Brestenský, M.; Nitrayová, S.; Patráš, P.; Heger, J.; Nitray, J. Branched chain amino acids and their importance in nutrition. *JMBFS* **2015**, *5*, 197–202. [CrossRef]

24. Gannon, N.P.; Schnuck, J.K.; Vaughan, R.A. Bcaa metabolism and insulin sensitivity—Dysregulated by metabolic status? *Mol. Nutr. Food Res.* **2018**, *62*, e1700756. [CrossRef] [PubMed]

25. Guido, F.; Rita, R.; Michela, T.; Gianluca, D.; Umberto, B.; Giovanni Battista, F. Tryptophan-derived catabolites are responsible for inhibition of t and natural killer cell proliferation induced by indoleamine 2,3-dioxygenase. *J. Exp. Med.* **2002**, *196*, 459–468.

26. Fallarino, F.; Grohmann, U.; Vacca, C.; Bianchi, R.; Orabona, C.; Spreca, A.; Fioretti, M.C.; Puccetti, P. T cell apoptosis by tryptophan catabolism. *Cell Death Differ.* **2002**, *9*, 1069–1077. [CrossRef]

27. Rey, B.; Dégletagne, C.; Bodennec, J.; Monternier, P.-A.; Mortz, M.; Roussel, D.; Romestaing, C.; Rouanet, J.-L.; Tornos, J.; Duchamp, C. Hormetic response triggers multifaceted anti-oxidant strategies in immature king penguins (aptenodytes patagonicus). *Free Radic. Biol. Med.* **2016**, *97*, 577–587. [CrossRef]

28. Sakamoto, A.; Sulpice, R.; Hou, C.X.; Kinoshita, M.; Higashi, S.I.; Kanaseki, T.; Nonaka, H.; Moon, B.Y.; Murata, N. Genetic modification of the fatty acid unsaturation of phosphatidylglycerol in chloroplasts alters the sensitivity of tobacco plants to cold stress. *Plant Cell Environ.* **2010**, *27*, 99–105. [CrossRef]

29. Králová, S. Role of fatty acids in cold adaptation of antarctic psychrophilic flavobacterium spp. *Syst. Appl. Microbiol.* **2017**, *40*, 329–333. [CrossRef]

30. Mao, Z.-X.; Fu, H.; Nan, Z.-B.; Wang, J.; Wan, C.-G. Fatty acid content of common vetch (vicia sativa l.) in different regions of northwest china. *Biochem. Syst. Ecol.* **2012**, *44*, 347–351. [CrossRef]

31. Sobczyńska, M.; Blicharski, T.; Tyra, M. Relationships between longevity, lifetime productivity, carcass traits and conformation in polish maternal pig breeds. *J. Anim. Breed. Genet.* **2014**, *130*, 361–371.

32. Qiao, M.; Huang, J.; Wu, H.; Wu, J.; Peng, X.; Mei, S. Molecular characterization, transcriptional regulation and association analysis with carcass traits of porcine tcap gene. *Gene* **2014**, *538*, 273–279. [CrossRef] [PubMed]

33. Çlnar, M.U.; Fan, H.T. The mrna expression pattern of skeletal muscle regulatory factors in divergent phenotype swine breeds. *Kafkas Univ. Vet. Fak.* **2012**, *18*, 685–690.

34. Buys, N. Characterization of the complete porcine mstn gene and expression levels in pig breeds differing in muscularity. *Anim. Genet.* **2010**, *39*, 586–596.

35. Rahelic, S.; Puac, S. Fibre types in longissimus dorsi from wild and highly selected pig breeds. *Meat Sci.* **1981**, *5*, 439–450. [CrossRef]

36. Cho, E.S.; Lee, K.T.; Kim, J.M.; Lee, S.W.; Jeon, H.J.; Lee, S.H.; Hong, K.C.; Kim, T.H. Association of a single nucleotide polymorphism in the 5′ upstream region of the porcinemyosin heavy chain 4gene with meat quality traits in pigs. *Anim. Sci. J.* **2016**, *87*, 330–335. [CrossRef]

37. Larzul, C. Pig genetics: Insight in minipigs. In Proceedings of the Bilateral Symposium on Miniature Pigs for Biomedical Research in Taiwan and France, Hsinhua, Taiwan, 22–23 October 2013; pp. 1–6.

38. Li, X.; Xia, A.-Q.; Chen, L.-J.; Du, M.-T.; Chen, L.; Kang, N.; Zhang, D.-Q. Effects of lairage after transport on post mortem muscle glycolysis, protein phosphorylation and lamb meat quality. *J. Integr. Agric.* **2018**, *17*, 2336–2344. [CrossRef]

39. Legeard, D.; Marty-Mahe, P.; Camillerapp, J.; Marchal, P.; Leredde, C. Real-time quality evaluation of pork hams by color machine vision. *Proc. SPIE Int. Soc. Opt. Eng.* **1999**, *3652*, 138–149.

40. Gajewczyk, P.; Gajewczyk, B.; Akin´Cza, J.; Szman´Ko, T. Influence of crossing polish and foreign pig breeds on physicochemical traits of longissimus lumborum muscle. *Turk. J. Vet. Anim. Sci.* **2014**, *38*, 183–188. [CrossRef]

41. Zhou, W.; Sun-Waterhouse, D.; Xiong, J.; Cui, C.; Wang, W.; Dong, K. Desired soy sauce characteristics and autolysis of aspergillus oryzae induced by low temperature conditions during initial moromi fermentation. *J. Food Sci. Technol.* **2019**, *56*, 2888–2898. [CrossRef]

42. Gao, X.; Zhang, J.; Regenstein, J.M.; Yin, Y.; Zhou, C. Characterization of taste and aroma compounds in tianyou, a traditional fermented wheat flour condiment. *Food Res. Int.* **2018**, *106*, 156–163. [CrossRef]

43. Pallottini, A.C.; Sales, C.H.; Dads, V.; Marchioni, D.M.; Fisberg, R.M. Dietary bcaa intake is associated with demographic, socioeconomic and lifestyle factors in residents of são paulo, brazil. *Nutrients* **2017**, *9*, 449. [CrossRef]

44. Elroy, N.N.; Rogers, J.; Mafi, G.G.; VanOverbeke, D.L.; Hartson, S.D.; Ramanathan, R. Species-specific effects on non-enzymatic metmyoglobin reduction in vitro. *Meat Sci.* **2015**, *105*, 108–113. [CrossRef] [PubMed]

45. Mensink, R.P. Fatty acids: Health effects of saturated fatty acids. In *Encyclopedia of Human Nutrition*, 3rd ed.; Academic Press: London, UK, 2013; pp. 215–219.

46. Doychev, V.; Mihaylova, G. Effect of flaxsee d and alpha tocopherol supplementation of pig diets on fatty acid content and lipid oxidation stability of m. Longissimus. *Bulg. J. Agric. Sci.* **2013**, *19*, 1416–1424.

47. Tapiero, H.; Ba, G.N.; Couvreur, P.; Tew, K.D. Polyunsaturated fatty acids (pufa) and eicosanoids in human health and pathologies. *Biomed. Pharmacother.* **2002**, *56*, 215–222. [CrossRef]

48. Starkey, C.P.; Geesink, G.H.; Collins, D.; Hutton Oddy, V.; Hopkins, D.L. Do sarcomere length, collagen content, ph, intramuscular fat and desmin degradation explain variation in the tenderness of three ovine muscles? *Meat Sci.* **2016**, *113*, 51–58. [CrossRef]

49. Liu, L.; Ngadi, M.O. Predicting intramuscular fat content of pork using hyperspectral imaging. *J. Food Eng.* **2014**, *134*, 16–23. [CrossRef]

50. Li, W.Z.; Zhao, S.M.; Huang, Y.; Yang, M.H.; Pan, H.B.; Zhang, X.; Ge, C.R.; Gao, S.Z. Expression of lipogenic genes during porcine intramuscular preadipocyte differentiation. *Res. Vet. Sci.* **2012**, *93*, 1190–1194. [CrossRef] [PubMed]

51. Chen, Q.M.; Wang, H.; Zeng, Y.Q.; Chen, W. Developmental changes and effect on intramuscular fat content of h-fabp and a-fabp mrna expression in pigs. *J. Appl. Genet.* **2013**, *54*, 119–123. [CrossRef]

52. Jiang, Z.; Michal, J.J.; Tobey, D.J.; Daniels, T.F.; Rule, D.C.; Macneil, M.D. Significant associations of stearoyl-coa desaturase (scd1) gene with fat deposition and composition in skeletal muscle. *Int. J. Biol. Sci.* **2008**, *4*, 345–351.

53. Rogowski, M.P.; Flowers, M.T.; Stamatikos, A.D.; Ntambi, J.M.; Paton, C.M. Scd1 activity in muscle increases triglyceride pufa content, exercise capacity, and pparδ expression in mice. *J. Lipid Res.* **2013**, *54*, 2636–2646. [CrossRef]

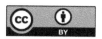

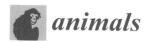 *animals*

Article

Effect of Replacement of Synthetic vs. Natural Curing Agents on Quality Characteristics of Cinta Senese Frankfurter-Type Sausage

Silvia Parrini [1,*], Francesco Sirtori [1], Anna Acciaioli [1], Valentina Becciolini [1], Alessandro Crovetti [1], Oreste Franci [1], Annalisa Romani [2], Arianna Scardigli [2] and Riccardo Bozzi [1]

1   Department of Agricultural, Environmental, Food and Forestry Science and Technology, University of Florence, Via delle Cascine 5, 50144 Firenze, Italy; francesco.sirtori@unifi.it (F.S.); anna.acciaioli@unifi.it (A.A.); valentina.becciolini@unifi.it (V.B.); alessandro.crovetti@gmail.com (A.C.); oreste.franci@unifi.it (O.F.); riccardo.bozzi@unifi.it (R.B.)
2   Pharmaceutical, Cosmetic, Food Supplement, Technology and Analysis, Department of Statistics Computer Science Applications "G. Parenti", University of Florence, Via U. Schiff, 6, 50019 Sesto Fiorentino, Firenze, Italy; annalisa.romani@unifi.it (A.R.); ari.scardigli@gmail.com (A.S.)
*   Correspondence: silvia.parrini@unifi.it; Tel.: +39-055-2755591

Received: 13 November 2019; Accepted: 18 December 2019; Published: 19 December 2019

Simple Summary: The increasing demand of natural and environmentally sustainable foods promotes the use of natural extract as curing agents in meat products. In this context, the extensive rearing system, characteristic of autochthonous pigs, could represent an added value for the consumers. Moreover, the introduction of new types of products to enhance the second-choice portion of meat can be economically important. The present study aims to test and to evaluate the quality traits during storage times of frankfurter-type sausages of Cinta Senese using natural extract to replace nitrites and nitrates as curing agents. Results of this study demonstrate that those products are safe for the human consumption, but some sensorial and physical traits could be improved. The implementation of a new product using meat of a local breed and agricultural by products as curing agents could be interesting both in terms of sustainability and valorization of the territory and of Cinta Senese products.

Abstract: Frankfurter-type sausages (called sausages) were manufactured using Cinta Senese meat. Two different formulations were considered: (i) nitrite and nitrate as curing agents (NIT), (ii) natural mixture (NAT) totally replacing the synthetic curing agents. Microbiological, chemical, and physical characteristics during three different storage times (7, 30, 60 days) were investigated, while sensorial traits were evaluated at the end of the period. The main foodborne pathogens (*Escherichia coli*, *Listeria monocytogenes*, coagulase positive *Staphylococcus* spp., *Salmonella* spp., total bacterium at 30 °C) were absent in both sausage groups. Both types of sausage had a high content of fat probably due to the high intramuscular fat of the local breed. The fatty acid composition of NAT sausages would seem slightly less efficient in the lipid oxidation control. Regarding color parameters, NIT sausages showed greater lightness and redness, while NAT ones were more yellow, thanks to the effect of nitrate on color. All texture parameters resulted higher in NIT, except for the springiness. Storage time mainly affected total microbial count, pH, and color. The addition of natural extract changed the perception of some sensorial properties above all in terms of taste and odor. Natural extract represented an alternative to synthetic additives in Cinta Senese sausages even if some attributes could be improved.

Keywords: natural extract; curing agents; sausages; Cinta Senese pig

1. Introduction

Cinta Senese is an Italian local pig breed characterized by the production of high-quality meat with specific regional identity, traditionally processed into pork products in order to allow the extension of shelf-life respect to the fresh meat. Among them, Frankfurter-type sausage does not represent a typical cured meat product but may be an opportunity of innovation in the specific framework and an improvement in the use of second-choice portion of meat. In Tuscany, Cinta Senese is often reared in marginal areas where farms usually support the animal rearing with other productions such as olives in hilly areas and chestnuts in mountain areas in order to have more sources of income. These types of agricultural systems are accompanied by the production of byproducts that could be used in the food sector to form additives in curing products, increasing the link between the breed and its origin.

Traditionally, curing agents included in processed meat products are sodium and potassium salts of nitrite and nitrate additives and their use is authorized by European Union within a safe level [1]. Their role includes the capacity to inhibit the growth of pathogenic bacteria and to delay oxidative rancidity [2], leading to high stability and increasing the product shelf-life. These curing agents are also involved in the stabilization of the sensory properties [3] and have a positive effect on color, cured cooked flavor, and aroma [4]. However, the nitrite-nitrate consumption may represent a risk for human health. Ingested sodium and potassium salts of nitrite and nitrate are in the major part excreted as nitrate except for a small portion that recirculates through salivary glands, and it is converted by mouth bacteria into nitrite [1]. The absorption of an excessive amount of nitrite could cause an oxidation of hemoglobin into methemoglobin leading a reduction of "the ability of red blood cells to bind and transport oxygen through the body" [1]. Nitrite in food (and nitrate converted to nitrite in the body) may also contribute to the formation of a group of compounds known as nitrosamines (also called *N*-nitrosamines) some of which are associated to the formation of carcinogenic and mutagenic compounds [5]. To the best of our knowledge, besides to the amount of nitrite added to products, a wide range of factors may potentially affect the formation of nitrosamine such as meat quality and its fat content, processing condition as heat applied during drying or smoking, packaging, and storage/maturation conditions [6,7].

The increasing demand of consumers for natural foods moved the food industry interest to include natural curing agents in foods and in processing foods [8]. The use of natural extracts as antioxidants and antimicrobials has advantages such as high consumer acceptance and healthiness, although some studies [8,9] reported disadvantages such as their higher cost and lower effectiveness.

The total antioxidant capacity of fruit and vegetable extracts is based on the concentration of some compounds, such as ascorbic acid, alpha-tocopherol, beta-carotene, flavonoids, and phenols. Furthermore, some authors [10,11] have highlighted that the antimicrobial and antioxidant properties were primarily associated to phenolic compounds content, including volatile compounds. The antioxidant activity of phenolic compounds is given by three mechanisms: free-radical scavenging activity, [12] transition-metal-chelating activity, and/or singlet-oxygen quenching capacity [12,13]. The antimicrobial activity is enabled thanks to the presence of hydroxyl groups and their relative position in the phenolic ring [8].

Some studies [14,15] proposed the addition of natural compounds to the traditional recipe, that foresees synthetic additive, in order to enhance the qualitative properties of products. Ayo et al. [16] studied the effect of replacement of pork backfat with vegetable fat on frankfurter sausages indicating a health improvement of nutritional profile with a 25% addition of walnuts. The main concern of the various studies remains to find an alternative to synthetic curing agents able to address the multiple activities covered by the latter considering that there is no current single substitute for such compounds, particularly for nitrite and nitrate. Sebranek et al. [17] and Eskandari et al. [14] reported successful nitrite/nitrate additive reduction in processed meat products. Alirezalu et al. [18] working on the substitution of curing agents in commercial frankfurter-type sausages of unspecified pork with natural antimicrobial compounds (nisin, ε-polylysine, or chitosan) and antioxidant mixture suggested further research to improve color stability, storage, and other physical properties. Moreover, as highlighted in a review of Velasco et al. [8], some experimental studies have been focused on factors affecting natural extracts' activity such as the specific extraction process or the measurement method. The extraction of natural extract could follow a green chemistry procedure using a sustainable and eco-friendly methodology as the case reported by Romani et al. [19]. In this context the use of natural antioxidant/antimicrobial obtained from agricultural byproducts which otherwise would be wasted could become a good alternative.

The use of grape seeds (*Vitis vinifera*), chestnut (*Castanea sativa*), and olive oil (*Olea europaea*) characterized by antioxidant and antimicrobial proprieties associated to a high content of phenolic compounds [15] as meat products curing agents could represent an example of circular economy. Nevertheless, more studies are needed to assess the feasibility of frankfurter-type sausage production by replacing sodium and potassium salts of nitrite and nitrate with natural antioxidants, trying both to maintain quality traits and antimicrobial proprieties during storage. The natural extracts were chosen both for their properties and for the link with territory. In fact, the great availability of agricultural byproducts (chestnut, grape seeds, and olive pomace) in Tuscany, where Cinta Senese pigs are reared, was considered.

The present study considers Cinta Senese frankfurter-type sausage, henceforth called sausage and aims to (i) test the use of grape seeds, chestnut, and olive oil as natural extracts to totally replace sodium and potassium salts of nitrite and nitrate; (ii) evaluate the microbiological, physical, and sensorial qualities traits during the storage time (7, 30, 60 days).

2. Materials and Methods

2.1. Natural Mixtures

The natural antioxidant and antimicrobial extracts used in the present study is based on:

- grape seeds condensed tannins;
- hydroxytyrosol, hy-derivatives, and tyrosol from olive oil pomace of *Olea europaea* L.;
- chestnut hydrolysable tannins.

The extraction of polyphenols from olive oil byproducts is based on a water extraction and membrane separation system. This methodology was instead implemented at an industrial level by using physical technology (PCT/IT/2009/09425529 "Process for producing concentrated and refined active substances from tissues and by-products of *Olea europaea* L. with membrane technologies") considered sustainable technologies defined by Best Available Technology (BAT) and recognized by the Environmental Protection Agency (EPA) [20,21].

The hydrolysable chestnut tannin extract was obtained following the technology described by Campo et al. [22] (2016), while the extraction of bioactive compounds from the grape seed production was obtained as described by Lucarini et al. [23].

Antioxidant and antiradical capacity and phenolic content of the different extracts were analyzed by HPLC/DAD/MS [19] on three samples of each natural extract and reported in Table 1. Total polyphenolic content of olive pomace extract, grape seed extract and chestnut extract was 38.64 g/L, 822,713 mg/g,, and 16,109 mg/g, respectively. The 1,1-diphenylpicrylhydrazil radical (DPPH) assay on the three components pointed out an antiradical activity (EC50) of 0.196 mg/mg for the olive pomace, 0.147 mg/mg for grape seed extract, 0.085 mg/mg for chestnut extract.

The three extracts were combined to the same amount of hydroxytyrosol and tocopherol (E307) to form a defatted mixture (mix NAT), but their relative amounts are currently under patent and will not be reported in this study.

Table 1. Phenolic profile of the extracts combined in the mixture (natural mixture—NAT) used in the trial.

Olive Oil Pomace	g/L	Grape Seed	mg/g	Chestnut Tannin	mg/g
OH-tyrosol	11.65	Catechin	11.07	Vescalin	9.34
OH-tyrosol derivatives	5.13	Epicatechin	13.62	Castalin	9.00
Tyrosol	16.02	Catechin dimers	10.21	Pedunculagin	3.88
Verbascoside	5.84	Catechin trimers	6.92	Galloil glucose derivatives	42.59
		Epicatechin gallate derivatives	726.02	Gallic Acid	18.50
		Tetramers	54.88	Roburin D	10.51
				Vescalagin	32.15
				Castalagin	31.03
				Ellagic Acid	4.08

2.2. Sample Manufacturing

Meat used in the trial was derived from 24 Cinta Senese barrows reared outdoors in "Azienda Agricola Savigni" farm (Pistoia, Italy), within the normal running of the farm. Animals were slaughtered at the same age of 15.5 months and at an average live weight of 160 ± 10 kg in a commercial slaughter house as the usual customs of the farmer.

According to the experimental design "2 Lot × 2 Treatment", the meat was divided in two parts in order to create two lots of products, each including the meat of 12 animals.

For each lot, portions of trimmed pork lean (16 kg) and subcutaneous backfat (4 kg) were used. The meat was chopped into cubes of approximately 3 cm, ground in a commercial food processor, and homogenized adding ice (13.45% of the total recipe) in a cutter (Laska Cutter KU65, Traun, Austria) for 6 min at maximum 10 °C. Following the traditional recipe condiments (salt 1.55%, sucrose 0.25%, black pepper 0.04%) and other seasoning additives (0.47%) were added and therefore the full dough was divided in two parts:

- one with addition of nitrite and nitrate (1%) as curing agents forming the first treatment (NIT);
- one with addition of "mix NAT" (1%) to replace nitrite and nitrate and forming the second treatment (NAT).

Each treatment dough was again homogenized with the same quantity of ice in a cutter for 6 min not exceeding 10 °C and then mechanically stuffed (Omet Foodtech, Siena, Italy) into edible collagen casings (Fcase, Myślenice, Poland) (28 mm diameter).

Sausages were steam cooked at 80 °C for 90 min achieving an internal temperature of 72 °C producing about 140 sausages for each treatment. Sausages were immediately chilled with cold water shower, vacuum packed, and stored under refrigeration (4 °C) for 7, 30, and 60 days.

2.3. Microbiological, Chemical, and Physical Analysis

Four sausages for each treatment were submitted to microbiological analysis performed at 7, 30, and 60 days of storage time.

Microbiological analyses were carried out in an external accredited laboratory to determine the product safety. The following bacteria were investigated: *Escherichia coli* [24], *Listeria monocytogenes* [25], coagulase positive *Staphylococcus* spp. [26], *Salmonella* spp. [27], total bacterium at 30 °C [28].

Moisture, total protein, and ash contents were determined following AOAC [29] methods. (ii) Total lipid content was analyzed using a modified method of Folch et al. [30] and fatty acid profile of total lipids using the modified technique of Morrison and Smith [31]. Fatty acids (FAs) methyl esters were determined by gas chromatography using a Varian 430 apparatus (Varian Inc., Palo Alto, CA, USA) equipped with a flame ionization detector. FAs separation occurred in a Supelco Omegawax TM 320 capillary column (30-m length; 0.32 mm internal diameter; 0.25 μm film thickness; Supelco,

Bellafonte, PA, USA). The individual methyl esters were identified by their retention time using an analytical standard (F.A.M.E. Mix, C8-C22 Supelco 18,920- 1AMP). Response factors based on the internal standard (C19:0) were used for quantification and results were expressed as g/100 g of sample. Six sausages for each treatment were analyzed for chemical composition and physical parameters at the considered storage time (7, 30, and 60 d).

All the physical parameters were assessed on three replications for each of six samples of the two treatments. pH was measured at room temperature (20 °C) using a pH meter Delta Ohm HD 8705 (Delta Ohm S.R.L., Caselle di Selvazzano, Padova, Italy) with a temperature probe TP870 and pH electrode Hamilton double pore. Water activity (aW) was determined by ISO21807:2004 methodology.

Color parameters CIE L* (lightness), a* (redness), and b* (yellowness) were measured immediately after slicing using a Minolta colorimeter CR-200 (Minolta Camera Co., Ltd., Osaka, Japan). Recalibration on white and red plates was performed at the start of each measuring session.

Warner–Bratzler shear force and texture profile analysis (TPA) was performed using a Zwick Roell Z2.5 apparatus (Ulm, Germany texture analyzer) with a 1 kN-load cell at the crosshead speed of 1 mm/s and working at room temperature (22 °C). Tenderness was carried out by Warner–Bratzler shear force applying a tangential cut to a segment of a whole sausage. TPA curve-forces were determined by a 100-mm-diameter compression plate on 10 × 10 ×10 mm slices. Relative to TPA parameters, hardness, springiness, cohesiveness were recorded while chewiness was calculated [32].

2.4. Sensory Analysis

Sensory analysis was carried out in an equipped laboratory by nine trained panelists using a quantitative-descriptive analysis method.

Eleven attributes (overall acceptability, color uniformity, lightness, odor, off odor, off flavor, flavor, bitter taste, tannic taste, juiciness, hardness) were evaluated; each attribute was scored in a 100 mm nonstructured line, anchored at the extremities [33]. The list of attributes and their definitions (Supplementary Table S1) were presented to selected panelists underwent an introductory session, where the testing procedures and the chosen sensory traits were discussed using two types of comparable commercial products. During three sessions, panelists evaluated a total of eight sausages (2 lot × 2 treatments × 2 samples) identified by an alphanumerical code. The sausages were divided in 5 mm thick pieces and two pieces of each sample were randomly served to judges at room temperature (20 °C).

The sausages' sensory characteristics were evaluated exclusively at the storage time of 60 days.

2.5. Statistical Analysis

Data were analyzed by MIXED Procedure of SAS Software (SAS, 2007) according to the following model (1):

$$Y_{ijkl} = \mu + T_i + S_{ij} + L_k + D_l + (T \times D)_{il} + \varepsilon_{ijkl,} \tag{1}$$

where μ was the mean, T was the ith treatment, L was the kth production lot, D was the lth day of storage, (T×D) was the interaction between treatment and day of storage, S was the effect of the sample within treatment and it is equal to the covariance between repeated measurements within samples; ε was the random error with mean 0 and variance σ^2, i.e., the variance between measurement within samples.

For the sensory data, GLM procedure including in the model the effect of panelist (P) was used as shown in the following Equation (2):

$$Y_{ijkl} = \mu + T_i + S_{ij} + L_J + P_k + \varepsilon_{ijkl}. \tag{2}$$

Level of significance was started at $p < 0.05$. Tukey test was used to statistically test the differences between the least squares means.

3. Results

3.1. Microbiological Characterization

Table 2 shows the microbiological population in sausages at 7, 30, and 60 days. In all samples considered, the major foodborne pathogens (*Escherichia coli*, *Listeria monocytogenes*, *Staphilococcus* spp., and *Salmonella* spp.) were absent or below the legal threshold limit (Reg CE/2073/05). The total microbial population showed the same starting point but, as expected, a slight increase was observed during the whole storage period for both sausage groups. Between treatments, differences occurred from 30 days onwards.

Table 2. Microbiological analysis on Cinta Senese sausages manufactured with natural antioxidant (NAT) in replacement of sodium nitrite (NIT).

Parameter	Treatment	Days of Storage			T × D
		7	30	60	
Escherichia coli	NAT	<1.0	<1.0	<1.0	n.s.
	NIT	<1.0	<1.0	<1.0	n.s.
Listeria monocytogenes	NAT	–	–	–	n.s.
	NIT	–	–	–	n.s.
Coagulase positive *Staphilococcus* spp.	NAT	<1.0	<1.0	<1.0	n.s.
	NIT	<1.0	<1.0	<1.0	n.s.
Salmonella spp.	NAT	–	–	–	n.s.
	NIT	–	–	–	n.s.
Total microbial count (30 °C)	NAT	7.04 [a]	8.14 [b,A]	10.20 [c,A]	n.s.
	NIT	7.04 [a]	8.32 [b,B]	10.32 [c,B]	n.s.

Results are expressed as log 10 colony forming units (CFU) per g of sausage; the symbol "−" indicates that the organism was not present. NAT = sausage with natural extracts, NIT = sausage with nitrite and nitrate as curing agents, [a,b,c] = different letters in the same row indicate significant differences ($p < 0.05$), [A,B] = different letters in the same column indicate significant differences ($p < 0.05$), T × D = interaction treatments × days of storage, n.s. = not significant.

3.2. Chemical Traits

Regarding chemical composition during storage (Table 3), data were reported as mean value between treatments considering that the same raw materials were used for all treatments and no difference appeared between the experimental groups. Moisture content showed a decreasing trend: differences were significant from 30 to 60 days and, consequently, protein, fat, and ash content appeared slightly increased at 60 days.

Table 3. Chemical composition of sausage during storage times (%).

Parameter	Days of Storage			T × D
	7	30	60	
Moisture	52.04 [b]	51.71 [b]	50.07 [a]	n.s.
Protein	15.26 [a]	15.36 [a]	15.97 [b]	n.s.
Lipid	30.26 [a]	30.51 [a]	31.42 [b]	n.s.
Ash	2.44 [a]	2.42 [a]	2.54 [b]	n.s.

[a,b] = Different letters in the same row indicate significant differences ($p < 0.05$). T × D = interaction treatments × days of storage, n.s. = not significant.

Regarding fatty acids profile (Table 4), the main fraction was represented by MUFA, followed by the SFA and PUFA in both types of sausage. In all samples, the predominant individual fatty acid was oleic acid (C18:1) followed by palmitic (C16:0), linoleic (C18:2n6), stearic (C18:0). PUFA/SFA value, useful to determine the nutritional quality of the food lipid fraction, was higher than 0.42 in both sausage types.

Table 4. Fatty acid profile during storage times in natural (NAT) and nitrite/nitrate (NIT) sausages.

Parameter	Treatment	Days of Storage			T × D
		7	30	60	
C16:0	NAT	23.17	23.09	23.19 [A]	n.s.
	NIT	23.31 [a]	23.27 [a]	23.61 [b,B]	n.s.
C16:1	NAT	2.63 [A]	2.64 [A]	2.64 [A]	n.s.
	NIT	2.70 [a,B]	2.70 [a,B]	2.75 [b,B]	n.s.
C18:0	NAT	12.17 [b]	11.96 [a]	12.06 [a,b]	n.s.
	NIT	12.16	12.09	12.07	n.s.
C18:1	NAT	41.85 [A]	42.16	41.94	n.s.
	NIT	42.62 [B]	42.40	42.31	n.s.
C18:2n6	NAT	14.44 [B]	14.45 [B]	14.44 [B]	n.s.
	NIT	13.58 [A]	13.80 [A]	13.65 [A]	n.s.
C18:3n3	NAT	0.94 [B]	0.94 [B]	0.94 [B]	n.s.
	NIT	0.88 [A]	0.90 [A]	0.89 [A]	n.s.
SFA	NAT	37.38	37.03	37.29	n.s.
	NIT	37.51	37.45	37.73	n.s.
MUFA	NAT	45.70 [A]	46.04 [A]	45.79 [A]	n.s.
	NIT	46.59 [B]	46.35 [B]	46.30 [B]	n.s.
PUFA	NAT	16.90 [B]	16.92 [B]	16.91 [B]	n.s.
	NIT	15.90 [A]	16.20 [A]	16.00 [A]	n.s.
n3PUFA	NAT	1.20 [B]	1.21 [B]	1.21 [B]	n.s.
	NIT	1.14 [A]	1.17 [A]	1.14 [A]	n.s.
n6PUFA	NAT	15.67 [B]	15.68 [B]	15.67 [B]	n.s.
	NIT	14.72 [A]	14.98 [A]	14.80 [A]	n.s.
PUFA/SFA	NAT	0.45 [B]	0.46 [B]	0.45 [B]	n.s.
	NIT	0.42 [A]	0.43 [A]	0.42 [A]	n.s.

NAT = sausages with natural extracts, NIT = sausages with nitrite and nitrate as curing agents, [a,b] = different letters in the same row indicate significant differences ($p < 0.05$), [A,B] = different letters in the same column indicate significant differences ($p < 0.05$), T × D = interaction treatments × days of storage, n.s. = not significant.

Relative to the storage times, the main categories of fatty acids did not show significative differences during the considered period. Some single fatty acid significantly changed their content at 60 days in NIT sausages (i.e., palmitic and palmitoleic acids), while in NAT sausages stearic acid decreased from 7 to 30 days.

NAT sausages obtained a slightly lower content of MUFA and a higher content of polyunsaturated, while for SFA no differences were shown. These differences reflected the behavior of the single fatty acids such as palmitoleic, oleic, and linoleic. Indeed, already at 7 days, PUFA content in NAT sausages was higher than MUFA ones. Consequently, the PUFA/SFA ratio showed significant differences between treatments: NIT sausages had always the lowest values.

3.3. Physical Traits

The pH showed a range between 5.39 and 6.19 and decreased from 7 to 60 days in both sausage types. Significant differences among treatments were found, with a slightly lower values observed for NAT groups respect to NIT (Table 5).

Table 5. Physical traits during storage times in natural (NAT) and nitrite/nitrate (NIT) sausages.

Parameter	Treatment	Days of Storage			T × D
		7	30	60	
pH	NAT	6.07 c,A	5.62 b,A	5.39 a,A	n.s.
	NIT	6.19 c,B	5.74 b,B	5.53 a,B	n.s.
Water activity (aW)	NAT	0.977	0.977	0.978	n.s.
	NIT	0.989	0.989	0.988	n.s.
L*	NAT	66.84 A	66.84 A	67.00 A	n.s.
	NIT	69.62 b,B	69.97 b,B	67.89 a,A	n.s.
a*	NAT	8.22 a,A	9.77 bA	11.22 c,A	*
	NIT	17.02 B	17.03 B	17.27 B	
b*	NAT	12.43 a,B	11.55 b,B	11.61 b	*
	NIT	11.17 a,A	11.13 a,A	11.46 b	
Warner–Bratzler shear force (kg)	NAT	29.48 A	30.54 A	31.22 A	n.s.
	NIT	37.78 B	39.86 B	39.55 B	n.s.
TPA hardness (N)	NAT	71.54 A	70.21 A	74.76 A	*
	NIT	78.02 a,B	86.20 a,b,B	93.28 b,B	
Cohesiveness	NAT	0.55 a,b,A	0.51 a,A	0.59 b	*
	NIT	0.67 B	0.66 B	0.62	
Springiness (mm)	NAT	7.59	7.69	7.33	n.s.
	NIT	7.65	7.69	7.67	n.s.
Chewiness (Nx mm)	NAT	300.03 A	284.77 A	300.05 A	n.s.
	NIT	398.97 B	434.53 B	441.85 B	n.s.

NAT = sausages with natural extracts, NIT = sausages with nitrite and nitrate as curing agents, a,b = different letters in the same row indicate significant differences ($p < 0.05$), A,B = different letters in the same column indicate significant differences ($p < 0.05$), T × D = interaction treatments × days of storage, n.s. = not significant, * = significant ($p < 0.05$).

Water activity (aW), showed a range between 0.977 to 0.988 and no differences were found both between treatments and storage times.

Regarding color data, lightness remained constant during the storage period in NAT sausages while decreased in NIT groups from 30 to 60 days. Redness progressively increased in NAT sausages as storage time increased, while in NIT sausages remained stable. Yellowness slightly decreased its value from 7 to 30 days in NAT, while in NIT the decline was from 30 to 60 days.

All color attributes were affected by treatment: L* showed significantly greater values in NIT samples than NAT ones excluding lightness at 60 days; a* was nearly twice as red in NIT, while b* was significantly higher in NAT at 7 and 30 days compared to the control. Regarding the tenderness performed by Warner–Bratzler (WB) there were no significant differences in storage times, whereas there were between treatments with NIT samples always less tender than NAT.

Considering texture profile analysis (TPA), hardness did not change over time in NAT sausages, while in NIT products showed a significant increase from 7 to 60 days. Storage time affected the cohesiveness in NAT sausages showing an increase from 30 to 60 days, while springiness and chewiness did not change over time in both sausage types.

Except for springiness, all TPA parameters are affected by treatment, being higher in NIT samples than NAT.

3.4. Sensory Characterization

The results of sensory evaluation (Figure 1) indicated that the major part of attributes was influenced ($p < 0.05$) by replacement of synthetic curing agents with natural extracts. The sensorial characteristics of the products showed that the color of NAT sausages was less uniform color and was two times less lightness compared to NIT ones. Differences between sausage types in odor and flavor attributes occurred with more intensity; NAT sausages also recorded higher average scores for off odor and off flavor, identified as bitter and tannic taste by panelists (data not reported).

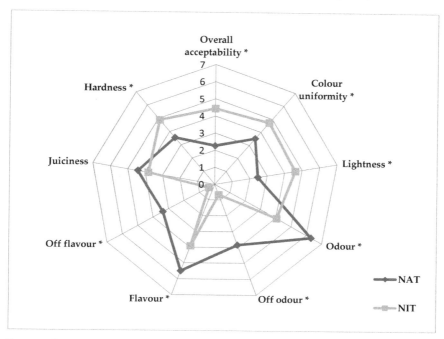

Figure 1. Sensorial traits of Cinta Senese sausages manufactured with natural extracts (NAT) as replacement of sodium nitrite (NIT), "*" indicates significant differences ($p < 0.05$).

According to TPA instrumental results, NAT sausages were evaluated more tender by panelists with respect to NIT, while no difference among samples were observed in juiciness.

The NIT sausages obtained a score evidently higher than NAT sausages.

4. Discussion

Sausages were safe for human consumption throughout the entire storage period and no visual spoilage was evident. Even if total microorganisms increase during the time, they did not cause alteration harmful for human consumption. Additionally, Rannucci et al. [34] observed an increase of total microorganisms during storage and in particular from 0 until 18 days in frankfurter sausages manufactured using an ancient recipe (pork meat from shoulder) but, even in this case, no pathogens were developed. Indeed, the antibacterial effect of some components included in NAT MIX was already documented, such as the effect of grape seed tannin against *Escherichia coli* [35] and of hydrolysable tannins against *Salmonella* and *Stafylococcus* [36].

The natural mixture seemed to be effective in terms of food safety showing lower values of total microbial count, probably because phenolic compounds chelate some metal ions of meat required for microbial growth [37]. A higher microbial growth could have played a role in degradation of different structural proteins, and, thus, tannins of natural mixtures, with their antioxidant and antimicrobial activity [38], prevented protein degradation of NAT products. The absence of main foodborne pathogens in natural curing agent sausages suggested that they provide the same antibacterial effect of synthetic curing agents. Hence, antimicrobial properties of natural curing agents could intervene in the delay of microbial spoilage as also suggested by Maqsood et al. [38] and Fasolato et al. [39].

However, further specified studies would be required to define the effectiveness of antimicrobial activity on products.

Water activity, often related with packaging and the sausages being a wet product, was always quite high, and this did not contribute to avoiding microbial growth. Ranucci et al. [34] obtained an aW value around 0.97 defining a high aW value that could promote the growth of such microbial populations even if samples were stored under vacuum refrigeration conditions. Alirezalu et al. [18] in frankfurter-type sausages with added nisin, polylysine, chitosan and natural extracts found similar aW values from 0.97 to 0.98 and, as in our case, the natural extract treatments did not affect this parameter.

Chemical composition of sausages suggested that they were less moist and more fat than similar products and even if stored under vacuum condition, they had lost part of the aqueous component up to 30 days. This could be probably due to Cinta Senese meat that had higher content of intramuscular fat than commercial breeds usually employed to produce sausages, as reported by Franci et al. [40]. Furthermore, the higher amount of fat in sausage products could negatively affect consumer opinion because a high daily fat intake is dangerous for human health, being a factor linked to the development of obesity, coronary heart disease, and arterial hypertension.

The fatty acid composition of sausages was characterized by lower level of SFA and higher levels of MUFA and PUFA compared to data reported in literature for pork frankfurter sausages [18,34,41]. As in this study, Škrlep et al. [42], in dry fermented sausages, recorded a PUFA amount of about one third of MUFA content and in parallel a low SFA content. This proportion of fatty acid groups can be associated to the outdoor rearing system, in particular to the availability of green feed. Additionally, lower fat saturation may be linked to higher physical activity of the pigs used in this study, as suggested by Daza et al. [43] who showed lower SFA in the backfat and higher PUFA in muscle of pigs reared outdoor than sedentary ones fed with the same diet.

The predominant individual fatty acids (oleic, palmitic, stearic, linoleic), typical of pork meat, were the same that occurred in the studies of Alirezalu et al. [18] and Fonseca et al. [44] in frankfurter and traditional Spanish sausages.

PUFA/SFA value was higher in both sausage types with respect to the threshold value indicated for healthiness of meat products (>0.40) reported by Wood et al. and with respect to other frankfurter sausages which reported values from 0.31 to 0.37 [16] and from 0.35 to 0.40 [18]. Additionally, Ranucci et al. [34], applying an ancient recipe for sausage preparation, showed a PUFA/SFA ratio above 0.40 associating these results with the lower value of saturated fatty acids.

The absence of differences in fatty acid composition and PUFA/SFA ratio during the storage time would seem to suggest that if process storage is conducted following the good practice, fatty acids do not change their profile. Furthermore, the lack of change of acidic profile during storage time, in particular of PUFA, denoted the positive influence of NAT and NIT curing agents on lipid oxidation. Both this lack of change together with the non-proliferation of pathogenic microorganisms are positive results in terms of product shelf-life.

Regarding the treatments, if the PUFA are considered as an indicator of meat oxidative status as proposed by Pateiro et al. [15], the slightly higher content in NAT already present at day 7 suggested that the natural curing agents employed had been less effective in the lipid oxidation control during the first part of the manufacturing process. Nevertheless, the addition of natural extract ingredients had only a "little impact" on fatty acid composition according to Alirezalu et al. [18].

The fatty acids results of this study seem to be linked to the use of Cinta Senese meat and consequently both to the genetic characteristic of the breed and to the specific outdoor rearing system, that included almost natural resources feeding. In fact, the fatty acid profile of local pigs is characterized to a greater deposition of MUFA, mainly oleic acid, than improved pigs whose fat contains higher quantities of saturated fatty acids. The highest level of monounsaturated fatty acids in native breeds is a consequence of differences in de novo lipid synthesis and their capacity to deposit monounsaturated fatty acids increases with age [45].

Regarding the physical traits, the pH showed values within the range obtained by other researches on frankfurter products [18,46]. The pH decline during the refrigerated vacuum package storage in both sausage types can be associated with meat intrinsic properties and/or microbial fermentation and in particular with the growth of lactic acid bacteria as suggested in study of Viuda-Martos et al. [47]. The pH differences recorded between treatments can be linked to the presence of *Lactobacillus* as observed by Hospital et al. [48] in low or nitrites-free sausages. This fact could be the cause of pH decline in NAT sausages. Nevertheless, the microbiota populations were not assessed in the present experiment and it is difficult to make any further conclusions. Regarding the color, higher redness of NIT sausages and its major stability was probably linked to the role of nitrites in nitrosyl-hemochrome formation which contributed both to characteristic red pigment of the commercial meat product and to its stability during storage times [4,7]. In addition, Özvur et al. [49] observed lower values of red color in products with added grape seed extract and they attributed the differences to natural color and emulsion properties of treatment. Ranucci et al. [34] obtained nitrate free frankfurter sausages with color parameter similar to this study (low a* and higher L* values) and they linked the result to the muscle and fat types that were different in their recipe.

Furthermore, in NAT sausages the lower color intensity could be associated to the oxidative reactions of lipids linked to the formation of yellow colored polymers [50] while the lower redness could be linked to the oxidation of muscle pigment myoglobin probably depending on lower pH [51].

It seems to be accepted that the main factors affecting the characteristic cured meat color is the nitrosylmyoglobin formation through the reaction of nitrite with myoglobin in the presence of endogenous or added reductants [52]. In absence of nitrites, natural extracts did not play this role and the sausages appear different.

The effect of treatments on sausages tenderness suggested that the NAT group were less hard than NIT, irrespective of the used method. The different result between Warner–Bratzler shear force and texture profile analysis could be associated to the different force that acts on the sample during the analysis. Novakovi et al. [32] in a review where they compared the two methods, suggested that the WB was less accurate because it has the highest coefficient of variability. Natural mixture also affected texture profile attributes—hardness, cohesiveness, and chewiness. Those results can be attributable basically to the differences in pH, which, when declining, causes the aggregation of myofibrillar proteins [53]. The higher pH of NIT samples could have led to the formation of a gel with myosin and entrapped water, leading to a stronger structure of sausages. In accordance with our results, Pateiro et al. [15] also reported that the hardness values significantly decreased with the addition of antioxidants. However, to the best of our knowledge, few data are available about frankfurter-type sausages with natural extract as single curing agents and the great variability of these traditional products makes comparisons difficult.

The sensory evaluation of sausages confirmed the differences in color and tenderness between products. Lower color uniformity and less lightness could be linked to the level of oxidation but also to the effect of nitrite on these attributes. Furthermore, in line with the results obtained from instrumental texture evaluation, NAT sausages were evaluated more tender by panelists. Odor and flavor were more intense in NAT sausages, even if these attributes were associated to off odor, off flavor, and other sensations. These results could be linked both to the remaining taste of the primary natural mixture constituents and to the effect of synthetic curing agents on products. In fact, Braghieri et al. [33] working on sensory evaluation of sausages suggested that, flavor being affected by several factors, differences in odor and flavor between products may be due to the inhibition of most activities as endogenous enzyme activities, microbial activities, and autoxidation in nitrate products. Regarding the overall acceptability, NIT samples obtained an evidently higher score than NAT sausages. Panelists considered synthetic curing agent sausages acceptable while the overall acceptability of natural extract product needs to be improved. This result was probably affected by many factors such as off flavor and off odor of NAT sausages but also by the consumers' habit of traditional taste and texture of synthetic curing agents' sausages. According to Alirezalu et al. [18] panelists preferred more compact sausages attributing higher scores to sausages with high hardness values. Similarly, Ribas-Agustí et al. [54] working on dry fermented sausages reported that panelists discarded the products with grape seed extract, because judged to be abnormal with respect to control samples. In addition, Özvural [55] observed a decrease in overall acceptability of frankfurters with grape seed extract added.

Sensory characteristics together with safety traits represent the primary attributes for consumers quality evaluation, followed by ethical and nutritional factors [33]. In terms of sensory properties, taste is the most important factor followed by color and texture. If these factors effectively influence the consumer intention to purchase [51], the results of sensory analysis of this study suggested that these attributes could be improved by a revaluation of the recipe of natural extracts sausages.

5. Conclusions

Nitrite/nitrate and natural frankfurter-type sausage was safety for the human consumption, as none of the main foodborne pathogens were found during the storage time considered.

Both types of sausages had a higher content of fat probably associated with the higher intramuscular fat of the Cinta Senese breed. Considering that the higher amount of daily lipid intake is considered negative for human health, manufacturers could re-evaluate the recipe and decrease the amount of fat.

The fatty acid composition showed that NAT treatment would seem slightly less efficient on lipid oxidation during the manufacturing, while in all storage times both treatments did not implicate remarkable impacts. Some differences in color suggested that further research is needed to improve color stability of natural extract sausages both during processing and storage. The replacements of natural extract as curing agents changed the perception of some sensorial properties overall in terms of taste and odor, recognized as "off" attributes and, as a whole, had a negative effect on the sensorial evaluation of NAT sausages.

Finally, the results so far indicated that natural extracts are an alternative to synthetic additives in Cinta Senese sausages even if some attributes could be improved.

The implementation of a new product using second-choice portion meat of a local breed and agricultural by products as curing agents could be interesting in terms both of sustainability and valorization of the territory and of Cinta Senese products.

Supplementary Materials: The following are available online at http://www.mdpi.com/2076-2615/10/1/14/s1, Table S1: List of attributes of sausage sensory profile.

Author Contributions: Conceptualization, S.P., A.A. and O.F.; methodology, S.P., F.S., A.R.; formal analysis S.P., F.S., V.B., A.C., A.S.; data curation, S.P., F.S., O.F.; writing—Original draft preparation, S.P.; writing—Review and editing, S.P., F.S., O.F.; supervision, R.B.; funding acquisition, A.A. All authors have read and agreed to the published version of the manuscript.

Funding: This research was funded by Tuscany Region (PSR 2014–2020) and was conducted as part of PIF Project "ValMonTi".

Acknowledgments: We acknowledge Dott.ssa Silvia Urciuoli, Arianna Scardigli and Phytolab-DiSIA (UNIFI), activity included in the BakeriInnov and ASTAMIBEN projects, GO Tuscany Region 2017–2021 for manufacturing and providing the antioxidant mixtures. Authors also acknowledge the support of Azienda Agricola Savigni (Pistoia, Italy).

Conflicts of Interest: The authors declare no conflict of interest.

References

1. European Food Safety Authority. *EFSA Explains Risk Assessment Nitrites and Nitrates Added to Food*; European Food Safety Authority: Parma, Italy, 2017; ISBN 978-92-9499-007-5.
2. Marco, A.; Navarro, J.L.; Flores, M. The influence of nitrite and nitrate on microbial, chemical and sensory parameters of slow dry fermented sausage. *Meat Sci.* **2006**, *73*, 660–673. [CrossRef]
3. Hammes, W.P. Metabolism of nitrate in fermented meats: The characteristic feature of a specific group of fermented foods. *Food Microbiol.* **2012**, *29*, 151–156. [CrossRef] [PubMed]

4. Honikel, K.-O. The use and control of nitrate and nitrite for the processing of meat products. *Meat Sci.* **2008**, *78*, 68–76. [CrossRef] [PubMed]

5. Mey, E.D.; Maere, H.D.; Paelinck, H.; Fraeye, I. Volatile N-nitrosamines in meat products: Potential precursors, influence of processing, and mitigation strategies. *Crit. Rev. Food Sci. Nutr.* **2017**, *57*, 2909–2923. [CrossRef] [PubMed]

6. Drabik-Markiewicz, G.; Dejaegher, B.; De Mey, E.; Kowalska, T.; Paelinck, H.; Vander Heyden, Y. Influence of putrescine, cadaverine, spermidine or spermine on the formation of N-nitrosamine in heated cured pork meat. *Food Chem.* **2011**, *126*, 1539–1545. [CrossRef]

7. Herrmann, S.S.; Granby, K.; Duedahl-Olesen, L. Formation and mitigation of N-nitrosamines in nitrite preserved cooked sausages. *Food Chem.* **2015**, *174*, 516–526. [CrossRef]

8. Velasco, V.; Williams, P. Improving meat quality through natural antioxidants. *Chil. J. Agric. Res.* **2011**, *71*, 313–322. [CrossRef]

9. Fasseas, M.K.; Mountzouris, K.C.; Tarantilis, P.A.; Polissiou, M.; Zervas, G. Antioxidant activity in meat treated with oregano and sage essential oils. *Food Chem.* **2007**, *106*, 1188–1194. [CrossRef]

10. Cosentino, S.; Tuberoso, C.I.; Pisano, B.; Satta, M.; Mascia, V.; Arzedi, E.; Palmas, F. In-Vitro antimicrobial activity and chemical composition of Sardinian Thymus essential oils. *Lett. Appl. Microbiol.* **1999**, *29*, 130–135. [CrossRef]

11. Rota, M.C.; Herrera, A.; Martinez, R.M.; Sotomayor, J.A.; Jordan, M.J. Antimicrobial activity and chemical composition of Thymus vulgaris, Thymus zygis and Thymus hyemalis essential oils. *Food Control* **2008**, *19*, 681–687. [CrossRef]

12. Mukai, K.; Nagai, S.; Ohara, K. Kinetic study of the quenching reaction of singlet oxygen by tea catechins in ethanol solution. *Free Radic. Biol. Med.* **2005**, *39*, 752–761. [CrossRef] [PubMed]

13. Andjelkovic, M.; Vancamp, J.; Demeulenaer, B.; Depaemelaere, G.; Socaciu, C.; Verloo, M.; Verhe, R. Iron-chelation properties of phenolic acids bearing catechol and galloyl groups. *Food Chem.* **2006**, *98*, 23–31. [CrossRef]

14. Eskandari, M.H.; Hosseinpour, S.; Mesbahi, G.; Shekarforoush, S. New composite nitrite-free and low-nitrite meat-curing systems using natural colorants. *Food Sci. Nutr.* **2013**, *1*, 392–401. [CrossRef] [PubMed]

15. Pateiro, M.; Bermúdez, R.; Lorenzo, J.M.; Franco, D. Effect of Addition of Natural Antioxidants on the Shelf-Life of "Chorizo", a Spanish Dry-Cured Sausage. *Antioxidants* **2015**, *4*, 42–67. [CrossRef]

16. Ayo, J.; Carballo, J.; Serrano, J.; Olmedilla-Alonso, B.; Ruiz-Capillas, C.; Jiménez-Colmenero, F. Effect of total replacement of pork backfat with walnut on the nutritional profile of frankfurters. *Meat Sci.* **2007**, *77*, 173–181. [CrossRef]

17. Sebranek, J.G.; Bacus, J.N. Cured meat products without direct addition of nitrate or nitrite: What are the issues? *Meat Sci.* **2007**, *77*, 136–147. [CrossRef]

18. Alirezalu, K.; Hesari, J.; Nemati, Z.; Munekata, P.E.S.; Barba, F.J.; Lorenzo, J.M. Combined effect of natural antioxidants and antimicrobial compounds during refrigerated storage of nitrite-free frankfurter-type sausage. *Food Res. Int.* **2019**, *120*, 839–850. [CrossRef]

19. Romani, A.; Campo, M.; Pinelli, P. HPLC/DAD/ESI-MS analyses and anti-radical activity of hydrolyzable tannins from different vegetal species. *Food Chem.* **2012**, *130*, 214–221. [CrossRef]

20. Romani, A.; Scardigli, A.; Pinelli, P. An environmentally friendly process for the production of extracts rich in phenolic antioxidants from Olea europaea L. and Cynara scolymus L. matrices. *Eur. Food Res. Technol.* **2017**, *243*, 1229–1238. [CrossRef]

21. Romani, A.; Pinelli, P.; Ieri, F.; Bernini, R. Sustainability, Innovation, and Green Chemistry in the Production and Valorization of Phenolic Extracts from Olea europaea L. *Sustainability* **2016**, *8*, 1002. [CrossRef]

22. Campo, M.; Pinelli, P.; Romani, A. Hydrolyzable tannins from sweet chestnut fractions obtained by a sustainable and eco-friendly industrial process. *Nat. Prod. Commun.* **2016**, *11*, 409–415. [CrossRef] [PubMed]

23. Lucarini, M.; Durazzo, A.; Romani, A.; Campo, M.; Lombardi-Boccia, G.; Cecchini, F. Bio-Based Compounds from Grape Seeds: A Biorefinery Approach. *Molecules* **2018**, *23*, 1888. [CrossRef] [PubMed]

24. ISO 16649-2:2001. Available online: http://store.uni.com/catalogo/index.php/iso-16649-2-2001 (accessed on 3 December 2019).

25. UNI EN ISO 11290-1:2005. Available online: http://store.uni.com/catalogo/uni-en-iso-11290-1-2005?__store=en&___from_store=it (accessed on 3 December 2019).

26. UNI EN ISO 6888-1:2004. Available online: http://store.uni.com/catalogo/index.php/uni-en-iso-6888-1-2004 (accessed on 3 December 2019).

27. UNI EN ISO 6579-1:2017. Available online: http://store.uni.com/catalogo/index.php/uni-en-iso-6579-1-2017 (accessed on 3 December 2019).

28. UNI EN ISO 4833-1:2013. Available online: http://store.uni.com/catalogo/index.php/uni-en-iso-4833-1-2013 (accessed on 3 December 2019).

29. AOAC. *Official Methods of Analysis*; AOAC: Rockville, MD, USA, 2019; Volume 1, p. 771.

30. Folch, J.; Lees, M.; Stanley, G.H.S. A Simple Method for the Isolation and Purification of Total Lipides from Animal Tissues. *J. Biol. Chem.* **1957**, *226*, 497–509. [PubMed]

31. Morrison, W.R.; Smith, L.M. PREPARATION OF FATTY ACID METHYL ESTERS AND DIMETHYLACETALS FROM LIPIDS WITH BORON FLUORIDE–METHANOL. *J. Lipid Res.* **1964**, *5*, 600–608.

32. Novaković, S.; Tomašević, I. A comparison between Warner-Bratzler shear force measurement and texture profile analysis of meat and meat products: A review. *IOP Conf. Ser. Earth Environ. Sci.* **2017**, *85*, 012063. [CrossRef]

33. Braghieri, A.; Piazzolla, N.; Carlucci, A.; Bragaglio, A.; Napolitano, F. Sensory properties, consumer liking and choice determinants of Lucanian dry cured sausages. *Meat Sci.* **2016**, *111*, 122–129. [CrossRef]

34. Ranucci, D.; Miraglia, D.; Branciari, R.; Morganti, G.; Roila, R.; Zhou, K.; Jiang, H.; Braconi, P. Frankfurters made with pork meat, emmer wheat (Triticum dicoccum Schübler) and almonds nut (Prunus dulcis Mill.): Evaluation during storage of a novel food from an ancient recipe. *Meat Sci.* **2018**, *145*, 440–446. [CrossRef]

35. Ahn, J.; Grün, I.U.; Mustapha, A. Effects of plant extracts on microbial growth, color change, and lipid oxidation in cooked beef. *Food Microbiol.* **2007**, *24*, 7–14. [CrossRef]

36. Taguri, T.; Tanaka, T.; Kouno, I. Antimicrobial activity of 10 different plant polyphenols against bacteria causing food-borne disease. *Biol. Pharm. Bull.* **2004**, *27*, 1965–1969. [CrossRef]

37. Nirmal, N.P.; Benjakul, S. Retardation of quality changes of Pacific white shrimp by green tea extract treatment and modified atmosphere packaging during refrigerated storage. *Int. J. Food Microbiol.* **2011**, *149*, 247–253. [CrossRef]

38. Maqsood, S.; Abushelaibi, A.; Manheem, K.; Al Rashedi, A.; Kadim, I.T. Lipid oxidation, protein degradation, microbial and sensorial quality of camel meat as influenced by phenolic compounds. *LWT Food Sci. Technol.* **2015**, *63*, 953–959. [CrossRef]

39. Fasolato, L.; Carraro, L.; Facco, P.; Cardazzo, B.; Balzan, S.; Taticchi, A.; Andreani, N.A.; Montemurro, F.; Martino, M.E.; Di Lecce, G.; et al. Agricultural by-products with bioactive effects: A multivariate approach to evaluate microbial and physicochemical changes in a fresh pork sausage enriched with phenolic compounds from olive vegetation water. *Int. J. Food Microbiol.* **2016**, *228*, 34–43. [CrossRef] [PubMed]

40. Franci, O.; Pugliese, C.; Acciaioli, A.; Bozzi, R.; Campodoni, G.; Sirtori, F.; Pianaccioli, L.; Gandini, G. Performance of Cinta Senese pigs and their crosses with Large White 2. Physical, chemical and technological traits of Tuscan dry-cured ham. *Meat Sci.* **2007**, *76*, 597–603. [CrossRef] [PubMed]

41. Estevez, M.; Ventanas, S.; Cava, R. Oxidation of lipids and proteins in frankfurters with different fatty acid compositions and tocopherol and phenolic contents. *Food Chem.* **2007**, *100*, 55–63. [CrossRef]

42. Škrlep, M.; Čandek-Potokar, M.; Tomažin, U.; Batorek Lukač, N.; Flores, M. Properties and aromatic profile of dry-fermented sausages produced from Krškopolje pigs reared under organic and conventional rearing regime. *Animal* **2018**, *12*, 1316–1323. [CrossRef] [PubMed]

43. Daza, A.; Rey, A.I.; Olivares, A.; Cordero, G.; Toldrá, F.; López-Bote, C.J. Physical activity-induced alterations on tissue lipid composition and lipid metabolism in fattening pigs. *Meat Sci.* **2009**, *81*, 641–646. [CrossRef]

44. Fonseca, S.; Gómez, M.; Domínguez, R.; Lorenzo, J.M. Physicochemical and sensory properties of Celta dry-ripened "salchichón" as affected by fat content. *Grasas y Aceites* **2015**, *66*, 059.

45. Pugliese, C.; Sirtori, F. Quality of meat and meat products produced from southern European pig breeds. *Meat Sci.* **2012**, *90*, 511–518. [CrossRef]

46. Horita, C.N.; Farias-Campomanes, A.M.; Barbosa, T.S.; Esmerino, E.A.; da Cruz, A.G.; Bolini, H.M.A.; Meireles, M.A.A.; Pollonio, M.A.R. The Antimicrobial, antioxidant and sensory properties of garlic and its derivatives in Brazilian low-sodium frankfurters along shelf-life. *Food Res. Int.* **2016**, *84*, 1–8.

47. Viuda-Martos, M.; Ruiz-Navajas, Y.; Fernández-López, J.; Pérez-Álvarez, J.A. Effect of added citrus fibre and spice essential oils on quality characteristics and shelf-life of mortadella. *Meat Sci.* **2010**, *85*, 568–576. [CrossRef]

48. Hospital, X.F.; Carballo, J.; Fernández, M.; Arnau, J.; Gratacós, M.; Hierro, E. Technological implications of reducing nitrate and nitrite levels in dry-fermented sausages: Typical microbiota, residual nitrate and nitrite and volatile profile. *Food Control* **2015**, *57*, 275–281. [CrossRef]

49. Özvural, E.B.; Vural, H. Which is the best grape seed additive for frankfurters: Extract, oil or flour? *J. Sci. Food Agric.* **2014**, *94*, 792–797. [CrossRef] [PubMed]

50. Ruiz, J.; García, C.; Muriel, E.; Andrés, A.I.; Ventanas, J. Influence of sensory characteristics on the acceptability of dry-cured ham. *Meat Sci.* **2002**, *61*, 347–354. [CrossRef]

51. Faustman, C.; Sun, Q.; Mancini, R.; Suman, S.P. Myoglobin and lipid oxidation interactions: Mechanistic bases and control. *Meat Sci.* **2010**, *86*, 86–94. [CrossRef] [PubMed]

52. Wakamatsu, J.; Akter, M.; Honma, F.; Hayakawa, T.; Kumura, H.; Nishimura, T. Optimal pH of zinc protoporphyrin IX formation in porcine muscles: Effects of muscle fiber type and myoglobin content. *LWT* **2019**, *101*, 599–606. [CrossRef]

53. Lücke, F.-K. Utilization of microbes to process and preserve meat. *Meat Sci.* **2000**, *56*, 105–115. [CrossRef]

54. Ribas-Agustí, A.; Gratacós-Cubarsí, M.; Sárraga, C.; Guàrdia, M.D.; García-Regueiro, J.-A.; Castellari, M. Stability of phenolic compounds in dry fermented sausages added with cocoa and grape seed extracts. *LWT Food Sci. Technol.* **2014**, *57*, 329–336. [CrossRef]

55. Özvural, E.B.; Vural, H. Grape seed flour is a viable ingredient to improve the nutritional profile and reduce lipid oxidation of frankfurters. *Meat Sci.* **2011**, *88*, 179–183. [CrossRef]

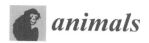

Article

Quality of Dry-Cured Ham from Entire, Surgically and Immunocastrated Males: Case Study on Kraški Pršut

Marjeta Čandek-Potokar [1,*], Martin Škrlep [1], Eliza Kostyra [2],
Sylwia Żakowska-Biemans [2], Klavdija Poklukar [1], Nina Batorek-Lukač [1], Kevin Kress [3],
Ulrike Weiler [3] and Volker Stefanski [3,*]

[1] Agricultural Institute of Slovenia, Hacquetova ul. 17, 1000 Ljubljana, Slovenia; martin.skrlep@kis.si (M.Š.); klavdija.poklukar@kis.si (K.P.); nina.batorek@kis.si (N.B.-L.)
[2] Institute of Human Nutrition Sciences, Warsaw University of Life Sciences (WULS-SGGW), ul. Nowoursynowska 159c, 02-787 Warsaw, Poland; eliza_kostyra@sggw.pl (E.K.); sylwia_zakowska_biemans@sggw.pl (S.Ż.-B.)
[3] Department of Behavioral Physiology of Livestock, Institute of Animal Science, University of Hohenheim, Garbenstraße 17, 70599 Stuttgart, Germany; kress.kevin@uni-hohenheim.de (K.K.); weiler@uni-hohenheim.de (U.W.)
* Correspondence: meta.candek-potokar@kis.si (M.Č.-P.); volker.stefanski@uni-hohenheim.de (V.S.); Tel.: +386-1-2805124 (M.Č.-P.)

Received: 13 December 2019; Accepted: 2 February 2020; Published: 3 February 2020

Simple Summary: The initiative to stop the surgical castration of piglets calls for the assessment of alternative solutions. The issue is particularly sensitive for the processing of traditional products. This study demonstrated important differences between male sex categories and showed that dry-cured ham from entire males presented distinct sensory depreciation and also differed in many other aspects important in dry-cured ham production. Under the conditions of the present study, i.e., standard slaughter age and weight and delay between immunocastration and slaughter, dry-cured ham from surgical castrates showed the most distinct properties, while immunocastrated pigs were more similar in many aspects to entire males, however, their main advantage was in their sensory attributes, i.e., absence of boar taint.

Abstract: Alternative solutions to the surgical castration of piglets need to be assessed because this is a particularly sensitive issue for the processing of traditional pork products. Currently, the available information about the advantages and drawbacks of castration for dry-cured products is limited; thus, the objective of this study was to evaluate the quality of Slovenian dry-cured ham (Kraški pršut) from entire males (EM), immunocastrates (IC) and surgical castrates (SC). Hams (12 per sex group) were processed for one year and physical-chemical, rheological and sensory analysis of the dry-cured hams was performed. With regard to processing aptitude, the main difference was in the subcutaneous fat thickness, which influenced the level of dehydration and salt intake. This was further reflected in the physical-chemical traits and the texture, which were measured instrumentally or assessed by panelists. Regarding the aforementioned traits, EM and IC were generally similar and different from SC. On the contrary, sensory profiling of odor, taste and flavor demonstrated that EM had the lowest overall sensory quality, different from both IC and SC, and presented odors and flavors described as sweat, manure, sharp and persistent. We confirmed that dry-curing did not eliminate the perception of boar taint in the product from EM. The IC were similar in many aspects to EM except for the odor, taste and flavor of dry-cured hams, in which case they were more similar to SC.

Keywords: immunocastration; entire male; castration; pig; dry-cured ham

1. Introduction

In pig production, it is a widespread practice to castrate male piglets in order to prevent an unpleasant off-flavor, the so-called boar taint, which can appear in the meat of sexually mature entire males. EU legislation allows the castration of male piglets without anesthesia/analgesia in the first seven days of life; however, this practice has been criticized from the animal welfare point of view [1]. Thus, in recent years, the European pig industry sector has considered ending this practice [2,3]. However, before this can happen, certain problems and alternative solutions must be assessed, not only because of the risk of boar taint but also due to the potential deterioration in the technological quality of the meat and its consequences for processed products needs to be evaluated [4]. The challenges are particularly relevant to traditional products, where the highest risks are associated with fat quantity and quality [5]. Boar taint (an unpleasant aroma attributed to the presence of two malodorous compounds, androstenone and skatole) is more apparent when fat content is high, no masking ingredients are used and the product is consumed warm [6]. It has been detected in dry-cured products, even if these were not consumed warm [7,8]. According to Tørngren et al. [9], androstenone levels must be below 0.4 ppm and the serving temperature must be below 23 °C for consumers to not detect it in the processed pork. A review of consumer studies [6] indicated the need for a better understanding of the risks related to the perception of boar taint in the case of different product types. However, there are not many studies available that compare the alternatives to surgical castration with regard to the processing aptitude of the meat and dry-cured product quality. The quality of the raw material is very important in dry-cured ham processing and is affected by many factors, including the sex of pigs [10]. Thus, the aim of the present study was to compare the effects of three male sex categories (immunocastrates, surgical castrates and entire males) on the production of dry-cured ham, more precisely, Kraški pršut, a Slovenian dry-cured ham that has protected geographical indication (PGI) status. Its manufacture is clearly defined with specific demands regarding the raw material (green ham weight, visual appearance, pH, fat thickness), and the minimum processing weight loss. A minimum curing period of 12 months is prescribed [11]. For this product, as is the case for many other similar PGI or unbranded dry-cured ham products, the origin of the raw material is not prescribed and provisions made with raw hams stem from standard pig production. In such situations, the probability of getting green hams from different castration methods is higher and raw material variability is increased. Due to differences in the physiological and metabolic characteristics of the three sex types of pigs, the raw material properties, i.e., its seasoning aptitude, may be altered. The question of interest is what are the consequences for the final product quality and the adaptations in processing that may be required. The present study covers the assessment of the raw material properties, processing yield and final product quality (chemical, rheological and sensory quality traits) as affected by the male sex group of pigs.

2. Materials and Methods

2.1. Origin and Processing of Hams

The hams for this study originate from a wider study evaluating immunocastration (for more details see [12]). We compared hams from surgical castrates (SC), immunocastrates (IC) and entire males (EM) of one crossbreed (Pietrain x German Landrace), which were fattened with the same diet ad libitum. Piglets of the SC group were surgically castrated within the first week of life, IC were vaccinated twice with Improvac® at an age of 12 (first vaccination—V1) and 22 weeks (second vaccination—V2). Pigs were slaughtered in an experimental slaughter unit (Landesanstalt für Schweinezucht Boxberg, Boxberg, Germany) using their standard procedures. For dry-cured ham processing, pigs (26 or 27 weeks old, with an average weight of 121.7 kg, $n = 36$) of one slaughter batch were included, one ham per pig was processed, giving a total of 12 hams for every sex group. A day after slaughter, the hams were cut from the carcasses between the 6th and 7th lumbar vertebra, shaped into the prescribed form for Kraški pršut and weighed. Subcutaneous fat thickness of the green ham was measured under the femoral head and pHu was measured in the semimembranosus muscle (SM) using a MP120 pH meter (Mettler-Toledo GmbH, Schwarzenbach, Switzerland).

Hams were submitted to a standard salting duration with dry salting for 12 days at 2–4 °C (first salting at 7 days and second salting 5 days later). After salting, the residual salt was removed and the hams were kept in a resting phase (4–6 °C and 70%–85% relative humidity (RH)) for 73 days. After this salt equilibration phase, the hams were dried for 87 days (at 20 °C and 60%–80% RH). Thereafter the open surface of the hams was coated with a mixture of pork fat, pepper and flour to prevent too strong desiccation, then, the hams were ripened for another 196 days, resulting in the final processing duration of 368 days. At each processing step, the hams were weighed in order to monitor processing losses. At the end of processing, samples were taken from the central part of the ham, vacuum packed and frozen at −20 °C until analyzed.

2.2. Color Measurements

Objective color parameters (CIE L*, a*, b*) were measured using a Minolta Chroma Meter CR-300 (Minolta Co. Ltd, Osaka, Japan) on the green ham muscle, gluteus medius (GM), on dry product muscles, the biceps femoris (BF), semitendinosus (ST), semimembranosus (SM), and the subcutaneous fat layer. The chroma (C*) value was calculated as $\sqrt{(a^{*2} + b^{*2})}$ and hue angle (h°) value as $\tan^{-1}(b^*/a^*)$, which denote color saturation and taint, respectively.

2.3. Chemical Analyses

Muscle samples (BF, SM, ST) were trimmed of superficial connective and fat tissue and pulverized in liquid nitrogen with a laboratory mill (Grindomix GM200, Retsch GmbH and Co., Haan, Germany). Total nitrogen, non-protein nitrogen (NPN) and salt (NaCl) contents were chemically determined as described by [13]. Briefly, the content of NaCl was determined by potentiometric titration using DL53 General Purpose Titrator (Mettler Toledo, Schwarzenbach, Switzerland), the proteolysis index (PI) was calculated as a ratio between NPN and total nitrogen content, while intramuscular fat (IMF) and dry-matter content were determined by near-infrared spectral analysis (NIR Systems 6500 Monochromator, Foss NIR System, Silver Spring, MD, USA) using internal calibrations. Water activity was measured with the HygroPalm AW1 SET instrument (Rotronic, Bassersdorf, Germany) using Aw Quick mode.

Thiobarbituric reactive substances (TBARS) of the BF muscle were determined according to the method described by Lynch and Frei [14]. Briefly, 0.5 g of sample was homogenized with 10 mL of 0.15 M KCl and 0.1 mM BHT, and an aliquot (0.5 mL) mixed with 1% (*w/v*) of 2-thiobarbituric acid in 50 mM NaOH and 2.8% (*w/v*) trichloroacetic acid, and incubated for 10 min at 100 °C in a thermostatic heating block. After cooling to room temperature, the pink chromogen was extracted into n-butanol and its absorbance was measured spectrophotometrically at 535 nm (BioSpectrometer Fluorescence, Eppendorf, Hamburg, Germany). TBARS concentration was expressed on a wet basis as µg malondialdehyde (MDA)/kg.

2.4. Texture Profile Measurements

Instrumental texture was measured in the SM, ST and BF muscles as previously described [13,15]. Two 15 mm thick pieces were taken from each ham and the muscles were excised, trimmed of fat and connective tissue. Six samples of defined dimensions (length × width × height = 20 mm × 20 mm × 15 mm) were submitted to stress relaxation (SR) and texture profile analysis (TPA) using a texture analyzer (Ametek Lloyd Instruments, Ltd., Bognor Regis, UK) with a 50 kg load cell and a 50 mm diameter compression plate. The SR test consisted of compressing the samples perpendicularly in the fiber-bundle direction to 25% of their initial height (crosshead speed of 1 mm/s). During compression for 90 s (speed of 50 points/s) the force was recorded and force decay coefficient (Y90) was calculated as Y90 = (F0 − F90)/F0, where F0 (N) is the initial force and F90 (N) is the force recorded after 90 s of relaxation. In the TPA test, the samples were compressed twice to 50% of their original height at a crosshead speed of 1 mm/s and the following parameters were calculated: hardness (N), cohesiveness, gumminess (N), springiness (mm), chewiness (N) and adhesiveness (N*mm).

2.5. Sensory Analysis

The sensory qualities of the dry-cured hams were assessed using the quantitative descriptive analysis method [16]. Thirty-seven attributes were chosen and defined according to the profiling procedure. Sample evaluation included: four appearance traits (fat, meat, color uniformity, marbling), thirteen odor traits (meat, fatty, smoky, acidic, sweet, bouillon-like, fermentation, yeast, sweat, manure, sharp, rancid, overall odor intensity), five texture attributes (hardness, gumminess, dryness, fibrousness, ease of fragmentation), fourteen taste/flavor traits (meat, fatty, smoky, sour, salty, sweet, bitter, bouillon-like, fermentation, yeast, sweat, manure, persistent, rancid) and overall sensory quality. The intensity of the descriptors was measured on a linear unstructured scale (0–10 cm) anchored at both extremes from "none" (on the left) to "very strong" (on the right). Overall sensory quality of the dry-cured hams was defined as the impression of the harmony of the examined attributes, with no or only slight intensity of negative notes.

The individual samples of dry-cured hams (one slice, 1 mm thick) were placed in coded (3-digit numbers) plastic containers (200 mL) and covered with lids. A meat slicer was used to cut the samples and the thickness of the first slice of dry-cured ham was additionally verified by a Vernier caliper. The samples were presented to the assessors in random order at room temperature (21 ± 2 °C) and under white bulb light. Unsweetened tea (at the temperature of approximately 50 °C) and a piece of matzah were used as a taste neutralizer between samples. The order of the samples presented to the panelists was balanced to minimize possible carry-over effects between dry-cured ham samples. The evaluations were conducted during the morning and afternoon hours, with two sessions per each set of three samples from EM, IC and SC pigs. The assessment of the samples was performed in an accredited sensory laboratory, equipped with 10 individual testing booths (ISO 8589:2007 [17]).

Ten trained and experienced assessors sensitive to boar compounds performed the profiling of the samples in two replications (ISO 8586:2012 [18]). Assessors were tested for their ability to qualitatively and quantitatively differentiate the odor of skatole and androstenone in low, high and very high concentrations on paper strips. Twenty individual results for each dry-cured ham sample were used for statistical analysis and interpretation of the sensory data according to the experimental design.

2.6. Statistical Analysis

To determine the effect of male sex group on green ham traits, ham processing weight losses, chemical properties and instrumental texture measurements, the results were submitted to one-way analysis of variance with a male sex group as fixed effect using the Mixed procedure of SAS statistical software (SAS Institute Inc., Cary, NC, USA). In the case of sensory traits, repeated measures analysis was performed with the model including male sex group and session as fixed and panelist as random effects. To assess differences between groups, the least squares means (LSM) were compared using Tukey's *t*-test. A cut-off *p*-value below 0.05 was considered significant.

3. Results

3.1. Green Ham Properties and Ham Processing Weight Loss

Table 1 presents the information on green ham properties and weight losses during the processing. There were no differences observed between EM, IC and SC in trimmed ham weight and pH value measured in SM muscle, whereas subcutaneous fat was significantly thicker in SC than in EM or IC hams ($p < 0.0001$). Color measurements exhibited differences for glycolytic GM but not oxidative GP muscle. IC had a higher L* value of GM muscle, i.e., lighter color than EM ($p = 0.02$), while SC had an intermediate position, and did not differ from EM or IC. Regarding processing weight loss, the hams from SC pigs exhibited significantly higher yields ($p < 0.01$) than IC or EM, which were similar in this respect.

Table 1. Effect of male sex group on green ham properties and ham processing weight loss.

Trait	EM	IC	SC	RMSE	p-Value
		Male Sex Group			
Ham trimmed, kg	11.1	11.2	11.8	0.947	0.1677
Fat thickness, mm	8.0 [a]	9.2 [a]	14.2 [b]	2.619	<0.0001
SM muscle pHu	5.55	5.53	5.57	0.061	0.3246
GM muscle color					
L*	47.5 [a]	50.1 [b]	48.8 [a,b]	2.181	0.0213
a*	9.8	9.8	9.5	1.429	0.8606
b*	6.1	6.7	6.4	0.9584	0.3932
c*	11.5	11.9	11.5	1.584	0.8096
H°	32.3	34.1	34.1	3.364	0.3260
GP muscle color					
L*	39.3	38.9	41.6	3.412	0.1293
a*	16.2	18.0	17.3	2.289	0.1998
b*	6.9	8.0	8.3	1.873	0.1792
c*	17.6	19.7	19.3	2.764	0.1917
H°	23.0	23.4	25.6	3.101	0.1055
Ham weight loss, %					
First salting	3.1 [b]	2.8 [a,b]	2.5 [a]	0.347	0.0022
Second salting	1.5 [b]	1.5 [b]	1.0 [a]	0.270	<0.0001
Resting	16.8 [b]	16.1 [b]	14.4 [a]	1.234	0.0002
Drying	9.3 [b]	9.0 [b]	7.7 [a]	0.724	<0.0001
Ripening	8.5 [b]	7.8 [b]	6.5 [a]	0.723	<0.0001
Total	39.2 [b]	37.2 [b]	32.2 [a]	2.669	<0.0001

Fat thickness was measured under the femoral head. SM semimembranosus; pHu denotes pH value measured 24 h post-mortem; GM gluteus medius; GP gluteus profundus; EM entire males; IC immunocastrates, SC surgical castrates, RMSE root-mean-square error. Values with different superscripts are significantly different ($p < 0.05$).

3.2. Physical-Chemical Properties of Dry-Cured Ham Muscles

Table 2 provides the results of the physical-chemical analysis for three dry-cured ham muscles, outer SM and inner ST and BF. There was a significant effect of male sex group ($p < 0.05$) on the proximate composition of all three muscles, showing that at the end of processing, muscles of SC retained more water and less salt. Consequently, water activity was higher in SC than EM or IC in all three muscles. Ham muscles from SC also had higher fat and lower protein content. Considering the index of proteolysis (ratio of non-protein to total nitrogen), the effect of male sex group differed according to muscle. It was not affected in the outer SM muscle, it was higher in SC and IC than EM in the inner ST, and it was higher in SC than IC or EM in the inner BF muscle.

Table 2. Effect of male sex group on physical-chemical properties of dry-cured ham muscles.

| | Male Sex Group | | | | |
Trait	EM	IC	SC	RMSE	*p*-Value
SM muscle					
Water (g/kg)	497.1 [a,b]	488.6 [a]	510.3 [b]	16.9	0.0126
IMF (g/kg)	34.6 [a]	40.7 [a,b]	48.2 [b]	8.9	0.0039
Salt (g/kg)	53.2 [b]	51.2 [a,b]	45.6 [a]	5.1	0.0037
Proteins (g/kg)	399.6 [a]	405.6 [a]	382.1 [b]	15.9	0.0031
PI, %	17.8	17.6	18.0	1.2	0.7330
aw	0.915 [a]	0.917 [a]	0.933 [b]	0.010	0.0003
ST muscle					
Water (g/kg)	561.1	563.9	569.8	17.7	0.6600
IMF (g/kg)	45.8 [a]	62.2 [a]	86.3 [b]	20.1	0.0001
Salt (g/kg)	58.8 [a]	57.7 [a]	49.3 [b]	6.0	0.0009
Proteins (g/kg)	316.6 [a]	302.4 [b]	282.1 [c]	13.5	<0.0001
PI, %	22.1 [a]	24.6 [b]	26.4 [b]	1.9	<0.0001
a_w	0.922 [a]	0.926 [a]	0.944 [b]	0.011	<0.0001
BF muscle					
Water (g/kg)	596.7 [a]	599.1 [a]	617.3 [b]	13.6	0.0014
IMF (g/kg)	21.6 [a]	26.7 [a,b]	32.5 [b]	7.6	0.0070
Salt (g/kg)	64.5 [a]	62.8 [a]	55.5 [b]	5.9	0.0017
Proteins (g/kg)	300.0 [a]	293.6 [a]	275.1 [b]	1.6	<0.0001
PI, %	23.6 [a]	24.4 [a]	27.7 [b]	1.6	<0.0001
a_w	0.917 [a]	0.922 [a]	0.941 [b]	0.010	<0.0001
TBARS (µg MDA/kg)	4.0	4.5	4.1	1.5	0.625

SM semimembranosus; ST semitendinosus; BF Biceps femoris; PI index of proteolysis; a_w water activity; TBARS thiobarbituric reactive substances; MDA malondialdehyde; EM entire males; IC immunocastrates, SC surgical castrates, RMSE root-mean-square error. Values with different superscripts are significantly different ($p < 0.05$).

3.3. Instrumental Texture Profile of Dry-Cured Ham Muscles

Instrumental measurements of the texture profile revealed the mechanical properties of dry-cured muscles and it can be observed that the majority of them were significantly affected by male sex group (Table 3). Based on texture profile traits depicted per muscle it can be summarized that dry-cured ham muscles from SC differ from IC and EM. Compared with EM and IC, SC dry-cured ham muscles are softer, less gummy, less springy and less chewy, but more adhesive. Dry-cured ham muscles of SC also have a higher stress relaxation coefficient, which denotes a more plastic structure.

Table 3. Effect of male sex group on measurements of texture profile of dry-cured ham muscles.

Trait	Male Sex Group			RMSE	*p*-Value
	EM	IC	SC		
SM muscle					
Hardness	128 [b]	112 [b]	67 [a]	31	0.0001
Cohesiveness	0.54	0.50	0.53	0.08	0.5848
Gumminess	68 [b]	56 [b]	37 [a]	17	0.0006
Springiness	4.7 [b]	4.7 [b]	4.1 [a]	0.53	0.0103
Chewiness	323 [b]	253 [b]	161 [a]	89	0.0005
Adhesiveness	−0.56 [b]	−0.72 [b]	−1.26 [a]	0.40	0.0005
Y90	0.611 [a,b]	0.601 [a]	0.631 [b]	0.022	0.0081
ST muscle					
Hardness	34 [b]	31 [a,b]	21 [a]	11	0.0140
Cohesiveness	0.42 [b]	0.39 [a,b]	0.36 [a]	0.06	0.0503
Gumminess	15 [b]	13 [a,b]	7 [a]	7	0.0282
Springiness	4.3	4.4	3.7	0.8	0.0532
Chewiness	70 [b]	54 [a,b]	28 [a]	35	0.0226
Adhesiveness	−2.2 [a]	−2.4 [a,b]	−3.0 [b]	0.6	0.0105
Y90	0.690 [a]	0.690 [a]	0.713 [b]	0.021	0.0132
BF muscle					
Hardness	46	52	40	12	0.0557
Cohesiveness	0.52 [b]	0.53 [b]	0.42 [a]	0.70	0.0011
Gumminess	24 [a,b]	29 [b]	17 [a]	10	0.0169
Springiness	4.3 b	4.1 [b]	3.5 [a]	0.48	0.0003
Chewiness	108 [a,b]	127 [b]	60 [a]	54	0.0128
Adhesiveness	−2.7 [b]	−2.6 [b]	−3.4 [a]	0.75	0.0026
Y90	0.694 [a]	0.692 [a]	0.728 b	0.023	0.0009

SM semimembranosus; ST semitendinosus; BF biceps femoris; Y90 stress relaxation parameter; EM entire males; IC immunocastrates, SC surgical castrates, RMSE root-mean-square error. Values with different superscripts are significantly different ($p < 0.05$).

3.4. Sensory Analysis of Dry-Cured Ham

Male sex group affected ($p < 0.05$) or tended to affect ($p < 0.10$) several sensory attributes of the examined dry-cured hams (Table 4). With regard to the appearance of the slices of ham, EM were leaner and less marbled than SC, with IC taking a somewhat intermediate position. With regard to the odor, EM had a slightly less meaty and bouillon-like odor ($p < 0.10$), but an intensely sharper odor with a strong sweat and manure taint. IC and SC were comparable with regard to odor. In the case of texture, EM and IC were similar (no significant differences) whereas SC exhibited significantly different texture from both IC and EM, i.e., it was softer, less gummy, less dry, less fibrous and the dry-cured ham slices had a more easily fragmentable texture. EM hams were different from SC and IC in the following taste and flavor attributes, i.e., meat, sweet, bouillon-like (lower), sweat, manure, persistence (higher) whereas IC hams were different from EM and SC in their saltiness (higher). The overall impression of sensory quality revealed that SC dry-cured ham were the most appreciated and EM dry-cured hams the least, and IC were in between, and different from both SC and EM.

Table 4. Effect of sex group on sensory traits of dry-cured hams.

Trait	EM	IC	SC	RMSE	*p*-Value
		Male Sex Group			
		Appearance attributes			
Fat visually	3.8	3.7	3.2	1.3	0.0587
Meat visually	6.3 [c]	5.4 [b]	4.6 [a]	1.3	<0.0001
Meat color uniformity	5.8	5.6	5.7	1.2	0.3950
Marbling visually	3.4 [a]	3.8 [a]	4.4 [b]	1.5	0.0002
		Odor attributes			
Meat	4.6	4.8	4.8	0.7	0.0739
Fatty	3.4	3.4	3.6	0.8	0.5055
Smoky	2.7	2.8	2.8	1.0	0.6830
Acidic	2.0	2.1	2.0	0.8	0.4956
Sweet	0.9	0.9	1.0	0.5	0.2040
Bouillon-like	1.6	1.7	1.8	0.7	0.0941
Fermentation	2.8	3.1	2.9	0.9	0.1856
Yeast	1.4	1.5	1.5	0.7	0.8739
Sweat	1.7 [b]	0.4 [a]	0.3 [a]	0.7	<0.0001
Manure	0.7 [b]	0.3 [a]	0.2 [a]	0.6	<0.0001
Sharp	2.4 [b]	1.7 [a]	1.6 [a]	0.9	<0.0001
Rancid	0.9	0.9	0.8	0.6	0.2466
Overall odor intensity	5.1	5.1	4.9	0.9	0.4286
		Texture attributes			
Hardness	4.2 [b]	3.8 [b]	2.8 [a]	1.0	<0.0001
Gumminess	4.3 [b]	4.1 [b]	3.3 [a]	1.1	<0.0001
Dryness	4.8 [b]	4.5 [b]	3.7 [a]	1.1	<0.0001
Fibrousness	4.1 [b]	4.0 [b]	3.4 [a]	1.2	<0.0001
Ease of fragmentation	5.8 [a]	6.3 [b]	6.9 [c]	1.2	<0.0001
		Taste and flavor attributes			
Meat	5.2 [a]	5.6 [b]	5.6 [b]	0.7	<0.0001
Fatty	3.3	3.2	3.4	0.9	0.6251
Smoky	2.8	3.0	2.9	1.0	0.4418
Sour	2.2	2.5	2.3	0.7	0.0645
Salty	5.0 [a]	5.4 [b]	5.0 [a]	0.9	0.0159
Sweet	0.8 [a]	1.0 [b]	1.0 [b]	0.6	0.0027
Bitter	0.6	0.7	0.6	0.6	0.7524
Bouillon-like	1.7 [a]	2.0 [b]	1.9 [a,b]	0.7	0.0312
Fermentation	2.6	3.0	2.8	1.0	0.0868
Yeast	1.4	1.5	1.3	0.8	0.3342
Sweat	2.8 [b]	0.3 [a]	0.3 [a]	0.8	<0.0001
Manure	0.9 [b]	0.2 [a]	0.2 [a]	0.6	<0.0001
Persistent	2.7 [b]	0.8 [a]	0.7 [a]	0.9	<0.0001
Rancid	0.7	0.7	0.6	0.6	0.4085
Overall sensory quality	4.2 [a]	5.9 [b]	6.2 [c]	0.9	<0.0001

EM entire males; IC immunocastrates, SC surgical castrates, RMSE root-mean-square error. Values with different superscripts are significantly different ($p < 0.05$).

4. Discussion

Due to their effect on dehydration, salt intake and biochemical changes during processing [10], green ham properties, which can be assessed without damage to further processing, were recorded. The main difference between male sex groups was in subcutaneous fat cover which was thicker in SC than EM or IC. As shown by meta-analytical studies, an absence of differences in subcutaneous fat thickness between EM and IC is generally observed [19,20]. Ham fat thickness is the principal factor affecting seasoning loss, with fatter hams exhibiting less and slower dehydration [21]. In agreement with this, lower processing loss was observed in SC than EM or IC hams (7% or 5%-point difference, respectively). In our recent study [22], we also observed a significant difference in processing weight loss between IC and EM, whereas in the present study, a 2%-point better yield in IC hams was not significant, but was consistent with insignificantly thicker fat cover and intramuscular fat of IC dry-cured ham muscles.

The observed physical-chemical properties of dry-cured ham muscles show that it was mainly SC that differed from EM and IC (which were similar in this respect). Higher water content and lower salt intake in SC than EM or IC corroborates the results for processing loss and the results in the literature on salt intake and water migration during processing, as monitored with computed tomography [23]. It is worth noting that due to lower dehydration, SC hams also had lower protein percentages than EM or IC. As a result, dry-cured ham muscle of SC presented higher water activity, which together with lower salt content may affect the proteolysis. It has been demonstrated that proteolysis is more pronounced in hams with reduced salt content or inversely, that protein breakdown is lower when salt concentration is higher [22,24,25]. High salt concentration inhibits muscle proteases responsible for the degradation of proteins to short peptides and free amino acids [26]. With regard to the index of proteolysis, the effect of male sex group differed according to the muscle. It was insignificant in SM muscle, which also exhibited lower PI values due to the fact that this muscle is exposed to air and salt and is thus submitted to more intense desiccation. In the case of ST and BF muscles, SC had higher PI than EM, whereas IC were SC-like in the ST muscle, and EM-like in the BF muscle. This inconsistency in IC response may indicate that IC behave differently from EM and SC in terms of proteolytic enzymes activity and protein breakdown. It has been suggested that EM have a higher degree of proteolysis than SC [27] and that higher androgenic potential (androstenone level) might be associated with increased proteolysis [28], which could not be confirmed in the present study. The only available relevant study including IC proteolytic potential [29] showed higher cathepsin B activity in green ham muscle of IC than SC, but showed the opposite trend for proteolysis (i.e., the highest PI was in SC hams).

The instrumentally assessed texture of dry-cured ham muscles also showed that it was mainly SC that differed from EM and IC, in line with the differences in physical-chemical properties. Dry-cured ham texture is due to dehydration, which causes hardening of the product [30] or to proteolysis [31], which increases the softness as a result of the cleavage of structural proteins. The absence of important differences in the rheological parameters of EM and IC have been reported previously [22]. The instrumentally assessed texture was consistent with the sensory evaluation by the expert panel, and confirmed that with respect to texture, dry-cured hams from IC are EM-like, while both were different from SC.

Visual assessment of dry-cured ham slices confirmed that EM are leaner than SC, and that IC were more EM-like with regard to fatness indicators, in line with results for the chemical composition of green ham or dry-cured ham. However, because of the potential interfering effect of boar taint presence in EM, the most important result of sensory analysis is the perception of odor, taste and flavor. Indeed, the results confirmed a clear, distinct profile for dry-cured hams from EM, while IC and SC exhibited similar sensory profiles. Significantly stronger perception of several sensory attributes (sweat, manure, sharp, persistent) that the literature describes for pork from EM [32], proves that boar taint did not diminish with processing and that panelists were able to detect the organoleptic defects in dry-cured hams from EM. Actually, 9 out of 12 EM hams presented androstenone levels above 1 μg/g while only 2 out of 12 hams presented skatole levels above 0.25 μg/g (data not shown), which are considered threshold levels for sensory perception. On the other hand, in hams from IC pigs the androstenone and skatole levels were below the detection level (0.24 and 0.03 μg/g liquid fat, respectively) [12]. Studies evaluating the effect of processing technologies on boar-tainted meat generally show that dry-curing does not eliminate its perception in the products [7,8]. It also seems that boar taint substances are neither degraded nor lost during the long dry-curing process [33].

5. Conclusions

The present investigation demonstrated that the quality of dry-cured ham is strongly affected by male sex group and that dry-cured ham from entire (uncastrated) males has sensory quality defects and also differs in other aspects that are important in dry-cured ham production (e.g., insufficient subcutaneous fat thickness). In the experimental conditions of the present study, the immunocastrates also produced hams with a fat thickness below the requirement for Kraški pršut PGI labelling, suggesting that to better meet the requirements for special products, the vaccination protocols (e.g., longer time delay between second vaccination and slaughter) and other management practices could be adapted or further optimized. Regarding the aptitude for processing into traditional dry-cured products, under the conditions of the present study, i.e., standard age and weight of pigs, lean type crossbreed, same diet, usual delay between effective immunocastration and slaughter, the immunocastrated pigs are more similar to entire males, however their main advantage is that they are free of boar taint, while the surgical castrates had the most appropriate raw hams for processing into traditional dry-cured products.

Author Contributions: Conceptualization, M.Č.-P. and M.Š.; methodology, M.Š., S.Ž.-B., E.K.; K.P., N.B.-L., formal analysis, M.Č.-P.; resources, K.K., V.S., U.W.; writing—original draft preparation, M.Č.-P.; writing—review and editing, M.Š., S.Ž.-B., E.K., K.P., N.B.-L., K.K., U.W., V.S.; funding acquisition, V.S., M.Č.-P. All authors have read and agreed to the published version of the manuscript.

Funding: This research is part of the ERA-NET SusAn, project SuSi (co-financed by the European Union's Horizon 2020 Research and Innovation Program and the German Federal Office for Agriculture and Food), grant number 696231 and also co-financed by the National Centre for Research and Development (NCBiR) in Poland (grant agreement SUSAN/I/SuSI/02/2017), Ministry of Agriculture, Forestry and Food of the Republic of Slovenia. Core financing by the Slovenian agency of research (grant P4-0133 and Z7-9416) is also acknowledged.

Acknowledgments: Collaboration between authors has also been enabled by participation within the project, COST-IPEMA 'Innovative Approaches for Pork Production with Entire Males' (CA 15215). The authors would also like to thank Urška Tomažin for chemical determination of TBARS.

Conflicts of Interest: The authors declare no conflict of interest.

References

1. Prunier, A.; Bonneau, M.; von Borell, E.H.; Cinotti, S.; Gunn, M.; Fredriksen, B.; Giersing, M.; Morton, D.B.; Tuyttens, F.A.M.; Velarde, A. A review of welfare consequences on surgical castration in piglets and the evaluation of non-surgical methods. *Anim. Welf.* **2006**, *15*, 277–289.

2. European Declaration on Alternatives to Surgical Castration of Pigs. 2010. Available online: http://ec.europa.eu/food/animals/welfare/practice/farm/pigs/castration_alternatives_en (accessed on 5 November 2019).

3. Boars on the Way. Available online: https://www.boarsontheway.com/ (accessed on 5 November 2019).

4. Candek-Potokar, M.; Skrlep, M.; Batorek Lukac, N. Raising Entire Males or Immunocastrates—Outlook on Meat Quality. *Procedia Food Sci.* **2015**, *5*, 30–33. [CrossRef]

5. Bonneau, M.; Čandek-Potokar, M.; Škrlep, M.; Font-i-Furnols, M.; Aluwé, M. The Castrum Network, Fontanesi, L. Potential sensitivity of pork production situations aiming at high-quality products to the use of entire male pigs as an alternative to surgical castrates. *Animal* **2018**, *12*, 1287–1295. [CrossRef] [PubMed]

6. Font-i-Furnols, M. Consumer studies on sensory acceptability of boar taint: A review. *Meas. Sci.* **2012**, *92*, 319–329. [CrossRef] [PubMed]

7. Bañón, S.; Gil, M.D.; Garrido, M.D. The effects of castration on the eating quality of dry-cured ham. *Meat Sci.* **2003**, *65*, 1031–1037. [CrossRef]

8. Corral, S.; Salvador, A.; Flores, M. Effect of the use of entire male fat in the production of reduced salt fermented sausages. *Meat Sci.* **2016**, *116*, 140–150. [CrossRef] [PubMed]

9. Tørngren, M.A.; Claudi-Magnussen, C.; Støier, S.; Kristensen, L. Boar taint reduction in smoked, cooked ham. In Proceedings of the 57th International Congress of Meat Science and Technology, Ghent, Belgium, 7–12 August 2011.

10. Čandek-Potokar, M.; Škrlep, M. Factors in pig production that impact the quality of dry-cured ham: A review. *Animal* **2012**, *6*, 327–338. [CrossRef]

11. Commission Implementing Regulation (EU) No. 506/2012 of 14 June 2012 Entering a Name in the Register of Protected Designations of Origin and Protected Geographical Indications (Kraški Pršut (PGI)). Available online: https://eur-lex.europa.eu/legal-content/EN/TXT/?uri=uriserv:OJ.L_.2012.154.01.0020.01.ENG&toc=OJ:L:2012:154:TOC (accessed on 2 February 2020).

12. Kress, K.; Weiler, U.; Schmucker, S.; Čandek-Potokar, M.; Vrecl, M.; Fazarinc, G.; Škrlep, M.; Batorek-Lukač, N.; Stefanski, V. Influence of housing conditions on success of immunocastration and consequences for growth performance in male pigs. *Animals* **2020**, *10*, 27. [CrossRef]

13. Škrlep, M.; Čandek-Potokar, M.; Žlender, B.; Robert, N.; Santé-Lhoutellier, V.; Gou, P. PRKAG3 and CAST genetic polymorphisms and quality traits of dry-cured hams–III. Associations in Slovenian dry-cured ham Kraški pršut and their dependence on processing. *Meat Sci.* **2012**, *92*, 360–365. [CrossRef]

14. Lynch, S.M.; Frei, B. Mechanisms of copper- and iron-dependant oxidative modification of human low-density-lipoprotein. *J. Lipid Res.* **1993**, *34*, 1745–1753.

15. Pugliese, C.; Sirtori, F.; Škrlep, M.; Piasentier, E.; Calamai, L.; Franci, O.; Čandek-Potokar, M. The effect of ripening time on chemical, textural, volatile and sensorial traits of biceps femoris and semimembranosus muscles of the Slovenian dry-cured ham Kraški pršut. *Meat Sci.* **2014**, *100*, 58–68. [CrossRef] [PubMed]

16. Stone, H.; Sidel, J.S. Descriptive analysis. In *Sensory Evaluation Practices*, 3rd ed.; Academic Press: San Diego, CA, USA, 2004; pp. 20–245.

17. ISO 8589: 2007: Sensory Analysis—General Guidance for the Design of Test Rooms; International Organization for Standardization: Geneva, Switzerland. 2007, p. 16. Available online: https://www.iso.org/standard/36385.html (accessed on 2 February 2020).

18. ISO 8586: 2012: General Guidelines for the Selection, Training and Monitoring of Selected Assessors and Expert Sensory Assessors; International Organization for Standardization: Geneva, Switzerland. 2007, p. 28. Available online: https://www.iso.org/standard/45352.html (accessed on 2 February 2020).

19. Batorek-Lukač, N.; Čandek-Potokar, M.; Bonneau, M.; Van Milgen, J. Meta-analysis of the effect of immunocastration on production performance, reproductive organs and boar taint compounds in pigs. *Animal* **2012**, *6*, 1330–1338. [CrossRef] [PubMed]

20. Pauly, C.; Luginbühl, W.; Ampuero, S.; Bee, G. Expected effects on carcass and pork quality when surgical castration is omitted—Results of a meta-analysis study. *Meat Sci.* **2012**, *92*, 858–862. [CrossRef] [PubMed]

21. Čandek-Potokar, M.; Škrlep, M. Dry ham ("kraški pršut") processing losses as affected by raw material properties and manufacturing practice. *J. Food Process. Pres.* **2011**, *35*, 96–111. [CrossRef]

22. Škrlep, M.; Čandek-Potokar, M.; Batorek Lukač, N.; Prevolnik Povše, M.; Pugliese, C.; Labusièrre, E.; Flores, M. Comparison of entire male and immunocastrated pigs for dry-cured ham production under two salting regimes. *Meat Sci.* **2016**, *111*, 27–37. [CrossRef]

23. Santos-Garcés, E.; Muñoz, I.; Gou, P.; Sala, X.; Fulladosa, E. Tools for studying dry-cured ham processing by using computed tomography. *J. Agric. Food Chem.* **2012**, *60*, 241–249. [CrossRef]

24. Martín, L.; Cordoba, J.J.; Antequera, T.; Timón, M.L.; Ventanas, J. Effects of salt and temperature on proteolysis during ripening of Iberian ham. *Meat Sci.* **1998**, *49*, 145–153. [CrossRef]

25. Ruiz-Ramírez, J.; Arnau, J.; Serra, X.; Gou, P. Relationship between water content, NaCl content, pH and texture parameters in dry-cured muscles. *Meat Sci.* **2005**, *70*, 579–587. [CrossRef]

26. Toldrá, F. Proteolysis and lipolysis in flavour development of dry-cured meat products. *Meat Sci.* **1998**, *49*, 101–110. [CrossRef]

27. Škrlep, M.; Tomažin, U.; Batorek Lukač, N.; Poklukar, K.; Čandek-Potokar, M. Proteomic Profiles of the Longissimus Muscles of Entire Male and Castrated Pigs as Related to Meat Quality. *Animals* **2019**, *9*, 74. [CrossRef]

28. Kaltnekar, T.; Škrlep, M.; Batorek Lukač, N.; Tomažin, U.; Prevolnik Povše, M.; Labussière, E.; Demšar, L.; Čandek-Potokar, M. Effects of salting duration and boar taint level on quality of dry-cured hams. *Acta Agric. Slov.* **2016**, *5*, 132–137.

29. Pinna, A.; Schivazappa, C.; Virgili, R.; Parolari, G. Effects of vaccination against gonadotropin-releasing hormone (GnRH) in heavy male pigs for Italian typical dry-cured ham production. *Meat Sci.* **2015**, *110*, 153–159. [CrossRef]

30. Serra, X.; Ruiz-Ramírez, J.; Arnau, J.; Gou, P. Texture parameters of dry-cured ham m. biceps femoris samples dried at different levels as a function of water activity and water content. *Meat Sci.* **2005**, *69*, 249–254. [CrossRef] [PubMed]

31. Ruiz-Ramírez, J.; Arnau, J.; Serra, X.; Gou, P. Effect of pH24, NaCl content and proteolysis index on the relationship between water content and texture parameters in biceps femoris and semimembranosus muscles in dry-cured ham. *Meat Sci.* **2006**, *72*, 185–194. [CrossRef] [PubMed]
32. Pauly, C.; Spring-Staehli, P.; O'doherty, J.V.; Kragten, S.A.; Dubois, S.; Messadène, J.; Bee, G. The effects of method of castration, rearing condition and diet on sensory quality of pork assessed by a trained panel. *Meat Sci.* **2010**, *86*, 498–504. [CrossRef] [PubMed]
33. Haugen, J.E.; Brunius, C.; Zamaratskaia, G. Review of analytical methods to measure boar taint compounds in porcine adipose tissue: The need for harmonised methods. *Meat Sci.* **2012**, *90*, 9–19. [CrossRef] [PubMed]

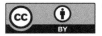

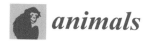 *animals*

Article

Effect of Free-Range and Low-Protein Concentrated Diets on Growth Performance, Carcass Traits, and Meat Composition of Iberian Pig

Juan F. Tejeda [1,2,*], **Alejandro Hernández-Matamoros** [1], **Mercedes Paniagua** [3] and **Elena González** [2,4]

1   Food Science and Technology, Escuela de Ingenierías Agrarias, Universidad de Extremadura, Avda. Adolfo Suárez s/n, 06007 Badajoz, Spain; fregepower@hotmail.com
2   Research University Institute of Agricultural Resources (INURA), Avda. de Elvas s/n, Campus Universitario, 06006 Badajoz, Spain; malena@unex.es
3   Centro de Investigaciones Científicas y Tecnológicas de Extremadura (CICYTEX-La Orden), Junta de Extremadura 06187 Guadajira, 06187 Badajoz, Spain; mercedes.paniagua@juntaex.es
4   Animal Production, Escuela de Ingenierías Agrarias, Universidad de Extremadura, Avda. Adolfo Suárez, 06007 Badajoz, Spain
*   Correspondence: jftejeda@unex.es; Tel.: +34 924 289 300

Received: 16 January 2020; Accepted: 9 February 2020; Published: 11 February 2020

Simple Summary: It is generally assumed in the Iberian pig sector that substitution of traditional free-range rearing, with acorns and grass, by mixed diets affects intramuscular fat content and fatty-acid composition, among others, causing a decrease in meat quality. As mixed diets are usually formulated with higher protein contents than those supplied by natural resources consumed by Iberian pig fed extensively, we hypothesized that the use of a low-protein diet in the final fattening period of pig could be a suitable strategy to improve meat and dry-cured product quality. However, it is also necessary to evaluate the effect of this strategy on performance and carcass traits of pigs. In this study, we found that Iberian pigs fed on low-protein diets had higher intramuscular fat content and different meat composition compared to pigs fed on concentrates with standard protein levels, which could be a suitable way of improving the Iberian pig meat and dry-cured product quality.

Abstract: The feeding system is one of the main factors influencing the Iberian pig meat quality. This experiment was undertaken to evaluate the influence of feeding diets containing different levels of protein on performance, carcass, and meat quality of Iberian pigs. To that aim, 24 castrated male Retinto Iberian pigs with an average weight of 116 kg were fed under free-range conditions with acorns and grass (FR), and on concentrated diets in confinement with standard (SP) and low protein content (LP). The crude protein content in acorns was lower than that in the grass and SP diet, but similar to that in the LP diet. FR pigs needed more time to achieve slaughter weight than LP and SP pigs. Iberian pigs fed on low-protein diet (FR and LP) had a higher intramuscular fat content in the musculus serratus ventralis than SP pigs. The influence of diet on the fatty-acid composition was reflected more markedly in subcutaneous fat than in muscles. FR pigs showed a higher level of C18:1 n-9 and total polyunsaturated fatty acids and lower total saturated fatty acids in subcutaneous fat than LP and SP. It is concluded that diets with low protein levels do not affect Iberian pig productive traits but change the meat composition, rendering them an interesting strategy to improve the quality of Iberian pig meat and dry-cured products.

Keywords: Iberian pig; extensive system; low-protein diet; carcass; meat quality; fatty-acid profile

1. Introduction

The Iberian pig is an autochthonous breed from the southwest Iberian Peninsula, characterized by its high-quality meat and dry-cured products (mainly hams, shoulders, and loins) [1]. This high quality is the consequence of several factors such as genetics, crossbreeding, rearing system, and processing conditions. Within the factors included under the rearing system, feeding seems to be the key one influencing Iberian product quality [2]. Originally, Iberian pigs were reared under free-range conditions in the *dehesa*, a Mediterranean forest system, based on natural resources, mainly fallen acorns and pasture, playing an important role in the agricultural and pastoral systems and, therefore, in the economy of these rural areas [3]. Unfortunately, an extensive traditional feeding production regime is not always feasible because the availability of natural resources is limited. In addition, an increase in demand for both fresh and dry-cured products from Iberian pigs currently involves the use of conventional mixed diets to produce a high proportion of Iberian pigs under intensive conditions. However, the replacement of free-range rearing and substitution of the natural feed by conventional mixed diets in Iberian pigs produce a markedly decrease in the sensory attributes of dry-cured products and, consequently, a lower acceptability [4]. It is well known that nutritional strategies are the main influential factors in meat quality of pigs. The acorn is an energy food rich in fat and carbohydrates; however, it has very low protein content and its amino-acid profile indicates that lysine is the main limiting amino acid [3]. On the other hand, although protein from pasture may be important to overcome the shortage in acorns, it is not enough to cover dietary requirements [5]. To increase pig chain sustainability, it is necessary to optimize the nutrient efficiency, since it may reduce nutrient excretion and production costs, making the reduction of the dietary protein content a priority objective in pig production [6,7]. In this sense, previous studies into intensive nutritional management were carried out to determine the influence of diets that differed widely in protein/energy ratio on performance, carcass, and meat quality traits of Iberian pig [8,9]. It is well known than the reduction of some nutrients, such as protein, could increase fat deposition in pigs [10,11]. With regard to Iberian pig, a high amount of intramuscular fat (IMF) was highlighted as one of the most relevant aspects of meat quality [12]. Thus, increasing the IMF levels is generally considered as a way of enhancing the quality of fresh pork and dry-cured products [12], and a low-protein diet could be considered as a strategy to increase fat deposition, allowing not only a decrease in feed costs, but also an increase in sustainability of pork production.

Thus, as free-range rearing of Iberian pigs, with a feed characterized by a high energy density and a low amount and quality of proteins, increases the IMF [13] and modifies the color of meat and dry-cured products [14], we hypothesized that feeding Iberian pigs with a low-protein diet during the final fattening period prior to slaughter under intensive conditions could be an adequate strategy to improve the meat quality. In addition, another purpose of this work was to study the influence of this type of a protein-restricted diet on the performance and carcass traits of Iberian pigs.

2. Materials and Methods

2.1. Animals and Diets

This study was carried out with 24 castrated Iberian male pigs of the Retinto variety. This variety belongs to the line Valdesequera (Extremadura Government, Badajoz, Spain), and it is recognized in Spain's official Iberian herd book (Spanish Association of Iberian Purebred Pig Breeders, AECERIBER). During the period prior to the experiment, the animals were kept from birth to the beginning of the fattening phase under intensive rearing conditions. Animals began the fattening phase with an average initial live weight of 116.0 kg (pooled SD = 5.9 kg) and age of 425 days. The pigs were divided into three groups ($n = 8$) according to feeding regime. One group was reared free range (FR), according to the traditional way, in which pigs are fed on natural resources, mainly acorns (*Quercus rotundifolia*) and grass, from November to January. The other two groups of pigs were raised on the experimental farm in confinement (housed outdoors, 230 m²/pig) and offered two different experimental diets, formulated to the same metabolizable energy (ME) value, 4100 kcal/kg dry matter (DM) (according to Fundación Española para el Desarrollo de la Nutrición Animal (FEDNA) [15]); one group was fed on a standard protein diet (SP) and the other one on a low-protein diet (LP). Standard protein diet was formulated to meet all the nutrient requirements for fattening the Iberian pigs; however, LP diet was designed as a protein-deficient diet, in order to obtain a low protein intake that simulates feeding of Iberian pigs reared free range. The main ingredients of the two diets were maize (150 g/kg), maize starch (400 g/kg), alfalfa meal (100 g/kg), and high-oleic sunflower oil (60 g/kg). The LP diet was also formulated with wheat (252 g/kg), resulting in a concentrated feed with 6.6 g/100 g DM of crude protein and 0.2 g/100 g DM of lysine, and the SP diet with wheat (55 g/kg) and soybean meal (44% crude protein), resulting in a concentrated feed with 12.8 g/100 g DM and 0.7 g/100 g DM of lysine. The diets contained also bicalcium phosphate (20 g/kg), sodium chloride (5 g/kg), vitamin and mineral premix (3 g/kg), and binder (10 g/kg). The chemical composition of diets (acorns, grass, and concentrated feed) was determined according to standard methods [16]: moisture (reference 935.29), crude protein (reference 954.01), crude fat (reference 920.39), crude fiber (reference 962.09), and ash (reference 942.05). The fatty-acid composition of diets was assayed by gas chromatography after lipid extraction according to the Bligh and Dyer [17] method and acidic transesterification [18].

2.2. Handling, Slaughtering, and Carcass Traits

Pigs from the three groups studied, FR, LP, and SP, had free access to water and feed throughout the trial. To achieve ad libitum feeding of pigs raised in confinement (LP and SP), a sufficient amount of feed was weighed and added to feed hoppers manually once a day, ensuring that feed was always available to the animals. Feed consumption was recorded weekly. Daily feed intake was calculated by weighing the feed leftovers, which were determined by weighing the entire feeder (the entire feeder included the feed hoppers) and subtracting the weight of the empty feeder. Pigs on the LP diet had a daily feed intake of 5161 g DM/pig versus 5088 g DM/pig in the SP group. As FR pigs were fed in freedom, with the resources that nature provides, it was not possible to measure their feed intake directly, but daily acorn pulp and grass intakes of 3600 and 655 g DM/pig, respectively, were estimated according to the previous studies published in Iberian pig (see Supplementary Materials) [3,19,20]. Pigs were weighed every week from the beginning of the fattening period to slaughter. The selection criterion for the slaughter of the pigs was weight increase. When the average weight of the batch increased by about 58 kg, all the pigs of a batch were transported to the abattoir. All the pigs were weighed unfasted 24 h before slaughter, and these weights were used to determine both final weight (174.2 kg and SD = 6.1) and carcass performance. Feed was withheld from animals for 12 h before slaughtering. FR pigs were locked in a pen and fed with acorns collected from the same place where they usually ate, until the pre-slaughter fasting. Pigs were slaughtered by electrical stunning and killed by exsanguination. Then, they were scalded, skinned, eviscerated, and split down both sides of the vertebral column according to the standard commercial procedures of the Iberian pig industry. Hot carcass weights without pelvic renal fat were recorded and used to calculate carcass yield. Hams and shoulders were removed from the carcasses and weighed 2 h postmortem. Serratus ventralis (SV) and longissimus thoracis and lumborum (LTL) muscles were also dissected from the carcasses, trimmed of external fat, and weighed within 45 min after slaughter. The weights of untrimmed hams and shoulders were recorded 2 h postmortem.

2.3. Meat Quality Traits and Fatty-Acid Profile of Samples

After collection of carcass data, a sample of subcutaneous adipose tissue at the level of the tailbone was chosen for lipid analysis. Then, a sample of approximately 300 g in the middle part of the SV and another one from the musculus longissimus lumborum (LL) was excised from all pigs. Meat samples were stored for chemical analysis in individual plastic bags and vacuum-packaged at −20 °C until subsequent analyses. The LL and SV samples were thawed inside the vacuum-packaged bags for 24 h at 4 °C, removed from packages, sliced, and exposed to light for 30 min before color measurement. The following color coordinates were determined: lightness (L*), redness (a*, red to green), and yellowness (b*, yellow to blue), according to CIELAB color space [21]. The color parameters were determined using a Minolta CR-300 colorimeter reflectance spectrophotometer (Minolta Camera Co., Osaka, Japan). Before use, the colorimeter was standardized using a white tile (mod CR-A43) using illuminant D65, 0° standard observer, and an 8 mm port/viewing area. The measurements were repeated at three randomly selected locations on each LL and SV slice and averaged for statistical analysis. The pH at 24 h of LL and SV samples was measured using a pH meter specific for meat products (model HI 99163, HANNA, Smithfield, RI, USA). Moisture (oven air-drying method), protein (Kjeldahl nitrogen), and ash (muffle furnace) were analyzed following official methods [16]. Lipids from subcutaneous fat samples were extracted in a microwave oven following the method described by De Pedro et al. [22]. IMF was extracted and quantified according to the method described by Bligh and Dyer [17]. Fatty-acid methyl esters from the lipids obtained were prepared by acidic transesterification in the presence of sodium metal (0,1 N) and sulfuric acid (5% sulfuric acid in methanol) [18], and they were analyzed by gas chromatography, using a Hewlett-Packard HP-4890 Series II gas chromatograph equipped with a split/splitless injector and a flame ionization detector (FID). Separation was carried out on a polyethylene glycol capillary column (30 m long, 0.25 mm inner diameter (id), 0.25 μm film thickness) (HP-INNOWax) maintained at 260 °C for 25 min. Injector and detector temperatures were 320 °C. The carrier gas was nitrogen at 1.8 mL/min. Individual fatty acids were identified by comparison of their retention times with those of reference standard mixtures (Sigma Chemical Co., St. Louis, MO, USA). Results were expressed as the percentage of total fatty acids present, considering a total of 16 fatty acids, none less than 0.1%.

2.4. Statistical Analysis

For descriptive data analysis, the mean and the standard error of the mean were used. The pig was used as the experimental unit. Significance of difference ($p < 0.05$) between dietary treatments was determined by one-way ANOVA followed by Tukey multiple comparison test. The general linear model procedure of the SPSS package (SPSS for Windows Ver. 19.0; SPSS Inc., Chicago, IL, USA, 2004) was used.

3. Results

3.1. Diets

Table 1 shows analysis of the chemical and fatty-acid composition of experimental diets, acorns, and grass. Acorns, the main component of FR Iberian pig diets, contain lower crude protein content (5.2% DM) than grass (19.1% DM) and the SP diet (12.8% DM), but similar content to the LP diet (6.6% DM). Acorns presented higher levels of fat (7.9% DM) than grass (4.6% DM), but similar levels to those found in LP and SP diets (8.3% and 8.0% DM, respectively). Acorns, LP, and SP diets exhibited higher proportions of oleic acid (64.0%, 72.5%, and 71.9%, respectively) than grass (13.2%). However, grass presented higher levels of linolenic acid (37.5%) compared to acorns, LP, and SP diets (1.0%, 0.6%, and 0.9%, respectively).

Table 1. Proximate composition (% dry matter, except for dry matter (%)) and fatty-acid profile (%) of the experimental diets (low-protein diet and standard protein diet), acorn, and grass.

Items	Diets			
Chemical Composition	LP diet	SP Diet	Acorn	Grass
Dry matter (DM)	91.6	91.3	60.5	19.4
Crude protein	6.6	12.8	5.2	19.1
Crude fat	8.3	8.0	7.9	4.6
Crude fibre	4.0	4.7	2.3	22.0
Ash	5.0	5.2	1.6	11.6
Free-nitrogen extractives	75.9	68.6	83.0	42.7
Lysine	0.2	0.7		
	Fatty acids [1]			
Palmitic acid (C16:0)	7.3	7.0	13.5	26.1
Stearic acid (C18:0)	2.9	2.7	3.3	6.1
Oleic acid (C18:1n-9)	72.5	71.9	64.0	13.2
Linoleic acid (C18:2n-6)	14.6	15.9	16.7	12.6
Linolenic acid (C18:3n-3)	0.6	0.9	1.0	37.5

LP diet = low-protein diet; SP diet = standard protein diet. [1] Of a total of 16 fatty acids, none less than 0.1%.

3.2. Pig Performance and Carcass Traits

Growth performance and carcass traits are shown in Table 2. Pigs from the FR group grew slower (1.05 kg/day) and needed more time (56.8 days) to get to the slaughter weight than pigs from LP and SP groups, which had significantly higher growth rates (1.27 and 1.24 kg/day, respectively) and only needed 45.4 and 46.3 days, respectively, to get to the slaughter weight. No significant differences were found between LP and SP groups in the average daily gain (ADG) and in the number of days to get to the final weight. Carcass weight and carcass yield were not influenced by production system or feed type. With regard to the cutting of pigs, the largest differences were in loin weight and yield. The three groups showed significant differences for LTL weight, with the highest value for SP (2.41 kg), followed by LP and FR (2.16 and 1.90 kg, respectively). Although SV showed the same behavior as LTL, statistically significant differences were not found. With respect to ham and shoulder weights, no differences were found among groups.

Table 2. Productive and carcass traits (kg) and yields (%) from Iberian pigs fed the experimental diets.

Productive and Carcass Traits	FR	LP	SP	SEM	*p*-Value
Initial weight	115.6	116.3	116.1	1.213	0.975
Final weight	175.2	174.0	173.5	1.243	0.859
Weight gain	59.6	57.7	57.4	0.734	0.445
Days	56.8 [a]	45.4 [b]	46.3 [b]	2.137	0.023
Carcass weight	137.2	137.3	135.2	1.169	0.721
ADG	1.05 [a]	1.27 [b]	1.24 [b]	0.062	0.049
LTL weight	1.90 [a]	2.16 [b]	2.41 [c]	0.054	0.000
SV weight	0.60	0.70	0.69	0.019	0.053
Ham weight	14.53	14.71	14.48	0.170	0.812
Shoulder weight	10.66	11.03	10.92	0.117	0.335
Carcass yield	78.35	78.97	77.91	0.344	0.558
LTL yield	2.82 [a]	3.19 [b]	3.66 [c]	0.084	0.000
Ham yield	21.15	21.40	21.44	0.213	0.894
Shoulder yield	15.44	15.96	16.11	0.129	0.063

[a,b,c] Values within a row with different superscripts differ significantly at *p* < 0.05. SEM, standard error of the mean. ADG, average daily gain. LTL, musculus longissimus thoracis and lumborum. SV, musculus serratus ventralis. Diets: FR, Iberian pigs reared in free-range conditions; LP, Iberian pig fed on experimental low-protein diet; SP, Iberian pig fed on experimental standard protein diet.

3.3. Meat Composition

The effect of feeding diet on proximate chemical composition, instrumental color coordinates, and pH of LL and SV is presented in Table 3. Significant differences between feeding diets were observed in SV muscle. SV from pigs fed on low levels of protein (FR and LP groups) had a higher IMF content (7.95 and 7.72 g/100 g, respectively) than pigs fed on standard levels of protein (SP group) (6.23 g/100 g). There were decreased pH levels measured at 24 h in FR pigs (5.73), as opposed to SP pigs (5.99), with the LP group showing intermediate values (5.87). With respect to color of SV, FR pigs had higher values of L* (39.53) than LP and SP (36.71 and 36.18, respectively). In LL muscle, the same trend was observed as in SV; however, the differences between feeding diets were not significant.

Table 3. Chemical composition (g/100 g of muscle), pH, and color of musculus longissimus lumborum and musculus serratus ventralis from Iberian pigs fed the experimental diets.

Items	Musculus Longissimus Lumborum					Musculus Serratus Ventralis				
	FR	**LP**	**SP**	**SEM**	*p*-Value	**FR**	**LP**	**SP**	**SEM**	*p*-Value
Moisture	69.56	70.15	71.39	0.362	0.104	71.17 [a]	71.78 [a,b]	72.77 [b]	0.242	0.016
Protein	22.44	21.92	22.16	0.143	0.350	19.54	19.15	19.61	0.129	0.296
IMF	6.60	6.57	5.06	0.363	0.141	7.95 [a]	7.72 [a]	6.23 [b]	0.298	0.030
Ash	1.10	1.05	1.09	0.011	0.228	1.03 [a]	1.06 [a,b]	1.09 [b]	0.009	0.037
pH 24 h	5.56	5.69	5.63	0.036	0.326	5.73 [a]	5.87 [a,b]	5.99 [b]	0.040	0.024
L*	43.22	40.41	41.39	0.559	0.111	39.53 [a]	36.71 [b]	36.18 [b]	0.563	0.025
a*	8.56	8.97	8.70	0.243	0.806	15.20	14.84	15.29	0.283	0.807
b*	6.86	6.84	6.83	0.190	0.999	9.61	9.22	8.89	0.209	0.388

[a,b] Values within a row with different superscripts differ significantly at *p* < 0.05. SEM, standard error of the mean. IMF, intramuscular fat. Diets: FR, Iberian pigs reared in free-range conditions; LP, Iberian pig fed on experimental low-protein diet; SP, Iberian pig fed on experimental standard protein diet. L*: lightness; a*: redness; b*: yellowness.

The influence of feeding diets on the fatty-acid composition of subcutaneous backfat is shown in Table 4. There were significant differences between Iberian pigs fed in free-range rearing conditions (FR) and pigs fed in confinement with experimental concentrated diets (LP and SP). FR pigs showed a higher percentage of C18:1 n-9, C18:2 n-6, C18:3 n-3, C20:4 n-6, and total polyunsaturated fatty acids (PUFA), and lower percentages of C16:0, C18:0, C20:0, and total saturated fatty acids (SFA) than LP and SP groups.

Table 4. Fatty-acid composition (%) of the subcutaneous fat from Iberian pigs fed the experimental diets.

Items	Subcutaneous Fat				
	FR	**LP**	**SP**	**SEM**	*p*-Value
C14:0	1.24	1.20	1.19	0.016	0.504
C16:0	19.60 [a]	20.77 [b]	20.51 [b]	0.163	0.004
C16:1	2.19	2.17	2.31	0.075	0.728
C17:0	0.30	0.26	0.29	0.010	0.227
C17:1	0.35	0.31	0.34	0.011	0.353
C18:0	8.58 [a]	10.36 [b]	9.94 [a,b]	0.264	0.009
C18:1 n-9	53.99 [a]	52.59 [b]	52.55 [b]	0.235	0.010
C18:2 n-6	9.95 [a]	8.43 [b]	8.93 [b]	0.195	0.002
C18:3 n-3	0.75 [a]	0.64 [b]	0.66 [b]	0.018	0.014
C20:0	0.16 [a]	0.20 [b]	0.20 [b]	0.006	0.019
C20:1 n-9	1.69	1.91	1.87	0.045	0.080
C20:2 n-9	0.70	0.68	0.72	0.015	0.543
C20:4 n-6	0.14 [a]	0.12 [b]	0.13 [a,b]	0.003	0.025
C20:3 n-3	0.27	0.26	0.27	0.008	0.896
SFA	29.89 [a]	32.79 [b]	32.13 [b]	0.404	0.004
MUFA	58.21	56.98	57.07	0.257	0.088
PUFA	11.90 [a]	10.22 [b]	10.80 [b]	0.219	0.002

[a,b] Values within a row with different superscripts differ significantly at *p* < 0.05. SEM, standard error of the mean. SFA, total saturated fatty acids; MUFA, total monounsaturated fatty acids; PUFA, total polyunsaturated fatty acids. Diets: FR, Iberian pigs reared in free-range conditions; LP, Iberian pig fed on experimental low-protein diet; SP, Iberian pig fed on experimental standard protein diet. Results are expressed as means in percentage of a total of 16 fatty acids, none less than 0.1%.

Considering the influence of diet on the fatty-acid composition of LL and SV (Table 5), the only significant differences were observed in the total PUFA of SV, mainly due to the differences in C18:2 n-6, C18:3 n-3, C20:2 n-9, and C20:3 n-3.

Table 5. Fatty-acid composition (%) of the musculus longissimus lumborum and musculus serratus ventralis from Iberian pigs fed the experimental diets.

Items	Musculus Longissimus Lumborum					Musculus Serratus Ventralis				
	FR	LP	SP	SEM	*p*-Value	FR	LP	SP	SEM	*p*-Value
C14:0	1.31	1.30	1.40	0.037	0.492	1.27	1.17	1.22	0.018	0.105
C16:0	24.19	24.48	23.46	0.386	0.562	23.47	24.25	23.24	0.262	0.266
C16:1	4.66	4.15	4.89	0.133	0.058	4.04	3.51	4.08	0.139	0.182
C17:0	0.14 [a]	0.12 [b]	0.16 [a]	0.007	0.044	0.19 [a]	0.15 [b]	0.19 [a]	0.006	0.011
C17:1	0.20	0.16	0.21	0.010	0.119	0.25 [a]	0.19 [b]	0.24 [a]	0.010	0.034
C18:0	10.22	11.41	10.38	0.271	0.152	10.24	12.21	10.40	0.376	0.053
C18:1 n-9	51.39	50.81	51.47	0.428	0.802	49.74	49.23	50.09	0.400	0.699
C18:2 n-6	5.41	4.96	5.33	0.179	0.576	7.88 [a]	6.39 [b]	7.52 [a]	0.210	0.006
C18:3 n-3	0.37 [a,b]	0.35 [a]	0.41 [b]	0.009	0.035	0.48 [a]	0.35 [b]	0.46 [a]	0.018	0.003
C20:0	0.17	0.18	0.17	0.005	0.529	0.17	0.20	0.17	0.008	0.094
C20:1 n-9	0.87	0.91	0.85	0.026	0.596	0.96	1.14	1.05	0.035	0.118
C20:2 n-9	0.21	0.19	0.22	0.007	0.364	0.30 [a]	0.25 [b]	0.31 [a]	0.008	0.002
C20:3 n-6	0.10	0.11	0.13	0.006	0.181	0.13	0.12	0.14	0.005	0.258
C20:4 n-6	0.67	0.78	0.82	0.046	0.400	0.79	0.72	0.76	0.032	0.708
C20:3 n-3	0.09	0.09	0.10	0.004	0.425	0.12 [a]	0.09 [b]	0.12 [a]	0.005	0.017
SFA	36.02	37.49	35.58	0.649	0.473	35.33	37.99	35.22	0.619	0.116
MUFA	57.13	56.03	57.42	0.521	0.538	54.98	54.08	55.47	0.507	0.546
PUFA	6.85	6.48	7.00	0.237	0.673	9.68 [a]	7.93 [b]	9.31 [a]	0.258	0.007

[a,b] Values within a row with different superscripts differ significantly at $p < 0.05$. SEM, standard error of the mean. SFA, total saturated fatty acids; MUFA, total monounsaturated fatty acids; PUFA, total polyunsaturated fatty acids. Diets: FR, Iberian pigs reared in free-range conditions; LP, Iberian pig fed on experimental low-protein diet; SP, Iberian pig fed on experimental standard protein diet. Results are expressed as means in percentage of a total of 16 fatty acids, none less than 0.1%.

4. Discussion

4.1. Experimental Diets

The chemical composition of the acorns and grass in this work showed similar values to those previously published [20,23]. These results show that the protein content in acorns consumed by Iberian pigs during the fattening period in free-range conditions is low compared to diets used in lighter pig systems. Moreover, acorn protein content is constrained by an unbalanced amino-acid profile, with lysine as the main limiting amino acid, according to Nieto et al. [8], who reported average values of 0.2 g lysine/100 g DM in the acorn kernel (Iberian pigs remove the acorn hull to ingest only the kernel). Even though the provision of supplementary protein via pasture could cause an increase in protein deposition in pigs, García-Valverde et al. [3] reported that the amount of protein supplied by pasture is not enough to supply the protein needed during the fattening phase in a free-range system. Thus, in our study, the experimental SP diet was designed to supply the total daily needs of Iberian pig in the fattening phase according to García-Valverde et al. [5], who stated that the maximum potential for the deposition of lean tissue in Iberian pigs during the fattening period is attained when the pigs are fed with a diet which provides 9.5 g crude ideal protein/100 g DM and 0.7 g lysine/100 g DM. On the other hand, the LP diet was designed to simulate, under controlled conditions, the nutrients received by the Iberian pigs in free-range conditions. For this, we took into account both the composition and the proportion of acorns and grass consumed by the pigs according to the studies of Rodríguez-Estévez et al. [24]. Total nutrient intake also depends on the amount of food consumed by the pigs in each treatment. In our study, confined pigs (SP and LP) had very high feed intake, far above that described by García Valverde et al. [5] and closer to that described by Dunker et al. [25] after a restricted feeding period. With respect to acorn and grass, the intakes estimated in our work (3.60 kg DM/day and 0.65 kg DM/day of acorn kernel and grass, respectively) are higher than (2.9 kg DM/day and 0.5 kg DM/day) [20] or similar to (3.6 kg DM/day and 0.38 kg DM/day) [24] those previously reported. Although the protein/energy ratio in LP pigs was much lower than recommended by García-Valverde et al. [5], the daily protein intake was not as low, due to the high daily feed intake. Thus, the estimated daily protein intake in FR pigs was 312 g crude protein/day (187 g from acorn and 125 g from grass), while, in LP and SP pigs, it was 340 and 651 g crude protein/day, respectively. Nevertheless, although the total protein intake between LP and FR could be similar, there may be a difference in the amount of available protein, due to the low protein retained/protein intake ratio in acorns and pasture (0.078 and 0.202, respectively) [3] and in concentrated feed (0.212) [5].

4.2. Pig Performance and Carcass Quality Traits

With respect to productive parameters, ADGs in our study were in general higher than those found in Iberian pigs fed during the fattening period on formulated diets in a confinement system [5,26] or fed with acorns and grass in a free-range system [27]. This could be explained by the pigs in our experiment being older at the beginning of the fattening period, as previously demonstrated [28], probably due to compensatory growth as a result of previous food restriction [27]. A significantly lower ADG was observed in FR compared to SP and LP pigs ($p < 0.05$). Several studies evidenced differences in ADG between free-range reared Iberian pigs and those raised in confinement, due to the effect of physical activity [29] and climatic conditions [30]. However, all pigs in this work had the same thermoregulation needs, given that SP and LP pigs were outdoors and near to those from the FR group. Thus, most of the differences could be due to the expenditure of energy for displacement. Although SP and LP pigs were confined outdoors within a large plot of 230 m^2/pig, they did not have to move to search for food; hence, this cost was higher in the FR animals. No dietary effect on ADG between LP and SP groups was observed, in accordance with previous studies in Alentejano (Iberian) pigs [31] and in heavy pigs [32–35]. In contrast, other authors found that feeding pigs ad libitum with protein- or lysine-deficient but adequate-energy diets during the finishing phase reduces ADG rate [36–38]. Differences between the abovementioned studies could be explained by the different growth rates of the pig breed [6], the pig body weight when the protein restriction is carried out [38], and the deficiencies in protein and essential amino-acid levels [31].

No differences in carcass yield were found in our work, in accordance with previous results in Iberian pigs [26] and in other pig breeds [35,39]. In contrast, Rey et al. [40] found higher carcass yield in pigs fed in confinement than in those fed under free-range conditions with acorn and grass, probably due to the greater fiber content in grass compared to concentrate diet, which could increase the development of the digestive system (mainly large intestine), as evidenced Roskosz et al. [41] in wild pigs fed on diets with a high cellulose content. However, the higher feed intake of intensively reared pigs increased the gut fill [19], which could compensate for the greater development of the digestive system from free range-reared pigs. Related to dietary protein content, our results are in agreement with previous papers [35,42], indicating that it is possible to reduce dietary crude protein without affecting growth performance and carcass composition as long as daily amino-acid supplies are adequate [34]. Only in loins were significantly lower levels of weight and yield detected in FR than in SP pigs, with intermediate values in LP. The effect of a different protein/energy ratio in the three diets studied could be more significant in loins compared to other cuts, such as ham or shoulder, due to loin being a leaner cut, and the reduction in the proportion of protein relative to energy in the diet consistently increases fat deposition and decreases muscle synthesis [43].

4.3. Meat Quality

The higher IMF content of Iberian pigs reared outdoors compared to those reared in intensive conditions and fed on concentrated diets is well known by farmers and dry-cured ham producers [44] and was previously reported [13,23]. This could be due to the high intake during the fattening period prior to slaughter of acorns which have a high caloric value (Rodríguez-Estévez et al. [20] estimated a daily feed intake of 2.92 kg DM acorn) and low protein content with an unbalanced amino-acid profile [8]. In the current study, there were no differences in IMF between FR pigs and LP pigs, but there were differences between both previous and SP pigs in SV. These results could be explained by the low protein content of the LP diet, which was similar to that of FR, and lower than that for the SP treatment. When insufficient dietary protein content is provided to pigs, excess energy is diverted to fat deposition [6]. Moreover, evidence suggests that, with low-protein diets, lipogenic enzymes are expressed more readily in muscle than in subcutaneous fat [45]. Therefore, diet composition, particularly the protein/energy ratio, can be used to increase fatness, with a consequent effect on performance [46]. Indeed, feeding pigs ad libitum with protein- or lysine-deficient but adequate-energy diets during the growing or finishing phases was shown to increase IMF proportion [36], which corroborates our results. In this sense, Schiavon et al. [47] found higher fat cover and thickness and marbling in hams from heavy pigs fed low-protein diets. More recently, Li et al. [38] evidenced the effects of low-protein diets on variations in the expression of two genes (*ACC* (acetyl-CoA carboxylase alpha) and *HSL* (hormone-sensitive lipase)) related to lipid metabolism, thereby promoting fat deposition in the muscle, which agrees with the results of the present study. The effect of feeding diets on chemical meat composition was only observed in SV. IMF content was lower in LL than in SV, which could be related to the type of muscle metabolism, as it is generally accepted that a higher proportion of oxidative fibers implies a greater IMF content [44].

With respect to color, the higher luminosity (L*) values in SV from pigs reared in the FR system than in that from pigs reared in intensive conditions (LP and SP) could be attributed to the combined effect of feed characteristics and the environment, and not only to the exercise of pigs, as demonstrated by López-Bote et al. [48] in studies with Iberian pigs. Thus, the higher L* value of SV from FR compared to LP and SP pigs could also be related to the higher IMF content in FR animals, in accordance with the results of Andrés et al. [44], who found a positive relationship between L* value and fat content in Iberian pork. In the same way, Tejerina et al. [14] found that pigs reared in extensive conditions with acorns and grass had higher L* and b* values in LL and SV than those from Iberian pigs raised in intensive conditions with concentrated diets. In our study, LL showed a same tendency as SV, albeit without significant differences, which could be related to the lower IMF content in LL than in SV, in accordance with Tejerina et al. [14].

4.4. Fatty-Acid Composition

It is well known that the fatty-acid composition of pig tissues is affected principally by the fatty-acid composition of feed [49]. In our study, the influence of feeding background on the fatty-acid composition of porcine tissues was reflected more markedly in subcutaneous fat than in LL and SV muscles. Even though pigs fed in confinement (SP and LP diets) had monounsaturated fatty-acid-enriched diets, a significant influence of FR on the four major fatty acids (C18:1 n-9, C16:0, C18:0, and C18:2 n-6) and SFA and PUFA of subcutaneous fat was found. FR pigs showed a higher C18:1 n-9 content at the level of the tailbone than SP and LP, reflecting the high concentration of oleic acid from acorns, in agreement with the results previously reported [50]. However, Ventanas et al. [13], studying the effect of extensive feeding vs oleic acid-enriched mixed diets in Iberian pigs, did not detect any effect on C18:1 n-9. Moreover, in our study, FR pigs exhibited a lower SFA and higher PUFA content than LP and SP, in accordance with previous studies comparing Iberian pigs fed on free-range and concentrated diets [23]. Nevertheless, the level of protein in the diet did not affect the fatty-acid composition of subcutaneous fat and LL. The greatest effect of the level of protein in diets was reflected in SV, with the biggest change being in C18:2 n-6, and subsequently total PUFA, with the LP regime exhibiting lower proportions than both FR and SP regimes. These results are in agreement with Wood et al. [6], who reported that C18:2 n-6 and C18:1 n-9 are the fatty acids whose concentrations are most affected by a reduction of protein in pig diets. Previous works showed that these two fatty acids are those most affected by changes in total fat deposition in pigs and other animal species [51]. Oleic acid is the main product of de novo fat synthesis in the pig, and it is logical that its concentration increases as the pig gets fatter. The linoleic acid obtained from the diet is then progressively diluted as fat synthesis increases, which explains the declining concentration of this fatty acid. Nevertheless, no significant effect of protein level in the diet was detected for C18:1 n-9 content in our study. The explanation of this aspect could be based on the fatty-acid composition of concentrated feed used in our study, which was rich in oleic acid. Hence, dietary protein content (and, more specifically, the protein/energy ratio) may be used to modify the degree of carcass fat and fatty-acid composition. It is generally accepted that the high sensory quality of Iberian pig meat products from pigs fed under extensive conditions when compared to those fed on mixed feeds is attributed to variation in the content and fatty-acid composition of intramuscular lipids [52,53].

5. Conclusions

The results of this trial show that low-protein diets during the final fattening period prior to slaughter, similar to a feeding regime in free-range conditions with acorns and grass, do not affect Iberian pig productive traits. Additionally, they increase IMF content, which is one of the quality parameters most appreciated by consumers. In this sense, there is growing interest in muscle tissue recently, owing to the effect of increasing IMF on meat quality. Thus, feeding Iberian pigs with LP diets should be an interesting strategy to improve the quality of Iberian pig meat and dry-cured products.

Supplementary Materials: Estimation of the intake of acorns and grass by Iberian pigs in extensive rearing system. The following are available online at http://www.mdpi.com/2076-2615/10/2/273/s1.

Author Contributions: Conceptualization, J.F.T. and E.G.; methodology, J.F.T., E.G., M.P., and A.H.-M.; data analysis, E.G.; animal management, E.G. and M.P.; writing—original draft preparation, J.F.T., E.G., and A.H.-M.; writing—review, J.F.T., E.G., A.H.-M., and M.P.; writing—editing, J.F.T.; project administration and funding acquisition, J.F.T. and E.G. All authors read and agreed to the published version of the manuscript.

Funding: The research was supported by the regional government of Extremadura and the European Social Fund (Research Project PRI08B091).

Acknowledgments: The authors gratefully acknowledge the workers at the Valdesequera farm (CICYTEX) for their technical assistance in animal management.

Conflicts of Interest: The authors declare no conflicts of interest. The funders had no role in the design of the study; in the collection, analyses, or interpretation of data; in the writing of the manuscript, or in the decision to publish the results.

References

1. Lopez-Bote, C.J. Sustained utilization of the Iberian pig breed. *Meat Sci.* **1998**, *49*, S17–S27. [CrossRef]

2. Carrapiso, A.I.; Bonilla, F.; García, C. Effect of crossbreeding and rearing system on sensory characteristics of Iberian ham. *Meat Sci.* **2003**, *65*, 623–629. [CrossRef]

3. García-Valverde, R.; Nieto, R.; Lachica, M.; Aguilera, J.F. Effects of herbage ingestion on the digestion site and nitrogen balance in heavy Iberian pigs fed on an acorn-based diet. *Livest. Sci.* **2007**, *112*, 63–77. [CrossRef]

4. García, C.; Ventanas, J.; Antequera, T.; Ruiz, J.; Cava, R.; Alvarez, P. Measuring sensorial quality of Iberian Ham by Rasch model. *J. Food Qual.* **1996**, *19*, 397–412. [CrossRef]

5. García-Valverde, R.; Barea, R.; Lara, L.; Nieto, R.; Aguilera, J.F. The effects of feeding level upon protein and fat deposition in Iberian heavy pigs. *Livest. Sci.* **2008**, *114*, 263–273. [CrossRef]

6. Wood, J.D.; Lambe, N.R.; Walling, G.A.; Whitney, H.; Jagger, S.; Fullarton, P.J.; Bayntun, J.; Hallett, K.; Bünger, L. Effects of low protein diets on pigs with a lean genotype. 1. Carcass composition measured by dissection and muscle fatty acid composition. *Meat Sci.* **2013**, *95*, 123–128. [CrossRef]

7. Dourmad, J.Y. Concept and application of ideal protein for pigs. *J. Anim. Sci. Biotechnol.* **2015**, *6*, 15. [CrossRef]

8. Nieto, R.; Rivera, M.; García, M.A.; Aguilera, J.F. Amino acid availability and energy value of acorn in the Iberian pig. *Livest. Prod. Sci.* **2002**, *77*, 227–239. [CrossRef]

9. Barea, R.; Nieto, R.; Aguilera, J.F. Effects of the dietary protein content and the feeding level on protein and energy metabolism in Iberian pigs growing from 50 to 100 kg body weight. *Animal* **2007**, *1*, 357–365. [CrossRef]

10. Pomar, C.; Pomar, J.; Dubeau, F.; Joannopoulos, E.; Dussault, J.P. The impact of daily multiphase feeding on animal performance, body composition, nitrogen and phosphorus excretions, and feed costs in growing-finishing pigs. *Animal* **2014**, *8*, 704–713. [CrossRef]

11. Andretta, I.; Pomar, C.; Rivest, J.; Pomar, J.; Lovatto, P.A.; Radünz Neto, J. The impact of feeding growing–finishing pigs with daily tailored diets using precision feeding techniques on animal performance, nutrient utilization, and body and carcass composition1. *J. Anim. Sci.* **2014**, *92*, 3925–3936. [CrossRef] [PubMed]

12. Ventanas, S.; Ventanas, J.; Ruiz, J.; Estévez, M. Iberian pigs for the development of high-quality cured products. *Recent Res. Devel. Agric. Food Chem* **2005**, *6*, 1–27.

13. Ventanas, S.; Tejeda, J.F.; Estévez, M. Chemical composition and oxidative status of tissues from Iberian pigs as affected by diets: Extensive feeding v. oleic acid- and tocopherol-enriched mixed diets. *Animal* **2008**, *2*, 621–630. [CrossRef] [PubMed]

14. Tejerina, D.; García-Torres, S.; Cabeza De Vaca, M.; Vázquez, F.M.; Cava, R. Effect of production system on physical-chemical, antioxidant and fatty acids composition of Longissimus dorsi and Serratus ventralis muscles from Iberian pig. *Food Chem.* **2012**, *133*, 293–299. [CrossRef] [PubMed]

15. FEDNA. *FEDNA Tables of Composition and Nutritive Value of Feeds for Feed Compounding*, 2nd ed.; De Blas, C., Mateos, G.G., Rebollar, P.G., Eds.; Fundación Española para el Desarrollo de la Nutrición Animal: Madrid, Spain, 2003; pp. 1–423.

16. Association of Official Analytical Chemists (AOAC). *Animal Feed*, 17th ed.; AOAC: Gaithersburg, MD, USA, 2000; pp. 69–90.

17. Bligh, E.G.; Dyer, W.J. A rapid method of total lipid extraction and purification. *Can. J. Biochem. Physiol.* **1959**, *37*, 911–917. [CrossRef]

18. Sandler, S.R.; Karo, W. *Sourcebook of Advanced Organic Laboratory Preparations*; Academic Press Harcourt Brace Jovanovich: New York, NY, USA, 1992; ISBN 0126185069.

19. Nieto, R.; Lara, L.; Barea, R.; García-Valverde, R.; Aguinaga, M.A.; Conde-Aguilera, J.A.; Aguilera, J.F. Response analysis of the iberian pig growing from birth to 150 kg body weight to changes in protein and energy supply. *J. Anim. Sci.* **2012**, *90*, 3809–3820. [CrossRef]

20. Rodríguez-Estévez, V.; Sánchez-Rodríguez, M.; García, A.; Gómez-Castro, A.G. Feed conversion rate and estimated energy balance of free grazing Iberian pigs. *Livest. Sci.* **2010**, *132*, 152–156. [CrossRef]

21. Cassens, R.; Demeyer, D.; Eikelemboom, G.; Honikel, K.; Johansson, G.; Nielsen, T.; Renerre, M.; Richardson, I.; Sakata, R. Recommendation of Reference methods for meat color. In Proceedings of the 41th ICoMST, San Antonio, TX, USA, 20–25 August 1995; pp. 410–411.

22. De Pedro, E.; Casillas, M.; Miranda, C.M. Microwave oven application in the extraction of fat from the subcutaneous tissue of Iberian pig ham. *Meat Sci.* **1997**, *45*, 45–51. [CrossRef]

23. Tejeda, J.F.; Gandemer, G.; Antequera, T.; Viau, M.; García, C. Lipid traits of muscles as related to genotype and fattening diet in Iberian pigs: Total intramuscular lipids and triacylglycerols. *Meat Sci.* **2002**, *60*, 357–363. [CrossRef]

24. Rodríguez-Estévez, V.; García, A.; Peña, F.; Gómez, A.G. Foraging of Iberian fattening pigs grazing natural pasture in the dehesa. *Livest. Sci.* **2009**, *120*, 135–143. [CrossRef]

25. Dunker, A.; Rey, A.I.; López-Bote, C.J.; Daza, A. Effect of the feeding level during the fattening phase on the productive parameters, carcass characteristics and quality of fat in heavy pigs. *J. Anim. Feed Sci.* **2007**, *16*, 621–635. [CrossRef]

26. Daza, A.; Menoyo, D.; López Bote, C.J. Carcass traits and fatty acid composition of subcutaneous, intramuscular and liver fat from iberian pigs fed in confinement only with acorns or a formulated diet. *Food Sci. Technol. Int.* **2009**, *15*, 563–569. [CrossRef]

27. Daza, A.; Lopez-Bote, C.J.; Olivares, A.; Menoyo, D.; Ruiz, J. Age at the beginning of the fattening period of Iberian pigs under free-range conditions affects growth, carcass characteristics and the fatty acid profile of lipids. *Anim. Feed Sci. Technol.* **2007**, *139*, 81–91. [CrossRef]

28. Rodríguez-Estévez, V.; Sánchez-Rodríguez, M.; García, A.R.; Gómez-Castro, A.G. Average daily weight gain of Iberian fattening pigs when grazing natural resources. *Livest. Sci.* **2011**, *137*, 292–295. [CrossRef]

29. Lachica, M.; Aguilera, J.F. Estimation of the energy costs of locomotion in the Iberian pig (Sus mediterraneus). *Br. J. Nutr.* **2000**, *83*, 35–41. [CrossRef]

30. López-Bote, C.J.; Rey, A.; Isabel, B. Alimentación del cerdo Ibérico en la dehesa. In *Porcino Ibérico: Aspectos Claves*; Buxadé, C., Daza, A., Eds.; Ediciones Mundi Prensa: Madrid, Spain, 2000; pp. 215–246.

31. Madeira, M.S.; Costa, P.; Alfaia, C.M.; Lopes, P.A.; Bessa, R.J.B.; Lemos, J.P.C.; Prates, J.A.M. The increased intramuscular fat promoted by dietary lysine restriction in lean but not in fatty pig genotypes improves pork sensory attributes. *J. Anim. Sci.* **2013**, *91*, 3177–3187. [CrossRef]

32. Galassi, G.; Colombini, S.; Malagutti, L.; Crovetto, G.M.; Rapetti, L. Effects of high fibre and low protein diets on performance, digestibility, nitrogen excretion and ammonia emission in the heavy pig. *Anim. Feed Sci. Technol.* **2010**, *161*, 140–148. [CrossRef]

33. Gallo, L.; Dalla Montà, G.; Carraro, L.; Cecchinato, A.; Carnier, P.; Schiavon, S. Growth performance of heavy pigs fed restrictively diets with decreasing crude protein and indispensable amino acids content. *Livest. Sci.* **2014**, *161*, 130–138. [CrossRef]

34. Monteiro, A.N.T.R.; Bertol, T.M.; De Oliveira, P.A.V.; Dourmad, J.; Coldebella, A. The impact of feeding growing- fi nishing pigs with reduced dietary protein levels on performance, carcass traits, meat quality and environmental impacts. *Livest. Sci.* **2017**, *198*, 162–169. [CrossRef]

35. Aquilani, C.; Sirtori, F.; Franci, O.; Acciaioli, A.; Bozzi, R.; Pezzati, A.; Pugliese, C. Effects of protein restriction on performances and meat quality of cinta senese pig reared in an organic system. *Animals* **2019**, *9*, 310. [CrossRef]

36. Lebret, B. Effects of feeding and rearing systems on growth, carcass composition and meat quality in pigs. *Animal* **2008**, *2*, 1548–1558. [CrossRef]

37. Ruiz-Ascacíbar, I.; Stoll, P.; Kreuzer, M.; Boillat, V.; Spring, P.; Bee, G. Impact of amino acid and CP restriction from 20 to 140 kg BW on performance and dynamics in empty body protein and lipid deposition of entire male, castrated and female pigs. *Animal* **2017**, *11*, 394–404. [CrossRef]

38. Li, Y.H.; Li, F.N.; Duan, Y.H.; Guo, Q.P.; Wen, C.Y.; Wang, W.L.; Huang, X.G.; Yin, Y.L. Low-protein diet improves meat quality of growing and finishing pigs through changing lipid metabolism, fiber characteristics, and free amino acid profile of the muscle. *J. Anim. Sci.* **2018**, *96*, 3221–3232. [CrossRef]

39. Presto Åkerfeldt, M.; Lindberg, J.E.; Göransson, L.; Andersson, K. Effects of reducing dietary content of crude protein and indispensable amino acids on performance and carcass traits of single-phase- and 2-phase-fed growing-finishing pigs. *Livest. Sci.* **2019**, *224*, 96–101. [CrossRef]

40. Rey, A.I.; Daza, A.; López-Carrasco, C.; López-Bote, C.J. Feeding Iberian pigs with acorns and grass in either free-range or confinement affects the carcass characteristics and fatty acids and tocopherols accumulation in Longissimus dorsi muscle and backfat. *Meat Sci.* **2006**, *73*, 66–74. [CrossRef]

41. Roskosz, T.; Kobrynczuk, F.; Brundnicki, W. The type of feed and the length of intestine in wild pig, Sus scrofa (L.). *Ann. Warsaw Univ. Live Sci. SGGW* **1990**, *16*, 13–17.

42. Dourmad, J.Y.; Jondreville, C. Impact of nutrition on nitrogen, phosphorus, Cu and Zn in pig manure, and on emissions of ammonia and odours. *Livest. Sci.* **2007**, *112*, 192–198. [CrossRef]

43. Ruusunen, M.; Partanen, K.; Pösö, R.; Puolanne, E. The effect of dietary protein supply on carcass composition, size of organs, muscle properties and meat quality of pigs. *Livest. Sci.* **2007**, *107*, 170–181. [CrossRef]

44. Andrés, A.I.; Cava, R.; Mayoral, A.I.; Tejeda, J.F.; Morcuende, D.; Ruiz, J. Oxidative stability and fatty acid composition of pig muscles as affected by rearing system, crossbreeding and metabolic type of muscle fibre. *Meat Sci.* **2001**, *59*, 39–47. [CrossRef]

45. Doran, O.; Moule, S.K.; Teye, G.A.; Whittington, F.M.; Hallett, K.G.; Wood, J.D. A reduced protein diet induces stearoyl-CoA desaturase protein expression in pig muscle but not in subcutaneous adipose tissue: Relationship with intramuscular lipid formation. *Br. J. Nutr.* **2006**, *95*, 609–617. [CrossRef]

46. Gómez, R.S.; Lewis, A.J.; Miller, P.S.; Chen, H.Y.; Diedrichsen, R.M. Body composition and tissue accretion rates of barrows fed corn-soybean meal diets or low-protein, amino acid-supplemented diets at different feeding levels. *J. Anim. Sci.* **2002**, *80*, 654–662. [CrossRef]

47. Schiavon, S.; Carraro, L.; Dalla Bona, M.; Cesaro, G.; Carnier, P.; Tagliapietra, F.; Sturaro, E.; Galassi, G.; Malagutti, L.; Trevisi, E.; et al. Growth performance, and carcass and raw ham quality of crossbred heavy pigs from four genetic groups fed low protein diets for dry-cured ham production. *Anim. Feed Sci. Technol.* **2015**, *208*, 170–181. [CrossRef]

48. López-Bote, C.J.; Toldrá, F.; Daza, A.; Ferrer, J.M.; Menoyo, D.; Silió, L.; Rodríguez, M.C. Effect of exercise on skeletal muscle proteolytic enzyme activity and meat quality characteristics in Iberian pigs. *Meat Sci.* **2008**, *79*, 71–76. [CrossRef]

49. Enser, M.; Richardson, R.I.; Wood, J.D.; Gill, B.P.; Sheard, P.R. Feeding linseed to increase the n-3 PUFA of pork: Fatty acid composition of muscle, adipose tissue, liver and sausages. *Meat Sci.* **2000**, *55*, 201–212. [CrossRef]

50. Pérez-Palacios, T.; Ruiz, J.; Tejeda, J.F.; Antequera, T. Subcutaneous and intramuscular lipid traits as tools for classifying Iberian pigs as a function of their feeding background. *Meat Sci.* **2009**, *81*, 632–640. [CrossRef]

51. De Smet, S.; Raes, K.; Demeyer, D. Meat fatty acid composition as affected by fatness and genetic factors: A review. *Anim. Res.* **2004**, *53*, 81–98. [CrossRef]

52. Antequera, T.; López-Bote, C.J.; Córdoba, J.J.; García, C.; Asensio, M.A.; Ventanas, J.; García-Regueiro, J.A.; Díaz, I. Lipid oxidative changes in the processing of Iberian pig hams. *Food Chem.* **1992**, *45*, 105–110. [CrossRef]

53. Ruiz-Carrascal, J.; Ventanas, J.; Cava, R.; Andrés, A.I.; García, C. Texture and appearance of dry cured ham as affected by fat content and fatty acid composition. *Food Res. Int.* **2000**, *33*, 91–95. [CrossRef]

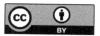

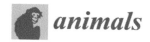

Article

Meat Quality, Amino Acid, and Fatty Acid Composition of Liangshan Pigs at Different Weights

Mailin Gan [1,2,†], **Linyuan Shen** [1,2,†], **Lei Chen** [1,2], **Dongmei Jiang** [1,2], **Yanzhi Jiang** [3], **Qiang Li** [4], **Ying Chen** [4], **Guihua Ge** [4], **Yihui Liu** [4], **Xu Xu** [4], **Xuewei Li** [1,2], **Shunhua Zhang** [1,2,*] and **Li Zhu** [1,2,*]

[1] College of Animal Science and Technology, Sichuan Agricultural University, Chengdu 611130, China; ganmailin@stu.sicau.edu.cn (M.G.); shenlinyuan@sicau.edu.cn (L.S.); chenlei815918@sicau.edu.cn (L.C.); jiangdm@sicau.edu.cn (D.J.); xuewei.li@sicau.edu.cn (X.L.)
[2] Farm Animal Genetic Resources Exploration and Innovation Key Laboratory of Sichuan Province, Sichuan Agricultural University, Chengdu 611130, China
[3] College of Life Science, Sichuan Agricultural University, Yaan 625014, China; 13526@sicau.edu.cn
[4] Sichuan Province General Station of Animal Husbandry, Chengdu 611130, China; B20050604@stu.sicau.edu.cn (Q.L.); S20163634@stu.sicau.edu.cn (Y.C.); S20163617@stu.sicau.edu.cn (G.G.); B20141408@stu.sicau.edu.cn (Y.L.); S20163644@stu.sicau.edu.cn (X.X.)
* Correspondence: 14081@sicau.edu.cn (S.Z.); zhuli@sicau.edu.cn (L.Z.)
† These authors contributed equally to this work.

Received: 27 March 2020; Accepted: 5 May 2020; Published: 9 May 2020

Simple Summary: The research on the quality of traditional pork can not only provide a reference for the thorough breeding and food development of pigs, but also make a reference for understanding the local history and social culture. The Liangshan pig is a traditional Chinese miniature pig breed. It is mainly raised in the Liangshan Yi area and is closely related to the dietary culture of the local people. The characteristics of, and changes in, the meat quality, amino acid composition and fatty acid composition of Liangshan pigs of different weights were revealed for the first time in this paper. It was found that as the weight of Liangshan pigs increased, the contents of marbling score, intramuscular fat, shear force, Met, Asp, Asn, C18: 0 and C20: 2 increased, and drip loss, Trp and C22: 6 decreased. Taken together, our findings serve as a reference for the development of the local Liangshan pig industry.

Abstract: Indigenous pig breeds are important biological resources and their diversity has been severely damaged. The Liangshan pig is a typical mountain-type local pig breed in southwest China. Here, the meat quality, amino acid, and fatty acid composition of Liangshan pigs were compared at seven stages within the weight range of 50–90 kg. A score for comprehensive factors of meat quality was maintained after rising and kept in a plateau within 74.9–91.5 kg of body weight. The total amount of amino acids in the longissimus dorsi muscle remained stable, and the total fatty acids showed an upward trend. Amino acid composition analysis revealed that as the body weight of Liangshan pigs increased, umami, basic, and acidic amino acid contents decreased, while the essential amino acids (EAA) content and the ratio of basic amino acids to acidic amino acids increased. Fatty acid composition analysis revealed that as body weight increased, the content of polyunsaturated fatty acids (PUFA) exhibited a downward trend, while the content of saturated fatty acids (SFA) exhibited an upward trend. This study is a primary step towards the development and utilization of Liangshan pigs and provides useful information for local pork processing and genetic improvement.

Keywords: Liangshan pig; meat quality; amino acid; fatty acid; traditional pig products

1. Introduction

Local pigs are important biological resources for new breeds and strains, the protection of animal diversity, and the realization of sustainable animal husbandry [1]. Pig production and breeding have rapidly entered globalization alongside economic globalization. Duroc, Yorkshire, Landrace, and Buckshire pigs represent the majority of breeds on the market, whereas many local pig breeds are endangered [2]. It is worth noting that pig breeding has long pursued high growth rates and high lean meat rates, which has led to a decline in pork quality, such as meat color, shear force and flavor [3]. However, consumers have recently begun to pursue pork of a higher quality and richer flavor. Therefore, local pig breeds are a resource that could meet the diverse needs of consumers [4].

The formation of local pig breeds is closely related to the local environment and people's consuming habits [5]. Pigs are an important part of local society and culture. In-depth studies of pork quality not only provide a reference for improved breeding and food development but can also provide insights into local history and social culture. The development and utilization of local pig breeds is an important way to protect local pig resources and diet culture and is of great significance for local economic development and national cultural heritage.

The Liangshan pig is a traditional small-sized Chinese indigenous pig breed, mainly reared in the Yi minority region of Liangshan, China. It has a strong resistance to cold and thrives on coarse feed. Like most local pigs, Liangshan pigs have strong adaptability and good meat quality. However, Liangshan pigs have a slow growth rate and low feed conversion rate; therefore, the population of Liangshan pigs has decreased rapidly in recent years [6]. Limited information exists on the Liangshan pig breed; therefore, the goal was to acquire basic information of different quality characteristics to be used a future reference in the development and utilization.

In the present study, the quality, and amino acid and fatty acid composition of meat from 140 slaughtered Liangshan pigs was measured. The analysis of these data will help towards understanding meat quality characteristics and change rules of Liangshan pigs, and to formulate optimal slaughter times and suitable food development strategies. The results of this study are also of reference value for the genetic improvement of other local pigs and the development of specialty foods.

2. Materials and Methods

The experimental protocol was approved by the Animal Care and Ethics Committee of Sichuan Agricultural University, Sichuan, China, under permit No. DKY-S20123030 and No. DKY-S20123138.

2.1. Animals

The experiment was organized and performed at the Liangshan pig conservation farm of Mabian Gold Liangshan Agriculture Development Co. Ltd. (Sichuan, China). A total of 140 pigs with a similar birth date and birth weight (half barrows and half gilts) were randomly selected from the farm. Based on the methods of previous reports, 140 pigs were slaughtered at 7 different weight stages (the difference between each stage was approximately 6 kg) between 160 and 260 days of age, with 20 pigs from each stage (Table 1). The ingredients of the basal experiment diets are shown in Table S1.

Table 1. Information of Liangshan pigs being slaughtered.

Group.	1	2	3	4	5	6	7
Number	20	20	20	20	20	20	20
Body weight, kg	53.2	59.5	67.4	74.9	80.4	86.7	91.5

2.2. Management

All pigs were fed the same commercial feedstuff. The pigs had ad libitum access to diet and water. All pigs were slaughtered following the method of Xiao et al. [7]. After transport to the abattoir, the pigs had no access to feed for 24 h before slaughter.

2.3. Meat Quality Trait Measurements

The determination of meat quality traits mainly refers to those used in our previous study [1]. The longissimus dorsi muscle samples used to measure meat quality traits were collected from the left side of the carcass adjacent to the last rib, within 45 min after slaughter. The penultimate 3–4 intercostal samples (the thickness is about 3 cm) of the longissimus dorsi muscle were used to measure pH, color and marbling scores (MS), and the samples (about 300–500 g) of the last rib of the longissimus dorsi muscle was used to measure drip loss, cooking loss and shear force (SF). The meat samples' pH was determined using a pH meter (model 720A; Orion Research Inc., Boston, MA, USA) according to the procedure of Alonso et al. [8]. The first measurement was to measure the central 1/3 location area of the meat sample at 45 min post-mortem (pH_1), and the second at 24 h (pH_2). Make 3 repetitions for each sample, take 3 readings for each repetition, and then calculate the average. Color parameters were measured using a Minolta CR-300 colorimeter (Minolta Camera, Osaka, Japan). Drip loss was calculated from the weight loss of a sample (approximately 30 g) wrapped in foil and placed on a flat plastic grid after storage for 24 h at 4 °C. Cooking loss was determined by cooking meat samples for 30 min, then, after cooling, measuring the weight loss relative to the uncooked weight. Marbling scores (MS) were determined using longissimus dorsi muscle 24 h after slaughter (colorimetric method, 5-point scale; the larger the score value, the richer the muscle fat content). Shear force (SF) was determined using a Texture Analyzer (TA.XT. Plus, Stable Micro Systems, Godalming, UK) equipped with a Warner-Bratzler shearing device.

2.4. Analysis of Free Amino Acids and Fatty Acids

Free amino acid (FAA) and fatty acid compositions were determined according to a previous article [1]. FAA composition was measured using liquid chromatography–mass spectrometry (Liquid phase: LC-20AD, Shimadzu, Japan; Mass Spectrometry: 5500 Q TRAP LC-MS/MS, AB SCIEX, Framingham, MA, USA), and gas chromatography–mass spectrometry (GC-MS 7890B-5977A, Agilent, Palo Alto, CA, USA) was used to detect fatty acid composition.

2.5. Meat Chemical Composition

Intramuscular fat (IMF), crude protein (CP) and ash contents were measured by the Nutrition Institute of Sichuan Agricultural University. CP was determined by the Kjeldahl method, and IMF content was determined by Soxhlet extraction [9].

2.6. Statistical Analyses

The ANOVA procedure was performed in SAS for Windows Release 8.0 (SAS Institute Inc., Cary, NC, USA) and was used to analyze the data collected. Duncan's test was used for comparing the mean values of the results. Mean values and standard errors are shown in the tables, with differences considered significant if $p < 0.05$. A comprehensive evaluation of Liangshan pigs at different bodyweight stages was performed using a factor analysis test.

3. Results

3.1. Meat Quality and Meat Crude Chemical Composition

The meat quality and crude chemical composition of Liangshan pig meat samples exhibited significant differences at different stages (Table 2). The first stage exhibited the highest L^*_2 and drip loss values, while the marbling score, shear force, crude protein, and intramuscular fat content were the lowest. At the seventh stage, meat samples' pH_1, shear force, and intramuscular fat content were the highest, while drip loss and ash value were the lowest.

Table 2. Meat quality of Liangshan pig at different stages.

Meat Quality	Group							S.E.	Significance
	1	2	3	4	5	6	7		
pH$_1$	6.40 ^{b}	6.34 ^{b}	6.60 ^{ab}	6.56 ^{ab}	6.60 ^{ab}	6.48 ^{b}	6.63 ^{a}	0.04	*
pH$_2$	6.02 ^{b}	5.89 ^{b}	6.11 ^{ab}	6.18 ^{a}	6.14 ^{ab}	5.92 ^{b}	6.16 ^{ab}	0.04	*
L*$_1$	41.49 ^{a}	41.50 ^{a}	39.01 ^{b}	39.91 ^{b}	40.56 ^{ab}	38.98 ^{b}	39.16 ^{b}	0.42	*
L*$_2$	44.58 ^{a}	44.05 ^{a}	42.41 ^{a}	43.78 ^{ab}	44.12 ^{a}	42.93 ^{b}	43.89 ^{ab}	0.28	*
Marbling score	2.25 ^{b}	2.75 ^{b}	3.33 ^{ab}	3.67 ^{a}	3.50 ^{a}	3.87 ^{a}	3.67 ^{a}	0.22	*
Shear force, kg	3.24 ^{b}	4.09 ^{b}	4.39 ^{ab}	4.99 ^{ab}	4.96 ^{ab}	4.90 ^{ab}	5.27 ^{a}	0.27	*
Drip loss, %	5.18 ^{a}	4.82 ^{ab}	4.43 ^{b}	4.31 ^{b}	4.35 ^{b}	4.32 ^{b}	4.24 ^{b}	0.13	*
Cooking loss, %	34.05 ^{b}	34.39 ^{b}	33.74 ^{b}	36.17 ^{a}	35.94 ^{ab}	34.68 ^{b}	35.75 ^{ab}	0.37	*
Crude protein, %	18.69 ^{c}	19.01 ^{bc}	19.25 ^{b}	19.36 ^{b}	19.49 ^{ab}	19.98 ^{a}	19.09 ^{bc}	0.15	*
Intramuscular fat, %	3.22 ^{b}	3.81 ^{b}	4.46 ^{ab}	4.49 ^{ab}	4.42 ^{ab}	4.71 ^{a}	5.02 ^{a}	0.76	*
Ash, %	1.19 ^{b}	1.21 ^{b}	1.16 ^{b}	1.20 ^{b}	1.15 ^{b}	1.11 ^{b}	1.05 ^{a}	0.27	*

pH$_1$ and L*$_1$ measured at 45 min postmortem; pH2 and L*$_2$ measured at 24 h postmortem. S.E. standard error, ^{a}, ^{b}, ^{c} and * mean significant difference.

With the increase in slaughter weight, meat samples' pH$_1$, pH$_2$, cooking loss, and crude protein increased slowly and fluctuated, while marbling score, shear force and intramuscular fat content rapidly and continuously increased (Figure 1A,B). As the slaughter weight increased, L*$_1$, L*$_2$ and ash decreased slowly and fluctuated, while drip loss rapidly and continuously decreased (Figure 1C,D). The overall analysis score for of Liangshan pig quality factors first increased and then remained at high levels with further increases in bodyweight (Figure 1E,F).

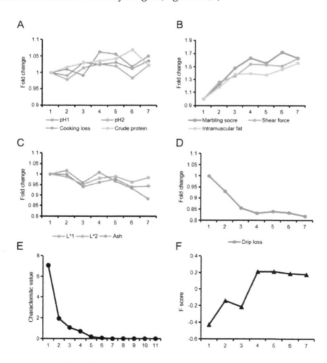

Figure 1. Change pattern of Liangshan pig meat quality traits. (**A**) Slowly increasing meat quality traits. (**B**) Rapidly increasing meat quality traits. (**C**) Slowly falling meat quality traits. (**D**) Rapidly falling meat quality traits. (**E**) Crushed stone graph for factor analysis of meat quality traits. (**F**) Comprehensive score for factor analysis of meat quality traits.

3.2. Free Amino Acid Contents

It can be seen in Table 3 and Figure 2A that the total amino acid (TAA) content in the longissimus dorsi muscle of Liangshan pigs slightly fluctuated (<30%) at different stages; the highest value was in the first stage and the lowest was in the second stage. Lys, Ile, Val, Trp, His, Arg, Glu, Tyr and Ala contents in Liangshan pig longissimus dorsi muscle were highest in the first stage, and Thr, Gln, Gly and Pro were the highest in the third stage (Table 3). Leu, Met, Ser and Asp contents were highest in the sixth stage, and Ile and Asn were the highest in the seventh stage.

The content of essential amino acids (EAA) in the longissimus dorsi muscle of Liangshan pigs in the seventh stage was the highest, reaching 28.13% (Figure 2A). Further analysis revealed that as the slaughter weight increased, the composition of basic amino acids and acidic amino acids in the longissimus dorsi muscle showed a downward trend and fluctuated, while the ratio of basic amino acids to acidic amino acids increased in fluctuation (Figure 2B). Sweet and umami amino acids were highest in the fifth stage, while bitter amino acids were highest in the sixth stage (Figure 2C).

3.3. Fatty Acid Levels

A total of 24 fatty acids were measured in the longissimus dorsi muscle of Liangshan pigs in the seven stages tested (Table 4). C16:0, C18:1, C18:2, C18:0, C20:4 and C14:0 are contained in more than 1%, and the cumulative proportion of these fatty acids exceeded 96% in the seven stages (Figure 3A). The C18:1 content was highest in the fourth stage, and the C16:0 content was highest in all stages other than stage six. The saturated fatty acids (SFA) was the lowest in the first stage and the highest in the fifth stage. Monounsaturated fatty acid (MUFA) content was highest in the fourth stage and lowest in the seventh stage. Polyunsaturated fatty acids (PUFA) content was highest in the first stage and lowest in the fifth stage (Figure 3B,C). Further analysis revealed that the overall n6 and n3 content showed a downward trend, while the n6:n3 values increased in volatility (Figure 3D).

Table 3. The amino acid content of longissimus dorsi muscle of Liangshan pig (mg/100g).

Amino Acid	Phase							S.E.	Significance
	1	2	3	4	5	6	7		
				EAA					
Lys	4.11 [a]	3.04 [b]	3.95 [a]	3.22 [b]	2.90 [b]	3.71 [ab]	3.96 [a]	0.19	*
Ile	2.39 [b]	2.13 [bc]	2.27 [b]	2.07 [bc]	1.73 [c]	2.92 [a]	2.39 [b]	0.14	*
Leu	4.09 [b]	3.54 [bc]	3.82 [bc]	3.70 [bc]	3.13 [c]	5.25 [a]	4.27 [b]	0.25	*
Val	4.05 [a]	3.30 [bc]	3.56 [b]	3.47 [b]	3.01 [c]	3.33 [bc]	3.67 [ab]	0.12	*
Thr	3.09 [ab]	2.64 [b]	3.22 [a]	2.68 [b]	2.44 [b]	3.57 [a]	3.05 [ab]	0.15	*
Phe	2.79 [b]	2.75 [b]	2.81 [ab]	2.43 [b]	2.46 [b]	3.19 [a]	3.10 [ab]	0.11	*
Met	1.62 [b]	1.49 [b]	1.51 [b]	1.76 [b]	1.55 [b]	2.80 [a]	2.61 [a]	0.21	*
Trp	0.57 [a]	0.35 [b]	0.48 [ab]	0.46 [ab]	0.21 [b]	0.28 [b]	0.23 [b]	0.05	*
				NEAA					
His	3.17 [a]	2.62 [b]	2.79 [b]	2.52 [b]	2.55 [b]	3.09 [ab]	2.60 [b]	0.10	*
Gln	19.76 [bc]	19.07 [bc]	25.13 [a]	17.88 [c]	21.23 [b]	22.31 [ab]	18.90 [bc]	0.94	*
Arg	3.38 [a]	2.31 [bc]	2.66 [b]	2.22 [bc]	1.87 [c]	3.19 [ab]	2.72 [ab]	0.20	*
Glu	4.60 [a]	3.22 [bc]	3.52 [b]	3.48 [b]	4.03 [b]	3.01 [bc]	2.63 [c]	0.25	*
Ser	3.71 [ab]	2.84 [b]	3.04 [b]	2.91 [b]	2.84 [b]	4.52 [a]	4.14 [a]	0.26	*
Asp	0.34 [b]	0.27 [b]	0.48 [a]	0.32 [b]	0.33 [b]	0.50 [a]	0.49 [a]	0.04	*
Gly	7.70 [ab]	6.29 [b]	7.88 [a]	6.01 [b]	6.77 [b]	6.25 [b]	6.02 [b]	0.30	*
Tyr	2.36 [a]	1.65 [b]	2.34 [a]	1.39 [b]	1.50 [b]	1.94 [ab]	1.72 [b]	0.15	*
Ala	21.39 [a]	15.17 [c]	19.15 [ab]	17.16 [bc]	17.08 [bc]	18.57 [b]	17.04 [bc]	0.75	*
Asn	1.52 [b]	1.68 [b]	1.59 [b]	1.25 [b]	1.26 [b]	1.94 [ab]	2.17 [a]	0.13	*
Pro	0.89 [b]	0.92 [b]	1.06 [a]	0.81 [b]	0.94 [ab]	1.01 [ab]	1.05 [a]	0.03	*
TAA	91.53 [a]	75.28 [b]	91.26 [a]	75.74 [b]	77.83 [b]	91.38 [a]	82.76 [ab]	2.87	*

[a], [b], [c] and * mean significant difference.

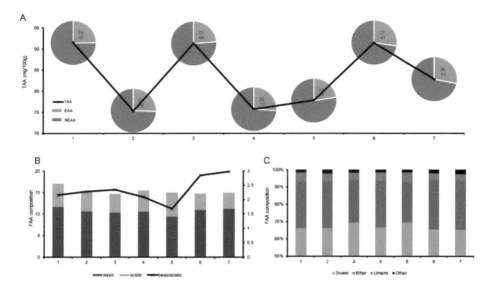

Figure 2. Analysis of amino acid composition in the longissimus dorsi muscle. (**A**) Changes in total amino acid (TAA) content and changes in essential amino acids (EAA) and non-essential amino acids (NEAA). (**B**) The content of basic and acidic amino acids. (**C**) The amino acid ratios of longissimus dorsi muscle with different flavors. Umami AA: Glu, Asp; Sweet AA: Gly, Ala, Ser, Thr, Pro, Gln, Lys; Bitter AA: Tyr, Arg, His, Val, Met, Ile, Leu, Trp, Phe.

Table 4. Fatty acid content of the longissimus dorsi muscle of the Liangshan pig (mg/100g).

FA	Phase							S.E.	Significance
	1	2	3	4	5	6	7		
C8:0	0.25 [b]	0.25 [b]	0.21 [b]	0.31 [a]	0.30 [ab]	0.30 [ab]	0.34 [a]	0.02	
C10:0	2.39 [b]	2.56 [b]	2.33 [b]	3.50 [a]	3.19 [a]	3.21 [a]	3.24 [a]	0.18	*
C12:0	1.93 [b]	2.23 [b]	1.74 [b]	2.67 [a]	2.89 [a]	2.63 [a]	2.47 [a]	0.16	*
C14:0	24.95 [b]	29.87 [a]	23.21 [b]	33.81 [a]	33.98 [a]	34.43 [a]	32.08 [a]	1.73	*
C15:0	1.23 [c]	1.37 [bc]	1.24 [c]	1.47 [bc]	1.85 [a]	1.43 [bc]	1.54 [b]	0.08	*
C15:1	0.69 [b]	0.88 [ab]	0.69 [b]	0.68 [b]	0.69 [b]	1.02 [a]	1.10 [a]	0.07	*
C16:0	391.56 [b]	453.18 [b]	397.11 [b]	491.12 [ab]	517.62 [ab]	534.75 [a]	490.13 [ab]	21.29	*
C17:0	4.18 [b]	5.02 [b]	4.31 [b]	5.47 [ab]	6.07 [a]	5.36 [ab]	5.84 [ab]	0.27	*
C17:1	3.03 [b]	4.26 [ab]	3.69 [b]	4.62 [ab]	5.03 [a]	4.78 [ab]	3.92 [b]	0.26	*
C18:0	165.32 [b]	301.69 [a]	275.60 [a]	337.06 [a]	350.95 [a]	356.85 [a]	344.99 [a]	25.73	*
C18:1	353.17 [b]	440.08 [ab]	393.2 [b]	513.13 [a]	463.96 [ab]	482.58 [a]	464.37 [ab]	19.75	*
C18:2	349.93 [b]	403.99 [ab]	340.86 [b]	443.20 [a]	341.58 [b]	458.11 [a]	455.98 [a]	20.59	*
C18:3	6.71 [b]	7.96 [a]	6.45 [b]	8.76 [a]	9.12 [a]	9.16 [a]	8.04 [ab]	0.42	*
C20:0	3.34 [b]	4.12 [ab]	3.48 [b]	4.74 [a]	4.98 [a]	4.91 [a]	4.91 [a]	0.27	*
C20:1	8.40 [b]	10.55 [ab]	8.40 [b]	11.77 [a]	10.96 [ab]	12.16 [a]	11.72 [a]	0.59	*
C20:2	9.33 [b]	12.16 [b]	9.54 [b]	13.15 [ab]	13.10 [ab]	13.12 [ab]	15.47 [a]	0.82	*
C20:3	1.45 [ab]	1.42 [ab]	0.99 [c]	1.39 [ab]	1.31 [b]	1.41 [ab]	1.61 [a]	0.07	*
C20:4	153.91 [b]	169.97 [ab]	126.87 [b]	197.36 [a]	158.14 [b]	190.68 [ab]	198.31 [a]	10.04	*
C20:5	3.11 [bc]	3.31 [b]	2.60 [c]	3.30 [b]	4.07 [a]	3.46 [b]	3.16 [bc]	0.17	*
C22:0	0.93 [b]	0.90 [b]	0.79 [b]	1.01 [b]	1.36 [a]	1.03 [b]	1.03 [b]	0.07	*
C22:1	0.54 [b]	0.60 [b]	0.54 [b]	0.57 [b]	0.75 [a]	0.56 [b]	0.57 [b]	0.03	*
C22:6	6.61 [ab]	6.02 [ab]	3.71 [b]	4.68 [b]	7.82 [a]	4.70 [b]	4.16 [b]	0.56	*
C23:0	0.14 [b]	0.12 [b]	0.10 [b]	0.15 [b]	0.26 [a]	0.13 [b]	0.14 [b]	0.02	*
C24:0	0.51 [b]	0.48 [b]	0.41 [b]	0.60 [b]	0.93 [a]	0.54 [b]	0.62 [b]	0.06	*
TFA	1493.61 [b]	1862.99 [ab]	1608.07 [b]	2084.52 [a]	1940.91 [ab]	2127.31 [a]	2055.74 [a]	92.93	*

[a], [b], [c] and * mean significant difference.

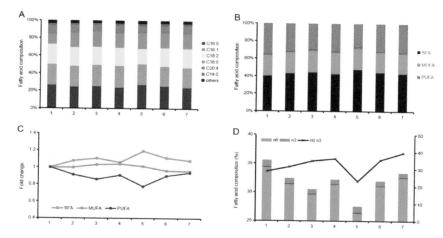

Figure 3. Analysis of fatty acid composition and characteristics in the longissimus dorsi muscle. (**A**) The content of the top 6 fatty acids. (**B**) A composition of saturated fatty acids (SFA), monounsaturated fatty acids (MUFA) and polyunsaturated fatty acids (PUFA) in longissimus dorsi muscle. (**C**) Changes in SFA, MUFA and PUFA contents. (**D**) The ratio of n6:n3 of longissimus dorsi muscle.

3.4. Comprehensive Meat Quality Evaluation of Liangshan Pigs at Different Bodyweight Stages

Correlation analysis was performed on meat quality indicators that changed by >50% of their values at the first stage. Mar bling score was significantly positively correlated with shear force, intramuscular fat, and C18:0 content. Shear force was significantly positively correlated with intramuscular fat and C18:0 content. Intramuscular fat content was significantly positively correlated with Asp and C18:0 content, and significantly negatively correlated with C22:6 content (Table 5).

Table 5. Correlation analysis of the indexes of longissimus dorsi in Liangshan pig.

	MS	SF	IMF	Trp	Met	Asp	Asn	C18:0	C20:2	C22:6
MS	1									
SF	0.95 *	1								
IMF	0.95 *	0.95 *	1							
Trp	−0.58	−0.65	−0.64	1						
Met	0.66	0.67	0.7	−0.62	1					
Asp	0.71	0.64	0.83 *	−0.55	0.68	1				
Asn	0.23	0.35	0.43	−0.53	0.71	0.52	1			
C18:0	0.79 *	0.83 *	0.80 *	−0.64	0.29	0.46	0.22	1		
C20:2	0.22	0.48	0.41	−0.6	0.54	0.3	0.67	0.23	1	
C22:6	−0.74	−0.67	−0.8 *	0.19	−0.61	−0.75	−0.49	−0.53	−0.1	1

* mean significant difference.

Through factor analysis, three characteristic values greater than 1 were obtained, and the cumulative contribution rate of the components reached 91.18% (Figure 4A). The component matrix results are shown in Table 6. The first principal component (PC) is mainly related to mar bling score, shear force and C18:0 content, the second principal component is mainly related to C22:6 content, and the third principal component is mainly related to C20:2 content (Table 6). As can be seen from Figure 4B, the comprehensive score shows a trend of first increasing, then decreasing (Figure 4B).

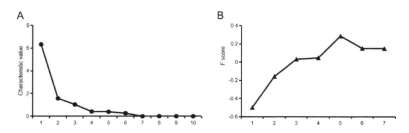

Figure 4. Results of the factor analysis. (**A**) A crushed stone graph. (**B**) A comprehensive score for factor analysis.

Table 6. Rotated component matrix.

PC [1]	MS	SF	IMF	Trp	Met	Asp	Asn	C18:0	C20:2	C22:6
1	0.811	0.833	0.749	−0.636	0.244	0.382	−0.051	0.919	0.193	−0.333
2	0.546	0.415	0.602	−0.028	0.637	0.751	0.486	0.174	−0.004	−0.911
3	0.073	0.277	0.25	−0.676	0.609	0.286	0.8	0.082	0.901	−0.004

PC: principal component. [1]: Only the principal components with feature values greater than 1 are displayed.

4. Discussion

The Liangshan pig is a typical small-sized mountain-type pig breed, which is mainly distri buted in the Yi Autonomous Prefecture of Liangshan. Like most of the world's local pig breeds, Liangshan pigs are endangered [10,11]. The natural environment of the Liangshan Yi area and the dietary culture of the local people have determined the characteristics of Liangshan pigs. However, little is known about the basic biological characteristics of the Liangshan pig. Many studies have shown that age and weight are the most important factors affecting meat quality [12,13]. Here, meat quality traits, and amino acid and fatty acid composition of the longissimus dorsi muscle of Liangshan pigs were measured at seven stages (between 50 and 90 kg bodyweight) and were analyzed for their characteristics and changes.

Studies on the development of animal tissues and organs have shown that fat deposition occurs later than muscle deposition, and fat deposition is rapid after the turning point in animal growth [14]. Our previous results showed that the Liangshan pig growth turning point was 193.4 days at 62.5 kg [6]. In the present study, mar bling score and IMF content increased rapidly with weight gain. As Liangshan pigs' weight increased, the shear force of the longissimus dorsi muscle rapidly increased, which may be due to the gradual growth of the muscle fi ber diameter and an increase in muscle connective tissue content [15]. Drip loss decreased as slaughter weight increased. The effect of weight on drip loss is consistent with the findings of other reports [13,16].

Amino acids are basic units that make up proteins required by animals [17]. EAAs must be o btained directly from food, which is extremely important for maintaining the body's nitrogen balance and health [18]. The total amount of amino acids in the longissimus dorsi muscle of Liangshan pigs at different weights remained relatively stable, but EAA content showed an upward trend. Amino acid composition is also related to the taste of meat. Amino acids are normally divided into sweet amino acids, bitter amino acids, and umami amino acids [19,20]. The sweet and bitter amino acid contents of Liangshan pigs were relatively sta ble at different bodyweights, but umami amino acid content gradually decreased. Approximately 30% of umami amino acids were lost by the seventh stage compared to the first stage.

Amino acids are also divided into neutral amino acids, basic amino acids, and acidic amino acids [21]. The acidity and basicity of amino acids are usually determined according to the num ber of car boxyl groups and amino groups. Amino acids with more car boxyl groups than amino groups per molecule are termed 'acidic' (Asp and Glu) [22], otherwise they are termed 'basic' (Arg, Lys and His) [23]. Interestingly, as the weight of Liangshan pigs increased in this study, basic and acidic amino acid contents decreased, while the ratio of basic to acidic amino acids increased. This may be a reason for the increase in Liangshan pig meat sample pH as weight increased.

As bodyweight increased, the total fatty acid content of Liangshan pig meat samples showed an upward trend, which was consistent with intramuscular fat content and mar bling score. Dietary fatty acids are closely related to cardiovascular health, and higher SFA content in meat products has been shown to affect cholesterol metabolism [24]. PUFAs possess many physiological functions [25], such as maintaining biofilm structures, treating cardiovascular diseases [26], anti-inflammation [27], and the promotion of brain development [28]. It is worth noting that as the weight of Liangshan pigs increased, SFA content showed an upward trend, while the changes of PUFA were symmetrical with SFA. Further analysis revealed that n6:n3 values in Liangshan pig meat samples showed a rising trend of volatility.

Among the 54 indicators measured in this study, 10 indicators changed by more than 50%. Among these indicators, three were of meat quality traits, four were amino acids, and three were fatty acids. Correlation analysis showed that as intramuscular fat was deposited, C18:0 and Asp content increased rapidly, while C22:6 content decreased rapidly. Although saturated fatty acids are associated with a higher risk of cardiovascular disease, C18:0 does not lead to an increase in blood cholesterol [24]. Asp is an umami amino acid, and an increase in Asp can improve the taste of pork [29]. Further factor analysis shows that, in the fourth to seventh stages, the comprehensive score was higher, which is consistent with the factor analysis results based on meat quality traits. A similar pattern was also found in other pig breeds [16].

5. Conclusions

The current results show that differences in meat quality, amino acid composition, and fatty acid composition are present in Liangshan pigs at different slaughter weights. As bodyweight increased, mar bling score, intramuscular fat, shear force, Met, Asp, Asn, C18:0, and C20:2 content increased, and drip loss, Trp and C22:6 content decreased. The comprehensive factor score first increased and then decrease with weight gain within 74.9–91.5 kg of bodyweight. When slaughtering between 74.9 and 80.4 kg, the meat quality of Liangshan pigs is the best. Slaughtering between 74.5 and 80.4 kg provides the best meat quality in Liangshan pigs. In addition, when slaughtered at 80.4 kg, pork had the highest sweet amino acid content and the lowest n6:n3 ratio. Therefore, considering the meat quality, amino acid composition and fatty acid composition, the suitable slaughter weight of Liangshan pigs is 74.9–80.4 kg. This study provides effective data for the genetic improvement and specialty food processing of Liangshan pigs and provides new insights and references for research into local high incidences of disease.

Supplementary Materials: The following are available online at http://www.mdpi.com/2076-2615/10/5/822/s1, Table S1: Ingredients of the basal experiment diets.

Author Contributions: Conceptualization: M.G., L.Z. and X.L.; Data curation: L.S. and L.C.; Funding acquisition: D.J., Q.L. and Y.J.; Methodology: Y.C. and G.G.; Project administration: L.C.; Supervision: X.X. and Y.L.; Validation: M.G. and S.Z.; Writing—original draft: M.G.; Writing—review & editing: L.S. and L.Z. All authors have read and agreed to the published version of the manuscript.

Funding: This study was supported by the National Natural Science Foundation of China (No. 31972524; No. 31530073), the Sichuan Science and Technology Support Program (No. 2016NYZ0050; No. SCCXTD-009SCSZTD-3-008), the earmarked fund for China Agriculture Research System (No. CARS-36-05 B).

Conflicts of Interest: The authors declare no conflict of interest. The funders had no role in the design of the study; in the collection, analyses, or interpretation of data; in the writing of the manuscript, or in the decision to publish the results.

References

1. Gan, M.; Shen, L.; Fan, Y.; Guo, Z.; Liu, B.; Chen, L.; Tang, G.; Jiang, Y.; Li, X.; Zhang, S.; et al. High altitude adaptability and meat quality in tibetan pigs: A reference for local pork processing and genetic improvement. *Animals* **2019**, *9*, 1080. [CrossRef] [PubMed]

2. Quan, J.; Gao, C.; Cai, Y.; Ge, Q.; Jiao, T.; Zhao, S. Population genetics assessment model reveals priority protection of genetic resources in native pig breeds in china. *Glob. Ecol. Conserv.* **2020**, *21*, e00829. [CrossRef]

3. Keenan, D.F. Pork meat quality, production and processing on. In *Encyclopedia of Food and Health*; Caballero, B., Finglas, P.M., Toldrá, F., Eds.; Academic Press: Oxford, UK, 2016; pp. 419–431.

4. Lebret, B.; Ecolan, P.; Bonhomme, N.; Méteau, K.; Prunier, A. Influence of production system in local and conventional pig breeds on stress indicators at slaughter, muscle and meat traits and pork eating quality. *Animal* **2015**, *9*, 1404–1413. [CrossRef] [PubMed]

5. Halimani, T.E.; Muchadeyi, F.C.; Chimonyo, M.; Dzama, K. Pig genetic resource conservation: The southern African perspective. *Ecol. Econ.* **2010**, *69*, 944–951. [CrossRef]

6. Luo, J.; Lei, H.; Shen, L.; Yang, R.; Pu, Q.; Zhu, K.; Li, M.; Tang, G.; Li, X.; Zhang, S.; et al. Estimation of growth curves and suitable slaughter weight of the liangshan pig. *Asian Australas. J. Anim. Sci.* **2015**, *28*, 1252–1258. [CrossRef]

7. Xiao, R.-J.; Xu, Z.-R.; Chen, H.-L. Effects of ractopamine at different dietary protein levels on growth performance and carcass characteristics in finishing pigs. *Anim. Feed Sci. Techmol.* **1999**, *79*, 119–127. [CrossRef]

8. Alonso, V.; Campo, M.D.M.; Español, S.; Roncalés, P.; Beltrán, J.A. Effect of crossbreeding and gender on meat quality and fatty acid composition in pork. *Meat Sci.* **2009**, *81*, 209–217. [CrossRef]

9. Cheng, C.; Liu, Z.; Zhou, Y.; Wei, H.; Zhang, X.; Xia, M.; Deng, Z.; Zou, Y.; Jiang, S.; Peng, J. Effect of oregano essential oil supplementation to a reduced-protein, amino acid-supplemented diet on meat quality, fatty acid composition, and oxidative stability of longissimus thoracis muscle in growing-finishing pigs. *Meat Sci.* **2017**, *133*, 103. [CrossRef]

10. Biermann, A.D.M.; Pimentel, E.C.G.; Tietze, M.; Pinent, T.; König, S. Implementation of genetic evaluation and mating designs for the endangered local pig breed 'bunte bentheimer'. *J. Anim. Breed. Genet.* **2014**, *131*, 36–45. [CrossRef]

11. Labroue, F.; Luquet, M.; Guillouet, P.; Bussiere, J.F.; Glodek, P.; Wemheuer, W.; Gandini, G.; Pizzi, F.; Delgado, J.V.; Poto, A. Gene banks for European endangered breeds of pigs. The situation in France, Germany, Italy and Spain. *Journées de la Recherche Porcine en France* **2000**, *32*, 419–427.

12. Čandek-Potokar, M.; Žlender, B.; Lefaucheur, L.; Bonneau, M. Effects of age and/or weight at slaughter on longissimus dorsi muscle: Biochemical traits and sensory quality in pigs. *Meat Sci.* **1998**, *48*, 287–300. [CrossRef]

13. Lo Fiego, D.P.; Macchioni, P.; Minelli, G.; Santoro, P. Lipid composition of covering and intramuscular fat in pigs at different slaughter age. *Ital. J. Anim. Sci.* **2010**, *9*, 200–205. [CrossRef]

14. Hocquette, J.-F.; Gondret, F.; Baeza, E.; Médale, F.; Jurie, C.; Pethick, D. Intramuscular fat content in meat-producing animals: Development, genetic and nutritional control, and identification of putative markers. *Anim. Int. J. Anim. Biosci.* **2010**, *4*, 303–319. [CrossRef] [PubMed]

15. Purslow, P.P. Contribution of collagen and connective tissue to cooked meat toughness; some paradigms reviewed. *Meat Sci.* **2018**, *144*, 127–134. [CrossRef] [PubMed]

16. Virgili, R.; Degni, M.; Schivazappa, C.; Faeti, V.; Poletti, E.; Marchetto, G.; Pacchioli, M.T.; Mordenti, A. Effect of age at slaughter on carcass traits and meat quality of italian heavy pigs. *J. Anim. Sci.* **2003**, *81*, 2448–2456. [CrossRef]

17. Vieillevoye, S.; Poortmans, J.R.; Carpentier, A. Effects of essential amino acids supplementation on muscle damage following a heavy-load eccentric training session. *Sci. Sports* **2019**, in press. [CrossRef]

18. Wang, Z.Y.; Duan, Y.H.; Li, F.N.; Yang, B.C.; Zhang, J.X.; Hou, S.Z. Dietary supplementation with lonicera macranthoides leaf powder enhances growth performance and muscle growth of Chinese tibetan pigs. *Livest. Sci.* **2017**, *206*, 1–8. [CrossRef]

19. Gao, X.; Zhang, J.; Regenstein, J.M.; Yin, Y.; Zhou, C. Characterization of taste and aroma compounds in tianyou, a traditional fermented wheat flour condiment. *Food Res. Int.* **2018**, *106*, 156–163. [CrossRef]

20. Chen, Z.-Y.; Feng, Y.-Z.; Cui, C.; Zhao, H.-F.; Zhao, M.-M. Effects of koji-making with mixed strains on physicochemical and sensory properties of chinese-type soy sauce. *J. Sci. Food Agric.* **2015**, *95*, 2145–2154. [CrossRef]

21. Absalan, G.; Akhond, M.; Sheikhian, L. Partitioning of acidic, basic and neutral amino acids into imidazolium-based ionic liquids. *Amino Acids* **2010**, *39*, 167–174. [CrossRef]

22. Tabuchi, N.; Akasaki, K.; Tsuji, H. Two acidic amino acid residues, asp (470) and glu (471), contained in the carboxyl cytoplasmic tail of a major lysosomal membrane protein, lgp85/limp ii, are important for its accumulation in secondary lysosomes. *Biochem. Biophys. Res. Commun.* **2000**, *270*, 557–563. [CrossRef] [PubMed]

23. Sakagami, H.; Yokote, Y.; Kochi, M.; Hara, E.I.; Akahane, K. Amino acid utilization during apoptosis in hl-60 cells. *Anticancer Res.* **1999**, *19*, 329–332. [PubMed]

24. Mensink, R.P. Fatty acids: Health effects of saturated fatty acids. In *Encyclopedia of Human Nutrition*; Allen, L.H., Prentice, A., Caballero, B., Eds.; Academic Press: Cambridge, MA, USA, 2013; pp. 215–219.

25. Tapiero, H.; Ba, G.N.; Couvreur, P.; Tew, K.D. Polyunsaturated fatty acids (pufa) and eicosanoids in human health and pathologies. *Biomed. Pharmacother.* **2002**, *56*, 215–222. [CrossRef]

26. Chang, J.P.-C.; Chang, S.-S.; Yang, H.-T.; Palani, M.; Chen, C.-P.; Su, K.-P. Polyunsaturated fatty acids (pufas) levels in patients with cardiovascular diseases (cvds) with and without depression. *Brain Behav. Immun.* **2015**, *44*, 28–31. [CrossRef]

27. de Bus, I.; Witkamp, R.; Zuilhof, H.; Albada, B.; Balvers, M. The role of n-3 pufa-derived fatty acid derivatives and their oxygenated metabolites in the modulation of inflammation. *Prostaglandins Other Lipid Mediat.* **2019**, *144*, 106351. [CrossRef]

28. Joffre, C.; Grégoire, S.; De Smedt, V.; Acar, N.; Bretillon, L.; Nadjar, A.; Layé, S. Modulation of brain pufa content in different experimental models of mice. *Prostaglandins Leukot. Essent. Fat. Acids* **2016**, *114*, 1–10. [CrossRef]

29. Moya, V.J.; Flores, M.; Aristoy, M.C.; Toldrá, F. Pork meat quality affects peptide and amino acid profiles during the ageing process. *Meat Sci.* **2001**, *58*, 197–206. [CrossRef]

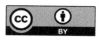

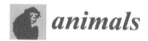

Article

Portuguese Local Pig Breeds: Genotype Effects on Meat and Fat Quality Traits

José Manuel Martins [1,*], **Rita Fialho** [2], **André Albuquerque** [2], **José Neves** [1], **Amadeu Freitas** [1], **José Tirapicos Nunes** [3] and **Rui Charneca** [3]

[1] MED—Mediterranean Institute for Agriculture, Environment and Development & Departamento de Zootecnia, Escola de Ciências e Tecnologia, Universidade de Évora, 7006-554 Évora, Portugal; jneves@uevora.pt (J.N.); aagbf@uevora.pt (A.F.)
[2] MED—Mediterranean Institute for Agriculture, Environment and Development, Universidade de Évora, 7006-554 Évora, Portugal; a.ritafialho@gmail.com (R.F.); andrealb@uevora.pt (A.A.)
[3] MED—Mediterranean Institute for Agriculture, Environment and Development & Departamento de Medicina Veterinária, Escola de Ciências e Tecnologia, Universidade de Évora, 7006-554 Évora, Portugal; jnunes@uevora.pt (J.T.N.); rmcc@uevora.pt (R.C.)
* Correspondence: jmartins@uevora.pt; Tel.: +351-266-760-817

Received: 19 March 2020; Accepted: 19 May 2020; Published: 22 May 2020

Simple Summary: Local breeds are generally associated with slower growth rates, higher slaughter weights, and fatter carcasses due to genetic and rearing system characteristics. When compared to intensive pig production systems, those based on European local breeds generally provide a more favourable response to the required increase in the production of high-quality pork and pork products in sustainable chains, meeting consumer demands. Reducing costs and improving the economic viability of production systems while preserving the quality of the products obtained is of vital importance. In this work, we propose that Portuguese local pig production chains could improve their performance and productivity without compromising the quality of the final product by crossing local breeds instead of crossing with modern breeds. This could help to maintain or increase local breed populations, supporting conservation of animal biodiversity.

Abstract: This work investigated the contribution of cross-breeding between two local Portuguese pig breeds to the conservation of animal biodiversity and income of local pig producers. Quality traits of semimembranosus (SM), gluteus medius (GM) and dorsal subcutaneous fat (DSF) were studied in Alentejano (AL), Bísaro (BI), AL × BI, and BI × AL (Ribatejano—RI) castrated male pigs. Pigs were reared outdoors, fed ad libitum, and slaughtered at ~65 (trial 1) and 150 kg BW (trial 2). In trial 1, AL pigs showed higher SM intramuscular fat, lower total collagen, and higher soluble collagen than BI pigs, while AL × BI and BI × AL pigs showed intermediate (NS) values. AL, AL × BI, and BI × AL pigs showed higher SM myoglobin content, and AL a more intense red colour than BI pigs. Finally, AL, AL × BI, and BI × AL showed higher total lipids in DSF than BI pigs. In trial 2, SM and DSF results were similar to those obtained in trial 1. In GM, AL and BI × AL showed higher intramuscular fat than BI and AL × BI pigs, while AL, AL × BI and BI × AL showed lower total collagen content than BI pigs. In conclusion, these results suggest that RI crosses are a productive alternative, with overall muscle and DSF traits statistically not different between AL × BI and BI × AL, and similar to those observed in AL pigs.

Keywords: swine; Alentejano; Bísaro; Ribatejano; meat quality; dorsal subcutaneous fat

1. Introduction

The increasing demand for pork products is leading to an international effort to save traditional pig breeds and develop new breeds [1]. In Portugal, the main local pig breeds are the Alentejano (AL), an Iberian type breed [2] with an extreme genetic closeness to the Iberian pig [3], and the Bísaro (BI) pig, from the Celtic type [2]. The AL pig is characterised by a low growth rate (except under "montanheira" regime) and precociously high adipogenic activity [4]. The BI pig presents a poor growth (although higher than AL), little backfat (although higher than that of industrial genotypes), and a high proportion of skin and bone [5]. These environmentally well-adapted local breeds are less productive than modern improved genotypes, and their production chains depend mainly on the marketing of meat, and fermented and dry-cured meat products with highly valued sensory characteristics [5–7]. Almost extinct in the 1980s [5,8], these two breeds and their traditional systems have recovered since the 1990s [6], driven by consumer concerns about animal welfare, sustainable production, and meat and meat product quality issues. Although still threatened (AL) and rare (BI) breeds [9], they currently have a high ecological, economic and social importance in their production regions [6,10,11]. Increased yields and reduced costs on these productive systems is a continuous challenge, and crossbreeding is one way of achieving it.

AL and BI breeds homelands, in the South and North of Portugal respectively [8], have contact zones in the Tagus River region. In these contact zones (e.g., Ribatejo region), crosses between the two breeds were common until the 1950s [12] and the meat and meat products obtained were highly appreciated. However, there are no data available regarding these crosses, popularly called Ribatejano (RI) pigs. This study, included in the TREASURE project dedicated to European local pig breeds, was the first to collect and analyse carcass, pork and fat data from crossbred RI pigs, using AL and BI pure animals as controls. It represents a potential new management strategy for these breeds' production chains, while attending to societal demands for environment preservation, sustainable local agro-economy, as well as to consumers demands for quality and healthiness on regional pork products. The recovery and commercial use of these crosses could also help to preserve the pure breed populations, maintaining animal biodiversity, essential for an efficient and sustainable world food production and to meet the different needs of modern human societies [13]. In fact, loss of biodiversity may lead to an impaired response to changing environments.

Following a previous work where growth, carcass traits and loin data were presented [14], this study evaluates meat and fat quality from AL, BI, and AL × BI and BI × AL (RI crosses) pigs, reared outdoors, fed ad libitum, and slaughtered at ~65 and 150 kg BW. Physicochemical traits of semimembranosus (SM), gluteus medius (GM), and dorsal subcutaneous fat (DSF) were determined.

2. Materials and Methods

2.1. Animals and Experimental Design

Experimental procedures and animal care were performed in compliance with the ethical guidelines and regulations of the Portuguese Animal Nutrition and Welfare Commission (DGAV—Directorate-General for Food and Veterinary, Portugal), following the 2010/63/EU Directive.

Composed by two sequential trials, this work had four experimental groups, with pure Alentejano (AL) and Bísaro (BI) pigs and their reciprocal crosses, AL × BI and BI × AL (Ribatejano (RI) pigs, the common name of these crossbred). Male pigs (n = 20 for each of the 4 genotypes) surgically castrated within the 1st week of age were reared outdoors from 28.6 ± 0.5 kg BW (mean ± SEM) until ~65 kg (trial 1) and from 65.2 ± 0.4 kg to ~150 kg (trial 2). In trial 1, pigs were group-fed with commercial diets (15.5–16.6 g/100 g crude protein, 12.4–12.7 g/100 g NDF, 4.5–5 g/100 g total lipids and 14.1–14.3 MJ/kg DE—Supplementary Table S1) at estimated ad libitum consumption [15], in a single daily meal (09:00 h). In trial 2, pigs were individually fed with commercial diets (15.4–16.6 g/100 g crude protein, 12.4–12.9 g/100 g NDF, 4.7–5 g/100 g total lipids and 14.1–14.3 MJ/kg DE—Table S1) and diet refusals were measured daily. All animals had free access to water and were weighed every fortnight.

Temperature and relative humidity data were registered throughout the experimental work. Average temperature, average minimal and maximal temperature, and average relative humidity were, respectively, 11.2, 6.5, 17.4 °C, and 75.0% in trial 1 (January–April), and 21.9, 13.7, 31.1 °C, and 56.3% in trial 2 (April–October).

Slaughtered at a commercial slaughterhouse in three batches per slaughter weight, animals had free access to water but were fasted for ~16 h during lairage. Ten animals from each genotype were slaughtered at the end of trial 1 (average BW of 64.2 ± 0.3 kg) and nine animals at the end of trial 2 (average of 150.6 ± 0.9 kg BW) by exsanguination following CO_2 stunning. Commercially reared local pigs are slaughtered at lighter weights for consumption as fresh meat or roasted pigs, or at heavier weights for the production of high quality traditional fermented and cured products [6,16] with PDO or PGI European certification.

2.2. Muscle and Adipose Tissue Sampling

Samples of SM muscle and of DSF were obtained from the left half carcasses at ~65 and 150 kg BW, while samples of GM muscle were collected only at ~150 kg. Samples were vacuum packaged and frozen (−20 °C) until analysis.

2.3. Muscles and Adipose Tissue Analyses

Leg (SM and GM) muscles represent a cut of greatest economic value and mass. Muscles ultimate pH (pH_u) was determined 24 h post-mortem by a pH-meter with a puncture electrode (LoT406-M6-DXK-S7/25, Mettler-Toledo GmbH, Germany).

Moisture was determined in muscles and DSF according to ISO-1442 [17]. Total nitrogen from muscle samples was determined in a Leco FP-528 (Leco Corp., St. Joseph, MI, USA) by the Dumas combustion method (method 992.15) and from DSF samples by the Kjeldahl method (method 928.08) [18]. Total protein content was estimated as total nitrogen × 6.25. Total lipids were determined in muscles according to Folch, et al. [19] and in DSF by Soxhlet extraction (method 991.36) [18]. Muscles myoglobin and total collagen were determined as previously described [20] and soluble collagen according to Hill [21].

Surface colour measurements [22] of raw SM and GM samples were recorded with a CR-400 colorimeter (Konica Minolta Sensing Europe B.V., Nieuwegein, Netherlands) with a D65 illuminant, after blooming for 30 min. Individual CIE (Commission Internationale de l'Éclairage) L^* (lightness), a^* (redness) and b^* (yellowness) values were averaged out of six random readings across muscle surface. The same procedure (without blooming) was applied to DSF samples. Chroma $\left(C^* = \sqrt{a^{*2} + b^{*2}}\right)$, hue angle $\left(H = tan^{-1}(b^*/a^*)\right)$, and saturation (C^*/L^*) were calculated.

2.4. Statistical Analysis

All data were tested for normality by the Shapiro-Wilk test. Results are presented as mean ± rSD. Data were analysed by one-way analysis of variance (ANOVA) with SPSS Statistics software (IBM SPSS Statistics for Windows, v24.0, IBM Corp., Armonk, NY, USA). Mean differences were considered statistically significant when $p < 0.05$, and p values between 0.05 and 0.10 were considered trends.

3. Results

3.1. Trial 1: Pigs Slaughtered at ~65 kg BW

Pigs were slaughtered at an average age of 186.2 ± 2.9 days.

3.1.1. Muscle Tissue Analyses

SM physico-chemical data were affected by genotype (Table 1). Moisture was lower ($p < 0.05$) in AL and AL × BI than in BI pigs, while total intramuscular fat (IMF) was higher ($p < 0.05$) in AL than in

BI pigs. Myoglobin content was higher ($p < 0.01$) in AL pigs and Ribatejano (RI) crosses than in BI pigs, whereas total collagen was lower ($p < 0.05$) in AL than in BI pigs, with their crosses showing intermediate values. Regarding soluble collagen, as a % of total collagen, values were higher ($p < 0.05$) in SM from AL than BI pigs. SM pH_u values were not affected by genotype, but significant differences were observed in colour parameters (Table 1). Lightness (L^*) was lower and redness (a^*) higher ($p < 0.05$) on AL than BI pigs, again with their crosses showing intermediate values. These results affected hue angle (H°) and saturation, respectively lower ($p < 0.01$) and higher ($p < 0.05$) in AL than BI pigs (Table 1).

Table 1. Chemical composition, pH, and CIE colour values of *Semimembranosus* muscle from Alentejano (AL), Bísaro (BI), AL × BI and BI × AL pigs slaughtered at ~65 kg BW ($n = 10$ for each genotype).

Traits	AL	BI	AL × BI	BI × AL	rSD	*p*-Values
Moisture (g/100 g)	71.8 [b]	74.0 [a]	72.2 [b]	72.8 [a,b]	1.9	0.049
Total protein (g/100 g)	23.8	22.8	23.3	23.2	1.1	0.272
Total intramuscular fat (g/100 g)	5.9 [a]	4.7 [b]	5.3 [a,b]	5.2 [a,b]	1.0	0.040
Myoglobin content (mg/g)	0.42 [a]	0.18 [b]	0.40 [a]	0.33 [a]	0.13	0.002
Total collagen (mg/g DM)	15.7 [b]	19.0 [a]	17.2 [a,b]	17.7 [a,b]	1.9	0.010
Soluble collagen (% total collagen)	11.5 [a]	9.2 [b]	10.0 [a,b]	10.0 [a,b]	2.1	0.044
pH (24 h *post-mortem*)	5.42	5.52	5.48	5.50	0.14	0.468
Lightness (Cie L^*)	43.0 [b]	46.6 [a]	45.1 [a,b]	44.8 [a,b]	2.9	0.043
Redness (Cie a^*)	13.5 [a]	11.7 [b]	12.1 [a,b]	13.1 [a,b]	1.5	0.049
Yellowness (Cie b^*)	6.6	7.1	6.8	7.0	0.8	0.568
Chroma (C^*)	15.1	13.8	13.9	14.8	1.6	0.214
Hue angle (H°)	26.3 [c]	31.4 [a]	29.5 [a,b]	28.3 [b,c]	2.8	0.004
Saturation	0.36 [a]	0.30 [b]	0.31 [a,b]	0.33 [a,b]	0.05	0.046

CIE—Commission Internationale de l'Éclairage. AL × BI and BI × AL represent the reciprocal crosses of the commonly known Ribatejano pig. DM—Dry matter. [a,b,c] Values in the same row with different superscript letters are significantly different ($p < 0.05$).

3.1.2. Adipose Tissue Analyses

Chemical composition of DSF was also affected by genotype (Table 2). Moisture content was lower ($p < 0.001$) in AL than in BI pigs, with RI crosses showing intermediate values. Total lipids, inversely related to moisture content, were higher ($p < 0.001$) in AL and RI crosses than in BI pigs (Table 2).

Table 2. Chemical composition, and CIE colour values of dorsal subcutaneous fat from Alentejano (AL), Bísaro (BI), AL × BI and BI × AL pigs slaughtered at ~65 kg BW ($n = 10$ for each genotype).

Traits	AL	BI	AL × BI	BI × AL	rSD	*p*-Values
Moisture (g/100 g)	7.3 [c]	11.0 [a]	8.5 [b,c]	9.0 [b]	1.4	<0.001
Total protein (g/100 g)	1.42	1.59	1.42	1.48	0.32	0.811
Total lipids (g/100 g)	85.0 [a]	71.5 [b]	81.4 [a]	81.6 [a]	4.6	<0.001
Lightness (Cie L^*)	82.3	80.7	81.1	80.6	2.5	0.459
Redness (Cie a^*)	2.91	3.50	3.18	3.29	0.6	0.257
Yellowness (Cie b^*)	4.84	5.17	4.92	4.97	1.1	0.937
Chroma (C^*)	5.7	6.2	5.9	6.0	1.2	0.788
Hue angle (H°)	58.3	55.9	56.7	56.4	4.3	0.551
Saturation	0.07	0.08	0.07	0.07	0.01	0.590

AL × BI and BI × AL represent the reciprocal crosses of the commonly known Ribatejano pig. [a,b,c] Values in the same row with different superscript letters are significantly different ($p < 0.05$).

3.2. Trial 2: Pigs Slaughtered at ~150 kg BW

Pigs were slaughtered at an average age of 353.6 ± 2.6 days.

3.2.1. Muscle Tissues Analyses

Physicochemical data from SM samples were less affected by genotype in the fattening period. IMF was higher in AL and BI × AL than in BI pigs, but this difference did not attain statistical significance (Table 3). Total collagen was lower ($p < 0.05$) in AL pigs and RI crosses than in BI pigs, with soluble collagen (% total collagen) following the opposite trend without attaining statistical difference. SM pH_u was higher ($p < 0.05$) in AL than in BI pigs (Table 3). Regarding colour, genotype only tended to affect lightness (L^*) ($p = 0.067$) and yellowness (b^*) ($p = 0.059$) values, and therefore hue angle (H°) ($p < 0.05$) was lower in AL and AL × BI than in BI pigs (Table 3).

Table 3. Chemical composition, pH, and CIE colour values of *Semimembranosus* muscle from Alentejano (AL), Bísaro (BI), AL × BI and BI × AL pigs slaughtered at ~150 kg BW (*n* = 9 for each genotype).

Traits	AL	BI	AL × BI	BI × AL	rSD	*p*-Values
Moisture (g/100 g)	73.7	73.7	73.6	73.5	0.9	0.968
Total protein (g/100 g)	22.4	22.8	22.7	22.3	0.7	0.410
Total intramuscular fat (g/100 g)	5.0	4.5	4.6	5.1	0.7	0.326
Myoglobin content (mg/g)	1.93	1.75	1.82	1.80	0.36	0.786
Total collagen (mg/g DM)	15.5 [b]	20.7 [a]	17.1 [b]	17.0 [b]	3.5	0.029
Soluble collagen (% total collagen)	8.2	6.8	7.4	7.8	2.1	0.518
pH (24 h *post-mortem*)	5.76 [a]	5.51 [b]	5.67 [a,b]	5.66 [a,b]	0.16	0.027
pH fall (45min to 24 h)	0.55	0.65	0.65	0.56	0.29	0.833
Lightness (Cie *L**)	35.4	38.4	35.0	35.6	2.7	0.067
Redness (Cie *a**)	14.5	14.3	14.0	15.0	1.3	0.434
Yellowness (Cie *b**)	6.7	8.0	6.5	8.0	1.4	0.059
Chroma (C*)	16.0	16.5	15.5	17.0	1.6	0.241
Hue angle (H°)	24.6 [b]	29.1 [a]	24.5 [b]	27.8 [a,b]	3.8	0.039
Saturation	0.46	0.43	0.44	0.48	0.04	0.102

AL × BI and BI × AL represent the reciprocal crosses of the commonly known Ribatejano pig. [a,b] Values in the same row with different superscript letters are significantly different ($p < 0.05$).

IMF from GM muscle was higher ($p < 0.01$) in AL and BI × AL than in BI and AL × BI pigs, while total collagen was lower ($p < 0.01$) in AL pigs and RI crosses than in BI pigs. However, soluble collagen (% total collagen) and colour parameters of GM were not affected by genotype (Table 4).

Table 4. Chemical composition, pH, and CIE colour values of *Gluteus medius* muscle from Alentejano (AL), Bísaro (BI), AL × BI and BI × AL pigs slaughtered at ~150 kg BW (*n* = 9 for each genotype).

Traits	AL	BI	AL × BI	BI × AL	rSD	*p*-Values
Moisture (g/100 g)	69.9	70.6	70.2	69.9	1.2	0.529
Total protein (g/100 g)	21.7	22.4	22.2	21.8	1.3	0.580
Total intramuscular fat (g/100 g)	9.0 [a]	6.2 [b]	7.0 [b]	8.7 [a]	1.6	0.002
Myoglobin content (mg/g)	1.63	1.34	1.38	1.56	0.32	0.205
Total collagen (mg/g DM)	15.2 [b]	17.9 [a]	15.7 [b]	15.3 [b]	1.4	0.002
Soluble collagen (% total collagen)	8.5	8.8	8.7	8.6	1.6	0.982
pH (24 h *post-mortem*)	5.62	5.58	5.65	5.61	0.14	0.748
pH fall (45min to 24 h)	0.95	0.89	0.72	0.87	0.28	0.274
Lightness (Cie *L**)	39.2	40.3	38.7	39.5	2.9	0.702
Redness (Cie *a**)	12.3	12.2	11.8	13.0	1.5	0.344
Yellowness (Cie *b**)	5.5	5.8	5.4	6.5	1.4	0.387
Chroma (C*)	13.4	13.6	13.0	14.6	1.8	0.333
Hue angle (H°)	23.9	25.1	24.3	25.9	3.4	0.807
Saturation	0.34	0.33	0.33	0.36	0.04	0.329

AL × BI and BI × AL represent the reciprocal crosses of the commonly known Ribatejano pig. [a,b] Values in the same row with different superscript letters are significantly different ($p < 0.05$).

3.2.2. Adipose Tissue Analyses

Chemical data from DSF were affected by genotype, with total protein lower ($p < 0.001$) in AL pigs and RI crosses than in BI pigs, and total lipids higher ($p < 0.05$) in AL than in BI and AL × BI pigs (Table 5). Finally, DSF colour parameters were also influenced by genotype. Redness (*a**), chroma (C*), and saturation were lower ($p < 0.05$) in AL than in BI pigs, while hue angle (H°) was higher ($p = 0.05$), with RI crosses showing intermediate values.

Table 5. Chemical composition and CIE colour values of dorsal subcutaneous fat from Alentejano (AL), Bísaro (BI), AL × BI and BI × AL pigs slaughtered at ~150 kg BW (*n* = 9 for each genotype).

Traits	AL	BI	AL × BI	BI × AL	rSD	*p*-Values
Moisture (g/100 g)	5.1	5.8	5.6	5.4	0.9	0.519
Total protein (g/100 g)	0.91 [b]	1.29 [a]	0.98 [b]	0.94 [b]	0.14	<0.001
Total lipids (g/100 g)	88.9 [a]	83.7 [c]	85.5 [b,c]	87.1 [a,b]	3.3	0.012
Lightness (Cie *L**)	79.3	79.1	79.5	78.8	1.1	0.495
Redness (Cie *a**)	2.25 [b]	3.36 [a]	2.70 [a,b]	2.70 [a,b]	0.9	0.042
Yellowness (Cie *b**)	4.47	4.91	4.36	4.69	0.6	0.291
Chroma (C*)	5.0 [b]	6.0 [a]	5.2 [a,b]	5.5 [ab]	0.9	0.048
Hue angle (H°)	63.3 [a]	56.4 [b]	59.0 [a,b]	60.7 [a,b]	6.2	0.049
Saturation	0.06 [b]	0.08 [a]	0.07 [a,b]	0.07 [a,b]	0.01	0.050

AL × BI and BI × AL represent the reciprocal crosses of the commonly known Ribatejano pig. [a,b,c] Values in the same row with different superscript letters are significantly different ($p < 0.05$).

4. Discussion

Sustainability and animal welfare policies are increasingly being adopted by the food industry in response to consumer demands. These changes can help strengthen pork niche markets and broaden the target audience for small farmers practicing outdoor swine production [23]. However, farmers and researchers must find a way to improve productivity and product quality, and scientifically support product differentiation [23,24]. One way to improve the performance of outdoor finishing pigs is through crossbreeding. AL and (mainly) BI genotypes are not sufficiently studied, namely in the case of muscles other than longissimus lumborum. In addition, currently available information was obtained in trials with very different or not even described rearing and feeding conditions, as well as age/slaughter weights, among other aspects. Therefore, additional studies are required to evaluate different production stages, in controlled experimental environments.

In order to evaluate meat and fat quality from AL and BI pigs, as well as their reciprocal crosses reared outdoors and fed ad libitum with commercial diets, animals were slaughtered at ~65 and 150 kg BW.

4.1. Trial 1: Pigs Slaughtered at ~65 kg BW

Growth and carcass data from this trial were previously presented and discussed by Martins et al. [14]. Briefly, AL pigs had a shorter carcass length and lower bone cuts weight than BI, while Ribatejano (RI) crosses showed intermediate values. AL pigs also showed low lean and high fat cuts proportions, while in BI pigs lean cut proportions were more important. This agrees with the presence in both genotypes of the LEPR c.1987T allele, usually associated with higher fatness, that is almost fixed in the fatty AL when compared to the leaner BI pig breed (0.98 vs. 0.26 frequencies, respectively) [3]. The lower lean and higher fat cuts of the carcasses from AL pigs led to a 12.1% lower commercial yield and 44.7% higher fat cuts proportion than those observed for BI. These differences were due to changes in untrimmed shoulder (−9.7%), loin (−15.8%) and untrimmed ham (−13.7%), and in belly (+24.4%) and backfat (+89.5%) cuts. Meanwhile, although RI crosses showed overall intermediate values, their fat cuts proportions were not significantly different from those of BI pigs. These differences led to lower lean-to-fat cuts ratio and higher backfat thickness and ZP ("Zwei punkte") fat depth in AL than in BI pigs [14].

Muscle physicochemical traits were affected by genotype. In SM, IMF content was 25.5% higher in AL than in BI pigs, confirming the precociously high adipogenic activity in the AL pig [4]. Strongly influenced by genotype, IMF is positively correlated with the sensory properties, juiciness and palatability of meat [25–27]. Meanwhile, compared to IMF values observed in 100 kg AL pigs fed at 85% ad libitum [20,28], and BI pigs [29], those observed in our trial were slightly higher in AL and similar in BI. The differences in the AL breed results, were probably due to different feeding conditions used in both trials.

Myoglobin content has been suggested as a genotype-related characteristic [30]. In our trial, myoglobin showed higher values in the SM muscle from AL pigs and RI crosses when compared to BI pigs. On the other hand, SM total and soluble collagen were respectively 17.4% lower and 25% higher in AL than BI pigs, with RI crosses showing intermediate values. Collagen proteins are the predominant constituents of skeletal muscle connective tissue network and a contributing factor to meat's texture [27,31]. Likewise, IMF content affects muscle cut resistance, with higher fat corresponding to lower shear force values [27,32]. Therefore, differences observed in IMF and collagen content of SM suggest a more tender meat in growing AL pigs, and tenderness is described as the most important factor for the perceived sensory quality of pork [33]. This trend was also observed in the longissimus lumborum (LL) samples from these animals [14]. Still, total collagen values were higher in SM than in LL, confirming that hindquarter muscles used for locomotion such as biceps femoris, semimembranosus, and semitendinosus, are inherently tougher than support muscles such as longissimus lumborum [27]. Finally, the pH_u values, not affected by genotype, were close to the lower value of the normal range in pork, which varies between 5.5 and 5.8 [34].

Consumer's critical first impression of meat depends mainly on colour, which is in turn largely associated to myoglobin concentration and its chemical form. Other factors, such as the physical state of meat, including pH value, protein state, denaturation degree, and water loss, are also important [30]. SM values for colour coordinates in the literature are scarce and vary widely among breeds (e.g., 36–57, 3–17, and 4–15, for L^*, a^*, and b^*, respectively) [7,20,29,35–37]. Values observed in this trial are within the above-mentioned ranges. In our trial, the SM lowest levels of L^* and H° and the highest levels of a^* and saturation were observed in AL pigs, indicating a darker and redder meat [27]. This agrees with the previously mentioned higher myoglobin content in this genotype. Thus, when compared to BI, AL pigs showed a more intense red SM muscle, as observed in LL [14], which is a distinctive feature for the consumer [38]. The higher L^* values observed in SM samples from BI pigs could be partially associated to a higher muscle water loss in these pigs, already noticed in LL muscle [14]. In fact, the higher amount of muscle free-water provides a more reflective surface for light and is positively correlated to lightness [27,39]. Finally, colour values detected in muscle samples from RI crosses were overall intermediate to those observed in AL and BI genotypes, except for H°, closer to the AL values in BI × AL and to the BI values in AL × BI pigs. The lower H° values observed in BI × AL pigs measure a colour closer to the true red axis and agree with a significantly high content in myoglobin in these pigs. Similar results were previously observed in biceps femoris from Duroc × Iberian pigs, when compared to Iberian × Duroc [40].

DSF chemical composition was also affected by genotype, with AL pigs showing a 33.6% lower moisture and an 18.9% higher total lipids content than BI pigs, confirming precociously high adipogenic activity of AL [4].

4.2. Trial 2: Pigs Slaughtered at ~150 kg BW

Growth and carcass data from this trial were presented and discussed by Martins et al. [14]. Briefly, in the fattening period AL pigs had a lighter bone structure and a more compact body than BI, presenting a shorter carcass, and lower bone cuts proportions. Carcass yields, higher in these older and heavier pigs, increased 1.16, 0.80, 1.17, and 0.97 percentage units for each 10 kg increase in BW from 65 to 150 kg in AL, BI, AL × BI, and BI × AL pigs, respectively. This confirms fat deposition as the main responsible for increasing carcass yield in older pigs [41,42]. AL pigs also showed a higher fat cuts proportion and a higher backfat thickness and ZP fat depth than BI, influencing the lean-to-fat cuts ratio, lower in AL pigs when compared to BI, and with RI crosses showing intermediate values.

SM muscle was only affected by genotype in total collagen content and pH_u parameters. IMF was 11% higher in AL than in BI pigs, however this difference did not attain statistical difference. When compared to BI, SM muscle samples from AL pigs also showed a higher percentage of IMF at 65 than at 150 kg BW (+23.4 and +11.1%, respectively). This was also observed in LL [14], suggesting that AL is an early maturing breed. Total protein values from AL were comparable to those previously reported for 100 kg castrated AL pigs fed at 85% ad libitum [20,28], but IMF values were higher, probably due to different feeding regimes and slaughter weight. Total protein and IMF values from BI pigs from our trial were identical to the ones reported by Carvalho [29].

Although the myoglobin content was 10.3% higher in SM from AL when compared to BI pigs, this difference did not attain statistical significance, contrary to what was observed in trial 1. Meanwhile, myoglobin content increased in all genotypes between 65 and 150 kg BW (186 and 354 days of age), showing that pork gained a more intense colour with age [27], as previously observed in Iberian pigs [43]. On the other hand, SM total collagen content observed in this trial in free-range AL pigs, was higher than the one in 100 kg confined AL pigs [20]. At 150 kg BW, SM total collagen and soluble collagen were also 25.1% lower and 20.6% higher in AL than in BI pigs, respectively. RI crosses also showed lower total collagen values than BI pigs. These differences suggest a higher tenderness of pork from AL pigs and RI crosses. Furthermore, ageing animals show a higher number of stable bonds between collagen molecules, with the corresponding decrease in its solubility [27,43,44], as observed in our pigs slaughtered at 65 and 150 kg. As animals age, meat becomes tougher, mainly due to an increase in the percentage of heat-insoluble collagen bonds [27]. This is a more important factor in local pig breeds than in industrial genotypes, because the former are slaughtered at physiologically older ages.

Ultimate pH (pH_u) of meat influences water-holding capacity, colour, tenderness, flavour and shelf life of meat [45] and therefore, is a main quality determinant [45,46]. The pH_u values observed in SM were within the normal range for pork [34], but were affected by genotype. As already observed in LL [14], pH_u values from SM samples were higher in AL than in BI pigs. This suggests a higher muscle glycogen content in BI pigs, positively correlated to lower pH values [47]. Generally, leaner animals have higher percentages of fast-contracting glycogen-rich type IIb or white fibres [48], with a glycolytic metabolism and higher ATP-ase activity, leading to lower pH_u values than those observed in slow-contracting oxidative type Ia or red fibres [46].

Meat colour, the major visual factor affecting meat quality [27], was influenced in a less expressive way by genotype in SM during fattening than during growth, as previously observed in LL [14]. Genotype only affected H°, which was significantly lower in SM samples from AL and AL × BI pigs. SM muscle from AL and AL × BI pigs also tended to show lower levels of *L** than BI pigs, but *a** values were not significantly different. A lower *L** and H°, as observed in AL and AL × BI pigs, is related to a darker and redder meat surface in terms of real colour perception [27]. Both darkness and redness can be enhanced at higher pH values, as observed in the SM muscle from AL pigs. In these conditions, reducing and oxygen-consuming enzymes are decreasing the percentage of myoglobin in the oxygenated form, and light scattering is minimized because hydrated muscle proteins are not releasing free water [39]. Overall, when comparing the two trials, an increase in age/weight led to a reduction of *L** and an increase of *a** values, generally associated to pork with a darker red colour [27]. This difference in *L** values from the SM muscle of AL and BI pigs was higher than two units in both trials, which could affect consumers preferences and influence the decision to purchase [49].

Chemical characteristics of GM muscle were slightly affected by genotype. IMF content was higher in AL and BI × AL pigs than in BI and AL × BI pigs, and was comparable to that previously observed in 103 kg BW Iberian pigs fed at 90% ad libitum [50]. Although the difference in IMF between AL and

BI was expected, due to the higher adipogenic activity of the former breed [4], IMF values observed in BI × AL, are interesting. In fact, when analysing the IMF values obtained in this trial, BI × AL pigs showed a fat content in both muscles numerically close to the one from AL pigs, suggesting a maternal effect. Since the technological quality of fresh meat and meat products is mainly determined by the lipid fraction, this higher IMF content in the two valuable ham muscles from BI × AL pigs, is very important. Similar results were obtained when comparing IMF content of biceps femoris from hams of Iberian pigs to those of Duroc boars × Iberian dams and of Iberian boars × Duroc dams [51]. Finally, GM total collagen observed in AL pigs and RI crosses was lower than the one in BI pigs. When associated to higher IMF values, as also observed in SM muscle (and in LL muscle—[14]), this suggests a higher tenderness of pork from AL pigs and RI crosses.

DSF chemical composition also varied among genotypes, with AL pigs showing a 29.5% lower total protein and a 6.2% higher total lipids content than BI. Such changes agree with the more adipogenic profile of AL when compared to the leaner BI pig [4,5]. However, histological studies are needed to clarify if the difference in protein content is related to collagen or fat deposition. The latter could be obtained either through an increased adipose cell number in BI pigs and/or by a cell hypertrophy in AL pigs (fewer cells per gram of subcutaneous tissue). When calculating the fat weight deposited in DSF ((DSF weight × % DSF lipids)/100) at 65 and 150 kg BW, the values were 2.88 and 6.31 kg, respectively. Once again, BI × AL pigs showed a total lipids content similar to that of AL, and higher than the one from BI and AL × BI pigs, which is important from a technological point of view. Finally, regarding DSF colour, AL pigs had a 33% lower $a*$ value than BI, which affected $C*$, $H°$, and saturation values. The higher lipid concentration in DSF of AL pigs may have contributed to the dilution of blood vessels in this tissue, leading to lower values of $a*$ and saturation, also observed in 65 kg pigs but without attaining statistical significance. In fact, haemoglobin, the major colour pigment in blood, can also affect tissue colour [27].

5. Conclusions

Data obtained at the growing period showed that Alentejano (AL) is a fatty breed, with lower lean and higher fat cut proportions than Bísaro (BI) [14]. SM muscle from AL pigs showed higher IMF, redder colour, and lower total collagen, features that could positively influence the consumer from a visual and/or an eating quality point of view. Ribatejano (RI) reciprocal crosses (AL × BI and BI × AL) showed overall intermediate features between AL and BI genotypes, but higher lean and lower fat cut proportions and backfat thickness than AL. On the other hand, they showed a SM muscle with a myoglobin content and colour characteristics in line with those observed in AL pigs. This suggests a redder and darker meat than the one from BI pigs, at a slaughter weight generally used for meat production. These features were overall similar in both muscles of pigs slaughtered at the end of the fattening period (~150 kg BW). At this slaughter weight, muscles from RI crosses also had a lower total collagen content, suggesting a darker, redder, and more tender meat for fresh and cured products than the one from BI pigs. Therefore, RI crosses have the potential to be sustainably reared outdoors and to produce high quality meat and fermented or dry-cured products. AL × BI, more easily reared in the north of Portugal (BI dams' homeland), could improve the meat and meat products quality when compared to the ones obtained with pure BI pigs. As to BI × AL, more easily reared in the south (AL dams' homeland), this cross has better commercial yield and primal cuts proportions, when compared to those obtained from pure AL pigs, without compromising meat and meat products quality. Finally, the production of high quality/certified products to attain better market prices can lead producers to increase animal and productivity numbers and therefore contribute to maintaining or increasing animal biodiversity.

Supplementary Materials: The following are available online at http://www.mdpi.com/2076-2615/10/5/905/s1, Table S1. Chemical composition (g/100 g) of the commercial diets fed to Alentejano (AL), Bísaro (BI), AL × BI and BI × AL pigs slaughtered at ~65 and 150 kg BW.

Author Contributions: Conceptualization, J.M.M., R.C. and J.T.N.; Methodology, J.M.M., R.F., A.A., J.N. and R.C.; Animal management, R.C., A.F., J.M.M. and J.N.; Data Analysis, J.M.M.; Writing—original draft preparation, J.M.M.; Writing—review, J.M.M., R.F., A.A., J.N., A.F., J.T.N. and R.C.; Writing—editing, J.M.M.; project administration and funding acquisition, R.C. and J.M.M. All authors have read and agreed to the published version of the manuscript.

Funding: The study was conducted within the project TREASURE, which has received funding from the European Union's Horizon 2020 research and innovation programme under grant agreement No. 634476. The content of this paper reflects only the author's view and the European Union Agency is not responsible for any use that may be made of the information it contains. This research was also funded by Portuguese national funds through FCT—Foundation for Science and Technology under Project UIDB/05183/2020, and a research grant SFRH/BD/132215/2017 to A. Albuquerque.

Conflicts of Interest: The authors declare no conflict of interest. The authors declare no conflict of interest. The funders had no role in the design of the study; in the collection, analyses, or interpretation of data; in the writing of the manuscript, or in the decision to publish the results.

References

1. Zhang, J.; Chai, J.; Luo, Z.; He, H.; Chen, L.; Liu, X.; Zhou, Q. Meat and nutritional quality comparison of purebred and crossbred pigs. *Anim. Sci. J.* **2018**, *89*, 202–210. [CrossRef] [PubMed]
2. Porter, V. Spain and Portugal. In *Pigs: A Handbook to the Breeds of the World*, 1st ed.; Porter, V., Mountfield, T.J., Eds.; Cornell University Press: Ithaca, NY, USA, 1993; pp. 137–140.
3. Muñoz, M.; Bozzi, R.; García, F.; Núñez, Y.; Geraci, C.; Crovetti, A.; García-Casco, J.; Alves, E.; Škrlep, M.; Charneca, R.; et al. Diversity across major and candidate genes in European local pig breeds. *PLoS ONE* **2018**, *13*, e0207475. [CrossRef] [PubMed]
4. Neves, J.A.; Sabio, E.; Freitas, A.; Almeida, J.A.A. Déposition des lipides intramusculaires dans le porc Alentejano. L'effet du niveau nutritif pendant la croissance et du régime alimentaire pendant l'engraissement. *Prod. Anim.* **1996**, *9*, 93–97.
5. Santos e Silva, J.; Ferreira-Cardoso, J.; Bernardo, A.; Costa, J.S.P.d. Conservation and development of the Bísaro pig. Characterization and zootechnical evaluation of the breed for production and genetic management. In *Quality of Meat and Fat in Pigs as Affected by Genetics and Nutrition*; Wenk, C., Fernández, A., Dupuis, M., Eds.; EEAP and Wageningen Pers: Zurich, Switzerland, 2000; Volume 100, pp. 85–92.
6. Freitas, A.B. A raça suína Alentejana: Passado, presente e futuro. In *Las Razas Porcinas Iberoamericanas: Un Enfoque Etnozootécnico*; Silva Filha, O.L., Ed.; Instituto Federal Baiano: Salvador, Brasil, 2014; pp. 55–80.
7. Neves, J.A.; Martins, J.M.; Freitas, A.B. Physicochemical characteristics of muscles from free-range reared pigs. In Proceedings of the 55th International Congress of Meat Science and Technology, Copenhagen, Denmark, 16–21 August 2009; p. 4.
8. Gama, L.T.; Martínez, A.M.; Carolino, I.; Landi, V.; Delgado, J.V.; Vicente, A.A.; Vega-Pla, J.L.; Cortés, O.; Sousa, C.O. Genetic structure, relationships and admixture with wild relatives in native pig breeds from Iberia and its islands. *Genet. Sel. Evol.* **2013**, *45*, 18. [CrossRef] [PubMed]
9. Ministério da Agricultura e do Mar. Portaria nº55/2015 de 27 de fevereiro. In *Diário da República n.º 41/2015, Série I de 2015-02-27*; INCM Ministério da Agricultura e do Mar: Lisboa, Portugal, 2015; pp. 1217–1222.
10. Pugliese, C.; Sirtori, F. Quality of meat and meat products produced from southern European pig breeds. *Meat Sci.* **2012**, *90*, 511–518. [CrossRef] [PubMed]
11. Santos Silva, J.; Araújo, J.P.; Cerqueira, J.O.; Pires, P.; Alves, C.; Batorek-Lukač, N. Bísaro Pig. In *European Local Pig Breeds–Diversity and Performance*; Candek-Potokar, M., Linan, R.M.N., Eds.; IntechOpen: London, UK, 2019; pp. 51–63. [CrossRef]
12. Miranda-do-Vale, J. Suínos. In *Gado Bissulco*; Miranda-do-Vale, J., Ed.; Livraria Sá da Costa: Lisboa, Portugal, 1949; Volume 17, pp. 35–78.
13. Food and Agriculture Organization of United Nations (FAO). *Biodiversity for Food and Agriculture*; FAO and Platform for Agrobiodiversity Research (PAR): Rome, Italy, 2011; p. 66.
14. Martins, J.M.; Fialho, R.; Albuquerque, A.; Neves, J.; Freitas, A.; Nunes, J.T.; Charneca, R. Growth, blood, carcass and meat quality traits from local pig breeds and their crosses. *Animal* **2020**, *14*, 636–647. [CrossRef]
15. Institut National de la Recherche Agronomique (INRA). *L' Alimentation des Animaux Monogastriques: Porc, Lapin, Volailles*; INRA: Paris, France, 1984; p. 282.
16. Álvarez-Rodríguez, J.; Teixeira, A. Slaughter weight rather than sex affects carcass cuts and tissue composition of Bisaro pigs. *Meat Sci.* **2019**, *154*, 54–60. [CrossRef]

17. International Organization for Standardization (ISO). *Meat and Meat Products—Determination of Moisture Content (Reference Method)*; ISO: Geneva, Switzerland, 1997; Volume 1442.

18. The Association of Official Analytical Chemists. *Official Methods of Analysis of AOAC International*, 18th ed.; AOAC: Gaithersburg, MD, USA, 2011; p. 2400.

19. Folch, J.; Lees, M.; Stanley, G.H.S. A simple method for the isolation and purification of total lipides from animal tissues. *J. Biol. Chem.* **1957**, *226*, 497–509.

20. Martins, J.M.; Neves, J.A.; Freitas, A.; Tirapicos, J.L. Effect of long-term betaine supplementation on chemical and physical characteristics of three muscles from the Alentejano pig. *J. Sci. Food Agric.* **2012**, *92*, 2122–2127. [CrossRef]

21. Hill, F. The Solubility of Intramuscular Collagen in Meat Animals of Various Ages. *J. Food Sci.* **1966**, *31*, 161–166. [CrossRef]

22. Commission Internationale de l'Éclairage. *CIE Publication 36, 18th Session*; CIE: London, UK, 1976.

23. Park, H.-S.; Min, B.; Oh, S.-H. Research trends in outdoor pig production—A review. *Asian Australas. J. Anim. Sci.* **2017**, *30*, 1207–1214. [CrossRef] [PubMed]

24. Čandek-Potokar, M.; Lukač, N.B.; Tomažin, U.; Škrlep, M.; Nieto, R. Analytical Review of Productive Performance of Local Pig Breeds. In *European Local Pig Breeds—Diversity and Performance*; Candek-Potokar, M., Linan, R.M.N., Eds.; IntechOpen: London, UK, 2019; pp. 281–303. [CrossRef]

25. Hocquette, J.F.; Gondret, F.; Baéza, E.; Médale, F.; Jurie, C.; Pethick, D.W. Intramuscular fat content in meat-producing animals: Development, genetic and nutritional control, and identification of putative markers. *Animal* **2010**, *4*, 303–319. [CrossRef] [PubMed]

26. Fernandez, X.; Monin, G.; Talmant, A.; Mourot, J.; Lebret, B. Influence of intramuscular fat content on the quality of pig meat. 1. Composition of the lipid fraction and sensory characteristics of *m. longissimus lumborum*. *Meat Sci.* **1999**, *53*, 59–65. [CrossRef]

27. Miller, R.K. 3 Factors affecting the quality of raw meat. In *Meat Processing*; Kerry, J.P., Kerry, J.F., Ledward, D., Eds.; Woodhead Publishing: Sawston, UK, 2002; pp. 27–63. [CrossRef]

28. Martins, J.M.; Neves, J.A.; Freitas, A.; Tirapicos, J.L. Rearing system and oleic acid supplementation effect on carcass and lipid characteristics of two muscles from an obese pig breed. *Animal* **2015**, *9*, 1721–1730. [CrossRef] [PubMed]

29. Carvalho, M.A.M.d. Estudo da Alometria Dos Ácidos Gordos Em Suínos da Raça Bísara. Ph.D. Thesis, Universidade de Trás-os-Montes e Alto Douro (UTAD), Vila Real, Portugal, 2009.

30. Honikel, K.O. Reference methods for the assessment of physical characteristics of meat. *Meat Sci.* **1998**, *49*, 447–457. [CrossRef]

31. Gregory, N.G.; Grandin, T. *Animal Welfare and Meat Science*; Grandin, T., Ed.; CABI Publishing: New York, NY, USA, 1998; p. 298.

32. Essén-Gustavsson, B.; Karlsson, A.; Lundström, K.; Enfält, A.C. Intramuscular fat and muscle fibre lipid contents in halothane-gene-free pigs fed high or low protein diets and its relation to meat quality. *Meat Sci.* **1994**, *38*, 269–277. [CrossRef]

33. Van Oeckel, M.J.; Warnants, N.; Boucqué, C.V. Pork tenderness estimation by taste panel, Warner–Bratzler shear force and on-line methods. *Meat Sci.* **1999**, *53*, 259–267. [CrossRef]

34. Bendall, J.R.; Swatland, H.J. A review of the relationships of pH with physical aspect of pork quality. *Meat Sci.* **1988**, *24*, 85–126. [CrossRef]

35. Tikk, K.; Lindahl, G.; Karlsson, A.H.; Andersen, H.J. The significance of diet, slaughter weight and aging time on pork colour and colour stability. *Meat Sci.* **2008**, *79*, 806–816. [CrossRef]

36. Lebret, B.; Meunier-Salaün, M.C.; Foury, A.; Mormède, P.; Dransfield, E.; Dourmad, J.Y. Influence of rearing conditions on performance, behavioral, and physiological responses of pigs to preslaughter handling, carcass traits, and meat quality. *J. Anim. Sci.* **2006**, *84*, 2436–2447. [CrossRef]

37. Charneca, R.; Martins, J.; Freitas, A.; Neves, J.; Nunes, J.; Paixim, H.; Bento, P.; Batorek-Lukač, N. Alentejano pig. In *European Local Pig Breeds—Diversity and Performance*; Candek-Potokar, M., Linan, R.M.N., Eds.; IntechOpen: London, UK, 2019; pp. 13–36. [CrossRef]

38. Muriel, E.; Ruiz, J.; Ventanas, J.; Petrón, M.J.; Antequera, T. Meat quality characteristics in different lines of Iberian pigs. *Meat Sci.* **2004**, *67*, 299–307. [CrossRef] [PubMed]

39. Brewer, M.S.; Zhu, L.G.; Bidner, B.; Meisinger, D.J.; McKeith, F.K. Measuring pork color: Effects of bloom time, muscle, pH and relationship to instrumental parameters. *Meat Sci.* **2001**, *57*, 169–176. [CrossRef]

40. Ventanas, S.; Ventanas, J.; Jurado, A.; Estévez, M. Quality traits in muscle biceps femoris and back-fat from purebred Iberian and reciprocal Iberian × Duroc crossbred pigs. *Meat Sci.* **2006**, *73*, 651–659. [CrossRef] [PubMed]

41. Serrano, M.P. A Study of Factors That Influence Growth Performance and Carcass and Meat Quality of Iberian Pigs Reared Under Intensive Management. Ph.D. Thesis, Universidad Politécnica de Madrid/Technical University of Madrid, Madrid, Spain, 2008.

42. Virgili, R.; Degni, M.; Schivazappa, C.; Faeti, V.; Poletti, E.; Marchetto, G.; Pacchioli, M.T.; Mordenti, A. Effect of age at slaughter on carcass traits and meat quality of Italian heavy pigs. *J. Anim. Sci.* **2003**, *81*, 2448–2456. [CrossRef] [PubMed]

43. Mayoral, A.I.; Dorado, M.; Guillén, M.T.; Robina, A.; Vivo, J.M.; Vázquez, C.; Ruiz, J. Development of meat and carcass quality characteristics in Iberian pigs reared outdoors. *Meat Sci.* **1999**, *52*, 315–324. [CrossRef]

44. Huff-Lonergan, E.; Lonergan, S.M. Mechanisms of water-holding capacity of meat: The role of postmortem biochemical and structural changes. *Meat Sci.* **2005**, *71*, 194–204. [CrossRef]

45. Pearson, A.M.; Young, R.B. *Muscle and Meat Biochemistry*; Academic Press: New York, NY, USA, 1989; p. 468.

46. Van Laack, R.; Kauffman, R.; Greaser, M. Determinants of ultimate pH of meat. In Proceedings of the 47th International Congress of Meat Science and Technology, Krakow, Poland, 26–31 August 2001; pp. 22–26.

47. Bidner, B.S.; Ellis, M.; Brewer, M.S.; Campion, D.; Wilson, E.R.; McKeith, F.K. Effect of ultimate pH on the quality characteristics of pork. *J. Muscle Foods* **2004**, *15*, 139–154. [CrossRef]

48. Solomon, M.B.; Laack, R.V.; Eastridge, J.S. Biophysical basis of pale, soft, exudative (PSE) pork and poultry muscle: A review. *J. Muscle Foods* **1998**, *9*, 1–11. [CrossRef]

49. Needham, T.; Hoffman, L.C. Physical meat quality and chemical composition of the Longissimus thoracis of entire and immunocastrated pigs fed varying dietary protein levels with and without ractopamine hydrochloride. *Meat Sci.* **2015**, *110*, 101–108. [CrossRef]

50. Seiquer, I.; Palma-Granados, P.; Haro, A.; Lara, L.; Lachica, M.; Fernández-Fígares, I.; Nieto, R. Meat quality traits in longissimus lumborum and gluteus medius muscles from immunocastrated and surgically castrated Iberian pigs. *Meat Sci.* **2019**, *150*, 77–84. [CrossRef]

51. Fuentes, V.; Ventanas, S.; Ventanas, J.; Estévez, M. The genetic background affects composition, oxidative stability and quality traits of Iberian dry-cured hams: Purebred Iberian versus reciprocal Iberian × Duroc crossbred pigs. *Meat Sci.* **2014**, *96*, 737–743. [CrossRef] [PubMed]

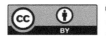

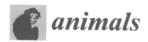

Article

A Newly Identified LncRNA LncIMF4 Controls Adipogenesis of Porcine Intramuscular Preadipocyte through Attenuating Autophagy to Inhibit Lipolysis

Yunmei Sun [†], Rui Cai [†], Yingqian Wang, Rui Zhao, Jin Qin and Weijun Pang [*]

Laboratory of Animal Fat Deposition and Muscle Development, Key Laboratory of Animal Genetics, Breeding and Reproduction of Shaanxi Province, College of Animal Science and Technology, Northwest A&F University, Yangling, Shaanxi 712100, China; sunyunmei@nwafu.edu.cn (Y.S.); cairui1663@nwafu.edu.cn (R.C.); Yingqianwang@126.com (Y.W.); ZR970510@163.com (R.Z.); qinjin19921026@sina.com (J.Q.)
* Correspondence: pwj1226@nwafu.edu.cn; Tel.: +86-029-87091893
† These authors contributed equally to this work.

Received: 9 April 2020; Accepted: 18 May 2020; Published: 26 May 2020

Simple Summary: Compared with lean-type pigs, the intramuscular fat content of fat-type Bamei pigs was greater. LncRNA, as a vital regular, plays an important role in numerous biological processes. However, there were a few studies on the role of lncRNAs during IMF development in pigs. Based on these, lncRNA sequencing in intramuscular adipocytes was performed to explore the effects of lncRNA on intramuscular fat deposition. RNA sequencing analysis of intramuscular adipocyte from Bamei pig (fat-type) and Yorkshire pig (lean-type) indicated that, a novel lncRNA, lncIMF4, was associated with intramuscular adipogenesis. In addition, further researches showed that knockdown lncIMF4 promoted proliferation and adipogenic differentiation of porcine intramuscular adipocytes, whereas inhibited autophagy. Moreover, knockdown lncIMF4 facilitated intramuscular adipogenesis through attenuating autophagy to repress the lipolysis. Our findings will contribute to better understand the mechanism of lncRNA controlling adipogenesis in pig. Furthermore, it also provides a new perspective to study the role of lncRNA in regulating porcine intramuscular adipogenesis for promoting pork quality.

Abstract: Intramuscular fat (IMF) is implicated in juiciness, tenderness, and flavor of pork. Meat quality of Chinese fat-type pig is much better than that of lean-type pig because of its higher IMF content. LncRNA is a vital regulator that contributes to adipogenesis. However, it is unknown about the regulation of lncRNA on IMF content. Here, by RNA sequence analysis of intramuscular adipocyte from Bamei pig (fat-type) and Yorkshire pig (lean-type), we found that a novel lncRNA, lncIMF4, was associated with adipogenesis. LncIMF4, abundant in adipose, differently expressed along with intramuscular preadipocyte proliferation and differentiation. Meanwhile, it is located both in cytoplasm and nucleus. Besides, lncIMF4 knockdown promoted proliferation and differentiation of porcine intramuscular preadipocytes, whereas inhibited autophagy. Moreover, lncIMF4 knockdown facilitated intramuscular adipogenesis through attenuating autophagy to repress the lipolysis. Our findings will contribute to understand better the mechanism of lncRNA controlling intramuscular adipogenesis for promoting pork quality.

Keywords: pork quality; lncIMF4; intramuscular preadipocyte; differentiation; autophagy

1. Introduction

Adipose tissue is essential for animals. It plays a vital role in the composition of living organisms and various metabolic processes. Among them, intramuscular adipose relates to meat quality.

Moderate intramuscular fat content can increase the tenderness and flavor of pork. The content of intramuscular fat (IMF) and its fatty acid composition play an important role in meat quality, affecting the sensory properties (juiciness, flavor, and tenderness), and nutritional value of meat [1]. The positive effects of IMF related to the quality of meat have been confirmed in pork [2], mutton [3], and beef [4]. The content depends not only on the amount of precursor fat cells converted to mature IMF cells but also on the deposition of lipid droplets in the IMF cells and lipid droplets in the myocytes [5].

LncRNA, a long noncoding RNA, participates in multiple life processes. They participated in many cellular biological processes, such as proliferation, differentiation, and apoptosis, by regulating the expression of their target genes [6–8]. There is some evidence demonstrated that lncRNAs regulated adipogenesis through multiple mechanisms. Hundreds of lncRNAs were involved in the regulatory network of adipogenesis [9,10]. More and more researchers are paying attention to study the influence of lncRNA on pig fat deposition and exploring its regulation for increasing meat quality. At present, many studies about lncRNA sequencing in adipose tissue from different pig breeds were performed. These sequencing analyses illustrated that many lncRNAs were involved in the development of porcine adipose tissue [11–13]. However, there were a few studies on the role of lncRNAs during IMF development in pigs. This exciting area needs to be further researched.

Autophagy is a process of phagocytizing its cytoplasmic protein or organelle and coating it into vesicles and fusing with lysosomes to form autophagosomes. Autophagy degrade the contents by autophagosomes to regulate cell metabolism. In addition, it updates to specific organelles; cell autophagy, like apoptosis and cell senescence, is an important biological phenomenon involved in the development and growth of organisms. Macroautophagy, is the best understood among the known autophagic pathways. It is characterized by forming a double-membrane structure called the autophagosome that fuses with the lysosome [14]. The study found that there was also the occurrence of macroautophagy in adipocytes. The lysosome contains various hydrolases; therefore, autophagy can degrade multiple cytoplasmic components and provide the resultant molecular building blocks, such as amino acids, glucose, nucleotides, and fatty acids [15]. Experiments in mouse models have shown that autophagy is required to maintain the levels of amino acids and glucose in blood and tissues of neonatal and adult mice during fasting [16–18]. Therefore, in order to investigate the mechanism of lncRNA on regulating adipose development, studies about the relationship between lipogenesis and autophagy require further exploration.

In our previous studies, we performed lncRNA sequencing in preadipocytes of porcine longissimus dorsi muscle during differentiation [19]. The data showed that lncIMF4 is a novel lncRNA. It was differentially expressed in different time groups. This inspired that lncIMF4 may be a potential target for adipogenesis. Additionally, bioinformatics analysis predicted that lncIMF4 participated in many biological processes including cell proliferation, differentiation, and autophagy. Therefore, this research on the function of lncIMF4 in intramuscular adipocytes was performed to better understand the mechanism of lncRNA controlling intramuscular adipogenesis for promoting pork quality.

2. Materials and Methods

2.1. Animal

Animal samples used in this study were approved by the Animal Care and Use Committee of Northwest A&F University. To investigate the expression pattern of lncIMF4 in pig, tissue samples from heart, liver, spleen, lungs, kidney, fat, and skeletal muscle (longissimus dorsi) of Bamei pigs at 3 days old (n = 4) and 180 days old (n = 4) were collected from experimental farm of Northwest A&F University (Yangling, China). All tissues for expression profile were immediately frozen in liquid nitrogen and then were kept at −80 °C until RNA isolation.

2.2. Cell Culture

The experiments refer to in vitro intramuscular adipocytes from Bamei and Yorkshire pigs. Intramuscular preadipocytes were isolated from longissimus dorsi muscle (LD) of 3-day-old piglets as described previously [19]. In brief, we used 0.2% collagenase I (270 U/mg; Gibco, Carlsbad, CA, USA) to digest samples at 37 °C in the water bath shaker for 2 h. Then, samples were sequentially filtered through 70 and 200 mesh filters to separate the cells. After washing twice with DMEM/F12, cells were seeded in dishes containing DMEM/F12 medium with 10% fetal bovine serum (Gibco, Australia). After 1.5 h, we rinsed off unattached cells. When density of cells reaches to approximately 100%, we used the cocktail method to induce adipocytes differentiation. The four differentiation stages were observed when cells were cultured in differentiation medium for 0 d (undifferentiated), 2 d (early differentiated), 4 d (middle differentiated), and 8 d (last differentiated). The autophagy was induced by a serum-free medium for 3 h after 6-day differentiation. Until that, preadipocytes were cultured in DMEM/F12 to proliferate. Briefly, we used OPTI to dilute negative control (NC) (or lncIMF4 siRNA to a concentration of 50 nM/mL), kept still for 5 min, then added Roche transfection reagent, gently blew, and further kept for 20 min. This mixed OPTI was added to the new medium.

2.3. Cell Transfection

For research on proliferation, 50 nM siRNA or negative control (NC) were transfected into cells by X-tremeGENE siRNA Transfection Reagent (Roche, San Francisco, USA) and Opti-MEM (Gibco, Grand Island, USA) when the density was 40%. After transfection for 24 h, the cells were harvested. For differentiation, when the density reached 80%, siRNA or NC were transfected, and differentiation medium was replaced with growth medium when the cells reached fusion. The siRNA and NC were obtained from RiboBio (Guangzhou, China).

2.4. Hematoxylin–Eosin Staining

The longissimus dorsi muscle tissue was taken from the fifth to sixth lumbar vertebrae of the 180-day-old Bamei pigs (n = 6) and the Yorkshire pigs (n = 6) and placed in the fixative. Longissimus dorsi muscle (LM) tissues were dehydrated by alcohol. The dehydrated tissues were made into paraffin sections. For HE staining, the sections were deparaffinized with xylene for 10 min. Then, the sections were washed with the distilled water and then were first placed in an aqueous solution of hematoxylin for several minutes. Then the sections were immersed in acid water and ammonia water for color separation for several seconds, respectively. Next, the sections were rinsed under the running water for 1 h, and then were immersed into distilled water for a while. Slices were dehydrated in 70% and 90% alcohol for 10 min, respectively, and then were dyed in eosin staining solution for 2–3 min. The stained sections were dehydrated with pure ethanol, and the sections were made transparent by xylene. The transparent slices were mounted with Canada Balsam and covered with a coverslip. Sample images were captured using a Nikon TE2000 microscope (Nikon, Tokyo, Japan).

2.5. Fluorescence in Situ Hybridization

Cell slide was placed on the bottom of the 12-well plate; cells were washed for 5 min and then were fixed at room temperature for 10 min with 4% paraformaldehyde. Briefly, 200 uL prehybrid solution was added to each well and they were blocked at 37 °C for 30 min. For prehybridization, the hybridization solution was preheated at 37 °C. To protect it from the light, 2.5 μL 20 uM lncRNA FISH Probe Mix stock solution or internal reference FISH Probe Mix stock solution was added to 100 μL hybridization solution. The prehybridization solution in each well was discarded and 100 μL of the probe hybridization solution containing the probe was added; the light was avoided, and then it was hybridized overnight at 37 °C. DNA staining is protected from light. Further, staining was done with DAPI staining solution for 10 min, avoiding light, and the cells were washed 3 times for 5 min each time. The cell slide was carefully removed from the well in dark and fixed on the loaded slide with a sealing tablet for fluorescence detection.

2.6. Cytoplasmic and Nuclear RNA Extraction

This method is referred to a previous research [20]. For the extraction of cytoplasmic and nuclear RNA fraction, intramuscular adipocytes were collected after 6-day differentiation. Cells were washed with PBS, suspended in lysis buffer (10 mM NaCl, 2 mM MgCl$_2$, 10 mM pH 7.8 Tris-HCL, 5 mM DTT, and 0.5% Igepal CA 630), and then incubated on ice for 5 min. After centrifuging at 8000 rpm for 5 min, the supernatant was transferred to a new microcentrifuge tube subjected to cytoplasmic RNA extraction, while the pellet was resuspended with lysis buffer and subjected to nuclear RNA extraction. For the RNA extraction, the fractions were first incubated with Proteinase K (10 mg/mL) at 37 °C for 20 min and then mixed with TRIzol. RNA was separated by chloroform and precipitated by ethanol with 3 M sodium acetate (pH 5.2, 1/10 volume). The extracted RNA was dissolved into ddH$_2$O and used for reversed transcribed and real-time PCR analysis.

2.7. RNA Extraction and Real-Time PCR

Total RNA was isolated by TRIzol reagent (Takara, Otsu, Japan). Afterwards, the reverse transcription of RNA was performed using kits (Takara, Otsu, Japan), following the manufacturer's instructions. Bio-Rad iQTM5 (Bio-Rad, Hercules, CA, USA) was used to perform RT-qPCR. Expression level of the listed genes and lncIMF4 were related to that of β-tubulin. The information of primers is shown in Table 1.

Table 1. Primers used for real-time quantitative PCR.

Name	Forward (5′→3′)	Reverse (5′→3′)
PPARγ	AGGACTACCAAAGTGCCATCAAA	GAGGCTTTATCCCCACAGACAC
AP2	GAGCACCATAACCTTAGATGGA	AAATTCTGGTAGCCGTGACA
C/EBPα	CGATGCTCTTAGCTGAGTGT	GGTCCAAGAATTTCACCTCT
SREBP1	GGAGCCATGGATTGCACATT	GGCCCGGGAAGTCACTGT
Cyclin B	AATCCCTTCTTGTGGTTA	CTTAGATGTGGCATACTTG
MyoD	TACACCGACAACTCCATCCG	GAGGGCGGGTTGGAAATGAA
Cyclin E	CAGAGCAGCGAGCAGGAGC	GCAAGCTGCTTCCACACCACAT
FAS	CCCCGAATCTGCACTACCAC	AGTTGGGCTGAAGGATGACG
ATGL	TCACCAACACCAGCATCCA	GCACATCTCTCGAAGCACCA
HSL	CACTGACTGCTGACCCCAAG	TCCTCACTGTCCTGTCCTTCAC
ATG7	GATTGCCTGGTGGGTGGTAA	CATGGCTTTCGATGAGCTGC
Beclin1	AGTAGGTGAAGGCTAGGCGA	AGCTCGTGTCCAGTTTCAGG
GAPDH	AGGTCGGAGTGAACGGATTTG	ACCATGTAGTGGAGGTCAATGAAG
LncIMF4	GTGGATTGGGAGCCTGCTAT	ACACTCCATGGCCTGGTAAAA

2.8. Western Blotting

The protocol of western blot was followed according to a previous study [10]. Briefly, adipocytes were split by radioimmunoprecipitation assay (RIPA) buffer (Beyotime, China) by adding protease inhibitor (Pierce, WA, USA). The total protein sample was separated in the SDS-polyacrylamide gel. Then, it was transferred into a PVDF membrane (Millipore, Bedford, MA, USA). Next, the membrane was blocked in 5% defatted milk for 2 h. After that, the membrane was incubated with primary antibodies at 4 °C overnight followed by a secondary antibody at room temperature for 1.5 h. The antibodies Cyclin B, Cyclin D, Cyclin E, PPARγ, and AP2 were purchased from Santa Cruz (CA, USA); C/EBPα and SREBP-1 were purchased from Abcam; p62, LC, ATGL, and HSL were purchased from CST (Boston, MA, USA); and β-tubulin was purchased from Sungene Biotech (Shanghai, China).

2.9. Cell Counting Kit (CCK8) and EdU Assays

The protocol of cell counting (CCK8) and EdU assays were performed following a previous study [6]. Adipocytes were cultured in 96-well plates with 2.5×10^3 cells per well. Cells were treated with NC or siRNA. The proliferation rates were tested by the Cell Counting Kit 8 (CCK-8) following manufacturer's instructions. For EdU assay, cells were incubated with EdU for 2 h after transfecting them with NC or siRNA. Subsequently, sample images were captured using a Nikon TE2000 microscope (Nikon, Tokyo, Japan).

2.10. Flow Cytometry

Cells were seeded in 6-well plates with 4×10^5 cells per well. After 24 h, cells were transfected with NC or siRNA. Next, cells were washed three times with PBS and fixed with 70% alcohol overnight at −20 °C. Cells were then treated with 1 mg/mL RNase at 37 °C for 40 min before being stained with 50 mg/mL propidium iodide (PI) at 4 °C for 1 h. Lastly, samples were detected with FACSCalibur flow cytometry (Franklin Lakes, NJ, USA).

2.11. Oil Red O Staining

Oil Red O Staining was performed according to a previously published method [12]. After being fixed in 4% paraformaldehyde solution, cells were incubated with 0.5% Oil Red O for 30 min and washed three times with PBS; adipocytes were visualized by phase-contrast microscopy (Tokyo, Japan). Oil Red O dissolved in lipid droplets was extracted with 100% isopropanol and its relative concentrations were determined by measuring the absorbance at 510 nm.

2.12. Monodansylcadaverine (MDC) Staining

The cells were digested with trypsin and centrifuged, and the cell pellet was collected. Then the cells were washed once with wash buffer and the supernatant was discarded. Next, the cells were resuspended by adding the appropriate amount of wash buffer to adjust the cell density to 10. Precisely, 90 uL of cell suspension was taken into the EP tube and 10 uL of MDC solution was added and mixed gently. The solution was stained at room temperature for 30 min, and the cells were collected by centrifugation. Then, the cells were washed twice with wash buffer, 300 uL DAPI solution was added to it, and stood still at room temperature. After 5 min, the cells were washed 3 times with PBS. The cells were resuspended in the collection buffer, the resuspended droplets were added to the slide, and the coverslip was attached. The slide was observed under a fluorescence microscope, and cells were counted and photographed. Autophagy staining detection kit was purchased from Solarbio.

2.13. Statistical Analysis

The diagrams were created by GraphPad Prism 6.0. SEM represents the variation between sample means. Group differences were analyzed with Student's *t* test or one-way ANOVA using PASW Statistics 20 (SPSS, Chicago, IL, USA) (*, $p < 0.05$; **, $p < 0.01$).

3. Results

3.1. LncIMF4 May be A Novel LncRNA Implicated in Intramuscular Fat Deposition

The meat quality of Bamei pig is better than Yorkshire pig probably highly influenced by the higher content of intramuscular adipocytes in Bamei pig. (Figure 1A,B). The lipid content in intramuscular adipocytes of Bamei pig was also more than Yorkshire (Figure 1C). Comparison of lncRNA sequences was performed between intramuscular adipocytes of Bamei pig and Yorkshire pig. The results showed that the level of lncIMF4 was higher in large white pig, and it presented rising first then falling pattern (Figure 1D). In addition, the alignment track showed that lncIMF4 is an unannotated lncRNA in the pig genome (Figure 1E). Interestingly, the result of Gene Ontology (GO) term analysis demonstrated that it was related with lipolysis and autophagy (Figure 1F). Therefore, further research was carried out following these pathways.

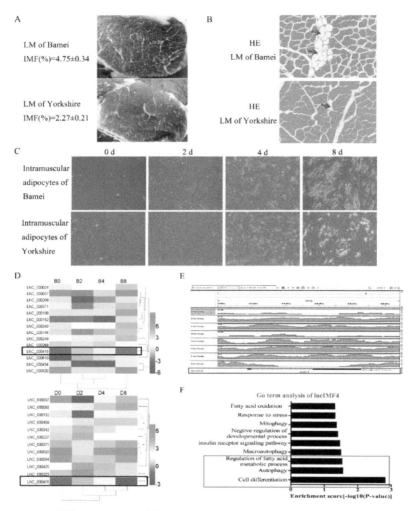

Figure 1. LncIMF4 may be a novel lncRNA implicated in intramuscular adipogenesis. (**A**) The intramuscular fat (IMF) content of longissimus dorsi muscle (LM) between Bamei and Yorkshire were analyzed by Soxhlet extraction method. (**B**) Hematoxylin–eosin (HE) staining of LM between Bamei and Yorkshire. (**C**) Porcine intramuscular adipocytes at 0, 2, 4, and 8 d after inducing differentiation (cell density reached 100%). (**D**) Heatmap depicting long noncoding RNA (lncRNA) having at least 2-fold change in intramuscular adipocytes between fat-type and lean-type pig at four differentiation stages; black fragments denote lncIMF4. (**E**) The alignment track of lncIMF4. (**F**) GO term of lncIMF4. The results were representative of means ± SEM of three independent experiments.

3.2. The Expression Pattern of LncIMF4 in Pig and Its Subcellular Location in Adipocyte

Based on the above results, we supposed that lncIMF4 was related to IMF content. We detected the levels of lncIMF4 during intramuscular adipocytes proliferation and differentiation. The expression patterns both showed a trend of rising first and then decreasing, reaching a peak on the second day, which was consistent with the sequencing results (Figure 2A,B). Tissue expression results demonstrated that lncIMF4 is highly expressed in adipose tissue, not only in 3-day-old piglets (Figure 2C) but also in 180-day-old pig (Figure 2D). To confirm the localization of lncIMF4 in intramuscular adipocytes, we performed the fluorescence in situ hybridization, showing that lncIMF4 was localized in both nucleus and cytoplasm (Figure 2E). The relative expression levels of LncIMF4 in the nucleus and cytoplasm were consistent with it (Figure 2F).

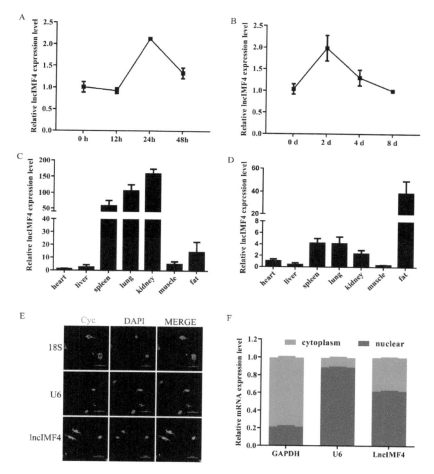

Figure 2. The expression pattern of lncIMF4 in pig and its subcellular location in adipocyte. (**A**) The levels of lncIMF4 during porcine intramuscular adipocytes proliferation. (**B**) The levels of lncIMF4 during adipocytes differentiation. (**C,D**) The levels of lncIMF4 in heart, liver, spleen, lung, kidney, muscle, and fat from 3-day-old piglets (**C**) and 180-day-old pig (**D**). (**E**) Subcellular localization of lncIMF4. (**F**) LncIMF4 expression in cytoplasm and nucleus. The results were representative of means ± SEM of three independent experiments.

3.3. LncIMF4 Knockdown Promoted the Proliferation of Porcine Intramuscular Preadipocytes

Proliferation is an important process for intramuscular adipose development. Therefore, we explored the function of lncIMF4 in the proliferation of intramuscular preadipocytes. We transfected siRNA into proliferating intramuscular preadipocytes to knockdown lncIMF4. The efficiency of siRNA meets the requirements of subsequent experiments (Figure 3A). CCK8 assay showed that the cell number was increased (Figure 3B). Furthermore, by cell cycle analysis, we found that knockdown of lncIMF4 increased the percentage of S phase cells and decreased the percentage of G1 and G2 phage cells (Figure 3C,D). The result of EdU assay was consistent with it (Figure 3E,F). Meanwhile, knockdown of lncIMF4 increased the levels of cell cycle-related genes compared with that of NC (Figure 3G,H). These results indicated that knockdown of lncIMF4 promoted the intramuscular adipocytes proliferation.

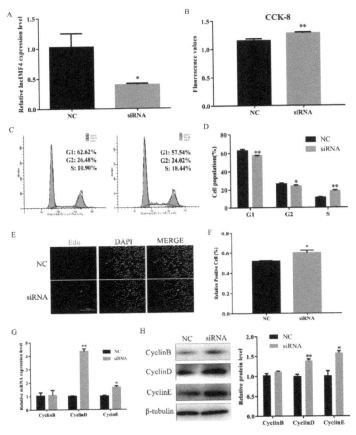

Figure 3. Knockdown of lncIMF4 promoted intramuscular adipocytes proliferation. LncIMF4 negative control (NC) or siRNA were transfected into cells at 40% density. (**A**) The inhibition efficiency of lncIMF4 in porcine intramuscular adipocytes treated with lncIMF4 siRNA. (**B**) Cell count was measured by Cell Counting Kit 8 (CCK8). (**C**) Cell cycle analyses. (**D**) The statistics results of cell cycle analysis. (**E**) EdU assay was performed after transfection for 24 h. (**F**) The percentage of EdU positive cells/DAPI positive cells was quantified. (**G**) RT-qPCR analyzed the cell cycle genes, cyclin B, cyclin D, and cyclin E after transfection for 24 h. (**H**) Western blot of the cell cycle genes, cyclin B, cyclin D, and cyclin E, after transfection for 24 h. The results were representative of means ± SEM of three independent experiments. *, $p < 0.05$; **, $p < 0.01$.

3.4. LncIMF4 Knockdown Promoted Intramuscular Adipogenic Differentiation

To explore the function of lncIMF4 during intramuscular adipocytes differentiation, we used the siRNA to knock down it, and the efficiency of siRNA reached the subsequence experiment requirement (Figure 4A). Oil Red O staining also showed a significant increase in intracellular lipid droplets in siRNA group (Figure 4B,C). Key genes of adipocytes differentiation were significantly increased after transfection with siRNA (Figure 4D). In addition, the protein levels of lipogenesis were upregulated (Figure 4E,F). Cumulatively, these results indicated that knockdown of lncIMF4 promoted adipocytes lipogenesis.

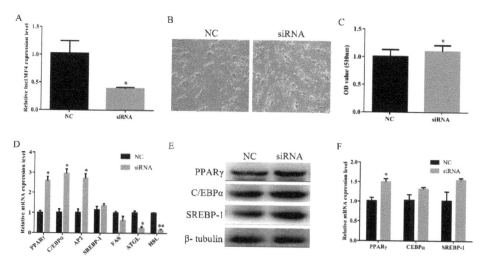

Figure 4. Knockdown of lncIMF4 promoted adipocytes lipogenesis. LncIMF4 siRNA or NC were transfected into cells at 70% density at 50 nM. (**A**) The inhibition efficiency of lncIMF4 in porcine intramuscular adipocytes after transfecting lncIMF4 siRNA with NC on 6 day of differentiation. (**B**) Oil Red O staining, scale bar = 100 μm. (**C**) Absorbance value at 510 nm after incubation with Oil Red O. (**D**) RT-qPCR analysis of adipogenic and lipolytic genes on 6 day of differentiation. (**E**) Western blot analysis of adipogenic genes on 6 day of differentiation. (**F**) The quantification of protein levels. The results were representative of means ± SEM of three independent experiments. *, $p < 0.05$; **, $p < 0.01$.

3.5. LncIMF4 Knockdown Inhibited Lipolysis by Attenuating Autophagy in Porcine Intramuscular Adipocytes

In this study, we constructed the autophagy model of porcine intramuscular adipocytes by using nonserum culture medium after 6 days. The results showed that the number of autophagy cell was increased (Figure 5A,B). The levels of ATG7 and Baclin1 were also upregulated (Figure 5C,D). These results indicated that the autophagy model was successfully constructed.

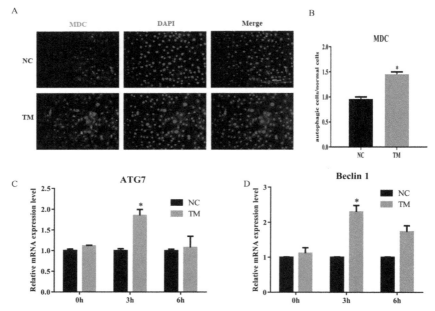

Figure 5. Autophagy model of porcine intramuscular adipocytes was constructed. (**A**) Monodansylcadaverine (MDC) staining of porcine intramuscular adipocytes after inducing autophagy by serum-free medium for 3 h. (**B**) The quantification of autophagic cells/normal cells. (**C,D**) RT-qPCR was carried out to detect the cell autophagic genes, ATG7 (**C**) and Beclin1 (**D**). Data were representative of means ± SEM of three independent experiments. *, $p < 0.05$. NC, negative control; TM, treatment.

We predict that lncIMF4 is related to autophagy according to the results of GO term, which showed that lncIMF4 was enriched in autophagy-related pathway. Therefore, lncIMF4 were knockdown to test whether adipocytes autophagy was regulated. After transfection with siRNA, cells with green fluorescent dot particles were less than in the control group (Figure 6A,B). This indicated that autophagy was decreased when lncIMF4 was knocked down. The mRNA and protein levels of ATG7 and Baclin1 were consistent with it (Figure 6C). Meanwhile, the markers of autophagy, p62 were significantly upregulated and the LC3 were downregulated (Figure 6D). Furthermore, Oil Red O staining revealed that lncIMF4 knockdown promoted porcine intramuscular adipocyte differentiation in autophagy model (Figure 6E). Protein levels of PPARγ and AP2 showed the same result (Figure 6F). Consistently, the mRNA and protein levels of ATGL and HSL, the key genes of lipolysis, were both decreased after transfection with siRNA (Figure 6G,H). These results demonstrated that knockdown of lncIMF4 promoted porcine intramuscular adipocyte adipogenesis by attenuating autophagy. The function of lncIMF4 is shown in Figure 6I.

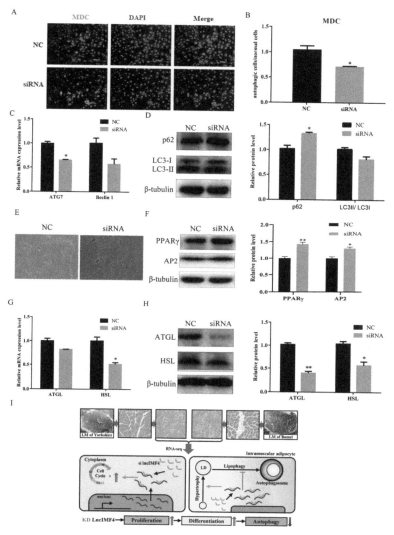

Figure 6. Knockdown of lncIMF4 inhibited lipolysis by downregulating autophagy. (**A**) MDC staining of porcine intramuscular adipocytes transfected into cells at 70% density at 50 nM after inducing autophagy by serum-free medium for 3 h. (**B**) The quantification of autophagic cells/normal cells. (**C**) RT-qPCR was carried out to detect the cell autophagic genes. (**D**) Western blot analysis of autophagic marker genes on 6 day of differentiation. (**E**) Oil Red O staining, scale bar = 100 μm. (**F**) Western blot analysis of adipogenic genes on 6 day of differentiation in autophagy model. (**G**) The mRNA expression level of lipolytic genes on 6 day of differentiation. (**H**) Western blot analysis and quantification of lipolytic protein levels. (**I**) The function of lncIMF4 in porcine intramuscular adipocytes. Data were representative of means ± SEM of three independent experiments. *, $p < 0.05$; **, $p < 0.01$.

4. Discussion

Higher intramuscular fat content in pork plays an important role in improving meat quality [21]. Many factors are included in the biological processes. The regulatory role of lncRNA is an essential part of it [22]. In our previous study, we performed the lncRNA sequencing and found some lncRNAs related to adipogenesis. lncIMF4 was a novel lncRNA, which is predicted to participate in cell differentiation and autophagy. These processes could affect fat content in adipocytes [23–25]. This indicated that lncIMF4 have an effect on lipid synthesis in porcine intramuscular adipocyte. Interestingly, further research demonstrated that lncIMF4 was located both in nucleus and cytoplasm, so the role of it may be complex. In this study, we used small interference to explore its function in adipocytes.

The development of adipose tissue includes adipocytes proliferation and differentiation [26]. Recently, studies reflected that lncRNAs affect cell proliferation through variety of signaling [27,28]. In this study, we found that the level of lncIMF4 changed regularly along with cell proliferation. Based on this, we suspected that lncIMF4 participated in the regulation of proliferation of porcine intramuscular adipocyte. Subsequent experimental results were consistent with this hypothesis. Further study showed that knockdown lncIMF4 promoted intramuscular adipocyte proliferation. It reflected that lncIMF4 was important for intramuscular adipose development. The adipocyte differentiation is an important process regulating lipid deposition in adipose tissue. Adipocytes hyperplasia arises in the early stage of differentiation. Then, small lipid droplets appear in the cells and merge into large droplets after many adipogenic factors are activated. Finally, adipocytes become hypertrophic. LncRNA has been known as a regulator to affect adipocyte differentiation [29–31]. However, there is little research on the role of lncRNA in porcine adipocyte differentiation. In our study, GO term analysis showed that lncIMF4 is associated with cell differentiation. Furthermore, the level of lncIMF4 is related to fat deposition closely. Therefore, we explored the effects of lncIMF4 on porcine intramuscular adipocyte. Consistently, the results demonstrated that knockdown lncIMF4 promoted adipogenic differentiation in porcine intramuscular adipocyte. It confirmed that lncIMF4 regulated porcine intramuscular adipocyte lipogenesis.

Autophagy is a biological process that maintains life survival by degrading organelles and proteins when there is lack of nutrition, energy, or imbalance of environment. Defective autophagy, is associated with numerous diseases, including neurological disorders, cancer, cardiomyopathies and metabolic disorders [32]. Autophagy has a dilution effect on high intracellular lipids and influences lipid metabolism in many ways, from lipogenesis to lipolysis [33,34]. The autophagosomes will wrap lipids to ablate if autophagy occurs in adipocytes. Autophagy and lipolysis are both decreased with enough food supply, while both are increased in nutrient deprivation [35]. In this research, bioinformatics analysis predicts that lncIMF4 may have a particular regulatory effect on autophagy. Autophagy can affect the differentiation and adipogenic processes of adipocytes. Many signaling pathways were involved in these processes [36]. Therefore, we hypothesized that lncIMF4 regulated lipolysis to affect lipid deposition through autophagy. This is a new insight to study the relationship between lncRNA and intramuscular adipose. The autophagy of normal cells is very weak. To explore this regulation, we firstly constructed an autophagy model of porcine intramuscular adipocyte. In recent years, the induction of autophagy has focused on the construction of nutrient-deficient environment and drug treatment. To reduce stress on cells and reduce cell loss, autophagy was induced by starvation treatment in this study. The appropriate induction time was determined to be 3 h after the addition of serum-free medium, which was more transient than the time in which the adipocytes induced autophagy in other literature. Further study showed that in autophagy model, knockdown lncIMF4 promoted lipogenesis and inhibited lipolysis. Moreover, it also attenuated autophagy in porcine intramuscular adipocyte. Generally, we confirmed that lncIMF4 knockdown promoted lipogenesis of porcine intramuscular preadipocyte through attenuating autophagy. The underlying mechanism will be the focus of our next experiment.

5. Conclusions

In conclusion, we identified lncIMF4 as a novel lncRNA, which is related to intramuscular fat deposition. lncIMF4, located in both nucleus and cytoplasm, knockdown promoted proliferation and differentiation of porcine intramuscular adipocytes, whereas inhibited lipolysis through attenuating autophagy. This research provides a new perspective to study the role of lncRNA in regulating porcine intramuscular adipogenesis for promoting pork quality.

Author Contributions: Conceptualization, W.P.; methodology, Y.S.; software, Y.W.; validation, R.Z.; investigation, R.C.; resources, W.P.; data curation, J.Q.; writing—original draft preparation, Y.S. and R.C.; writing—review and editing, Y.S. and R.C.; and funding acquisition, W.P. All authors have read and agreed to the published version of the manuscript.

Funding: This research was funded by following funding: the National Natural Science Foundation (31872979 and 31572366), the National Key Research and Development Program of China (2017YFD0502002), and the Key Research and Development Program of Shaanxi Province (2018ZDXL-NY-02-03).

Conflicts of Interest: The authors declare no conflicts of interest.

References

1. Hocquette, J.F.; Gondret, F.; Baéza, E.; Médale, F.; Jurie, C.; Pethick, D.W. Intramuscular fat content in meat-producing animals: Development, genetic and nutritional control, and identification of putative markers. *Animal* **2010**, *4*, 303–319. [CrossRef]
2. Gao, S.Z.; Zhao, S.M. Physiology, affecting factors and strategies for control of pig meat intramuscular fat. Recent. *Pat. Food Nutr. Agric.* **2009**, *1*, 59–74.
3. Watkins, P.J.; Frank, D.; Singh, T.K.; Young, O.A.; Warner, R.D. Sheep meat flavor and the effect of different feeding systems: A review. *J. Agric. Food Chem.* **2013**, *61*, 3561–3579. [CrossRef]
4. Mateescu, R.G.; Garrick, D.J.; Garmyn, A.J.; VanOverbeke, D.L.; Mafi, G.G.; Reecy, J.M. Genetic parameters for sensory traits in longissimus muscle and their associations with tenderness, marbling score, and intramuscular fat in Angus cattle. *J. Anim. Sci.* **2015**, *93*, 21–27. [CrossRef] [PubMed]
5. Lopes, P.A.; Costa, A.S.; Costa, P.; Pires, V.M.; Madeira, M.S.; Achega, F.; Pinto, R.M.; Prates, J.A. Contrasting cellularity on fat deposition in the subcutaneous adipose tissue and longissimus lumborum muscle from lean and fat pigs under dietary protein reduction. *Animal* **2014**, *8*, 629–637. [CrossRef]
6. Cai, R.; Tang, G.R.; Zhang, Q.; Yong, W.L.; Zhang, W.R.; Xiao, J.H.; Wei, C.S.; He, C.; Yang, G.S.; Pang, W.J. A novel lnc-RNA, named lnc-ORA, is identified by RNA-Seq analysis, and its knockdown inhibits adipogenesis by regulating the PI3K/AKT/mTOR signaling pathway. *Cells* **2019**, *8*, 477. [CrossRef]
7. Wei, G.H.; Wang, X. lncRNA MEG3 inhibit proliferation and metastasis of gastric cancer via p53 signaling pathway. *Eur. Rev. Med. Pharmacol. Sci.* **2017**, *21*, 3850–3856.
8. Yi, F.; Zhang, P.; Wang, Y.; Xu, Y.; Zhang, Z.X.; Ma, W.Z.; Xu, B.; Xia, Q.; Du, Q. Long non-coding RNA slincRAD functions in methylation regulation during the early stage of mouse adipogenesis. *RNA Biol.* **2019**, *19*, 1–13. [CrossRef] [PubMed]
9. Chen, L.; Yang, W.J.; Guo, Y.J.; Chen, W.; Zheng, P.; Zeng, J.S.; Tong, W.S. Exosomal lncRNA GAS5 regulates the apoptosis of macrophages and vascular endothelial cells in atherosclerosis. *PLoS ONE* **2017**, *12*, e0185406. [CrossRef]
10. Pang, W.J.; Lin, L.G.; Xiong, Y.; Wei, N.; Wang, Y.; Shen, Q.W.; Yang, G.S. Knockdown of PU.1 AS lncRNA inhibits adipogenesis through enhancing PU.1 mRNA translation. *J. Cell Biochem.* **2013**, *114*, 2500–2512. [CrossRef] [PubMed]
11. Wang, J.; Hua, L.S.; Chen, J.F.; Zhang, J.Q.; Bai, X.X.; Gao, B.W.; Li, C.J.; Shi, Z.H.; Sheng, W.D.; Gao, Y.; et al. Identification and characterization of long non-coding RNAs in subcutaneous adipose tissue from castrated and intact full-sib pair Huainan male pigs. *BMC Genom.* **2017**, *18*, 542. [CrossRef] [PubMed]
12. Wei, N.; Wang, Y.; Xu, R.X.; Wang, G.Q.; Xiong, Y.; Yu, T.Y.; Yang, G.S.; Pang, W.J. PU.1 antisense lncRNA against its mRNA translation promotes adipogenesis in porcine preadipocytes. *Anim. Genet.* **2015**, *46*, 133–140. [CrossRef] [PubMed]
13. Miao, Z.G.; Wang, S.; Zhang, J.Z.; Wei, P.P.; Guo, L.P.; Liu, D.Y.; Wang, Y.M.; Shi, M.Y. Identification and comparison of long non-conding RNA in Jinhua and Landrace pigs. *Biochem. Biophys. Res. Commun.* **2018**, *506*, 765–771. [CrossRef] [PubMed]
14. Saha, S.; Panigrahi, D.P.; Patil, S.; Bhutia, S.K. Autophagy in health and disease: A comprehensive review. *Biomed. Pharmacother* **2018**, *104*, 485–495. [CrossRef]
15. Kaur, J.; Debnath, J. Autophagy at the crossroads of catabolism and anabolism. *Nat. Rev. Mol. Cell Biol.* **2015**, *16*, 461–472. [CrossRef] [PubMed]

16. Carroll, B.; Korolchuk, V.I.; Sarkar, S. Amino acids and autophagy: Cross-talk and co-operation to control cellular homeostasis. *Amino Acids* **2015**, *47*, 2065–2088. [CrossRef]

17. Ha, J.; Guan, K.L.; Kim, J. AMPK and autophagy in glucose/glycogen metabolism. *Mol. Aspects Med.* **2015**, *46*, 46–62. [CrossRef]

18. Karsli-Uzunbas, G.; Guo, J.Y.; Price, S.; Teng, X.; Laddha, S.V.; Khor, S.; Kalaany, N.Y.; Jacks, T.; Chan, C.S.; Rabinowitz, J.D.; et al. Autophagy is required for glucose homeostasis and lung tumor maintenance. *Cancer Discov.* **2014**, *4*, 914–927. [CrossRef]

19. Sun, Y.M.; Chen, X.C.; Qin, J.; Liu, S.G.; Zhao, R.; Yu, T.Y.; Chu, G.Y.; Yang, G.S.; Pang, W.J. Comparative analysis of long noncoding RNAs expressed during intramuscular adipocytes adipogenesis in fat-type and lean-type pigs. *J. Agric. Food Chem.* **2018**, *66*, 12122–12130. [CrossRef]

20. Xiong, Y.; Yue, F.; Jia, Z.H.; Gao, Y.; Jin, W.; Hu, K.P.; Zhang, Y.; Zhu, D.H.; Yang, G.S.; Kuang, S.H. A novel brown adipocyte-enriched long non-coding RNA that is required for brown adipocyte differentiation and sufficient to drive thermogenic gene program in white adipocytes. *Biochim. Biophys. Acta. Mol. Cell Biol. Lipids* **2018**, *1863*, 409–419. [CrossRef]

21. Mo, D.L.; Yu, K.F.; Chen, H.; Chen, L.X.; Liu, X.H.; He, Z.Y.; Cong, P.Q.; Chen, Y.S. Transcriptome landscape of porcine intramuscular adipocytes during differentiation. *J. Agric. Food Chem.* **2017**, *65*, 6317–6328. [CrossRef] [PubMed]

22. Sarantopoulos, C.N.; Banyard, D.A.; Ziegler, M.E.; Sun, B.; Shaterian, A.; Widgerow, A.D. Elucidating the preadipocyte and its role in adipocyte formation: A Comprehensive Review. *Stem Cell Rev. Rep.* **2018**, *14*, 27–42. [CrossRef] [PubMed]

23. Green, C.R.; Wallace, M.; Divakaruni, A.S.; Phillips, S.A.; Murphy, A.N.; Ciaraldi, T.P.; Metallo, C.M. Branched-chain amino acid catabolism fuels adipocyte differentiation and lipogenesis. *Nat. Chem. Biol.* **2016**, *12*, 15–21. [CrossRef]

24. Khaldoun, S.A.; Emond-Boisjoly, M.A.; Chateau, D.; Carrière, V.; Lacasa, M.; Rousset, M.; Demignot, S.; Morel, E. Autophagosomes contribute to intracellular lipid distribution in enterocytes. *Mol. Biol. Cell* **2014**, *25*, 118–132. [CrossRef]

25. Sun, L.; Lin, J.D. Function and mechanism of long noncoding RNAs in adipocyte biology. *Diabetes* **2019**, *68*, 887–896. [CrossRef]

26. Galic, S.; Oakhill, J.S.; Steinberg, G.R. Adipose tissue as an endocrine organ. *Mol. Cell Endocrinol.* **2010**, *316*, 129–139. [CrossRef]

27. Chen, S.Z.; Chen, Y.; Qian, Q.F.; Wang, X.W.; Chang, Y.T.; Ju, S.H.; Xu, Y.D.; Zhang, C.; Qin, N.; Ding, H.; et al. Gene amplification derived a cancer-testis long noncoding RNA PCAT6 regulates cell proliferation and migration in hepatocellular carcinoma. *Cancer Med.* **2019**, *8*, 3017–3025. [CrossRef]

28. Tong, Y.X.; Wang, M.S.; Dai, Y.N.; Bao, D.J.; Zhang, J.J.; Pan, H.Y. LncRNA HOXA-AS3 sponges miR-29c to facilitate cell proliferation, metastasis, and EMT Process and activate the MEK/ERK signaling pathway in hepatocellular carcinoma. *Hum. Gene. Ther. Clin. Dev.* **2019**, *30*, 129–141. [CrossRef]

29. Nuermaimaiti, N.; Liu, J.; Liang, X.D.; Jiao, Y.; Zhang, D.; Liu, L.; Meng, X.Y.; Guan, Y.Q. Effect of lncRNA HOXA11-AS1 on adipocyte differentiation in human adipose-derived stem cells. *Biochem. Biophys. Res. Commun.* **2018**, *495*, 1878–1884. [CrossRef]

30. Xiao, T.F.; Liu, L.H.; Li, H.L.; Sun, Y.; Luo, H.X.; Li, T.P.; Wang, S.H.; Dalton, S.; Zhao, R.C.; Chen, R.S. Long noncoding RNA ADINR regulates adipogenesis by transcriptionally activating C/EBPalpha. *Stem Cell Reports* **2015**, *5*, 856–865. [CrossRef]

31. Zhu, E.D.; Zhang, J.J.; Li, Y.C.; Yuan, H.R.; Zhou, J.; Wang, B.L. Long noncoding RNA Plnc1 controls adipocyte differentiation by regulating peroxisome proliferator-activated receptor gamma. *FASEB J.* **2019**, *33*, 2396–2408. [CrossRef] [PubMed]

32. Levine, B.; Kroemer, G. Autophagy in the pathogenesis of disease. *Cell* **2008**, *132*, 27–42. [CrossRef] [PubMed]

33. Koga, H.; Kaushik, S.; Cuervo, A.M. Altered lipid content inhibits autophagic vesicular fusion. *FASEB J.* **2010**, *24*, 3052–3065. [CrossRef] [PubMed]

34. Chen, L.; Li, Z.; Zhang, Q.; Wei, S.; Li, B.W.; Zhang, X.; Zhang, L.; Li, Q.; Xu, H.; Xu, Z.K. Silencing of AQP3 induces apoptosis of gastric cancer cells via downregulation of glycerol intake and downstream inhibition of lipogenesis and autophagy. *Onco. Targets Ther.* **2017**, *10*, 2791–2804. [CrossRef] [PubMed]

35. Juarez-Rojas, J.G.; Reyes-Soffer, G.; Conlon, D.; Ginsberg, H.N. Autophagy and cardiometabolic risk factors. *Rev. Endocr. Metab. Disord.* **2014**, *15*, 307–315. [CrossRef] [PubMed]
36. Desjardins, E.M.; Steinberg, G.R. Emerging role of AMPK in brown and beige adipose tissue (BAT): Implications for obesity, insulin resistance, and type 2 diabetes. *Curr. Diab. Rep.* **2018**, *18*, 80. [CrossRef] [PubMed]

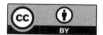

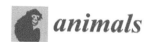 *animals*

Article

A Short Period of Darkness after Mixing of Growing Pigs Intended for PDO Hams Production Reduces Skin Lesions

Lieta Marinelli [1], Paolo Mongillo [1,*] , Paolo Carnier [1] , Stefano Schiavon [2] and Luigi Gallo [2]

[1] Department of Comparative Biomedicine and Food Science, Università degli Studi di Padova, Viale dell'Università 16, 35020 Legnaro, Padua, Italy; lieta.marinelli@unipd.it (L.M.); paolo.carnier@unipd.it (P.C.)
[2] Department of Agronomy, Food, Natural Resources, Animals and Environment, Università degli Studi di Padova, Viale dell'Università 16, 35020 Legnaro, Padua, Italy; stefano.schiavon@unipd.it (S.S.); luigi.gallo@unipd.it (L.G.)
* Correspondence: paolo.mongillo@unipd.it

Received: 11 August 2020; Accepted: 19 September 2020; Published: 23 September 2020

 check for updates

Simple Summary: Mixing unacquainted growing pigs is a common practice in commercial herds to adjust the group size to the pen dimensions and to balance the body weights of pigs within pens. Aggressive behavior following regrouping may include fights that can result in skin lesions and detrimental economic effects. Strategies aimed at limiting such issues can therefore improve animal welfare in practice. In the present study, we investigated the effects of darkness, maintained for 48 h after the formation of new social groups, on the expression of agonistic behavior and on the accumulation of skin lesions of growing pigs. The provision of 48 h of darkness significantly reduced the number of skin lesions on the mid- and rear thirds of pigs' body. However, no corresponding reduction was observed in agonistic behavior, suggesting that darkness decreases the efficacy of aggressions, rather than how often or for how long they are expressed. Furthermore, an analysis of the location of lesions indicates that aggressions towards a fleeing companion, rather than reciprocal ones, were those mostly affected by darkness. The present results identify in the provision of darkness an easily applicable and relatively inexpensive intervention, that leads to the reduction of one of the most problematic consequences of agonistic interactions, i.e., skin lesions.

Abstract: Agonistic behavior after the regrouping of unfamiliar pigs has been recognized as one of the major welfare issues for pig husbandry, as it may result in lesions, lameness, and health problems. One scarcely investigated strategy to curb agonistic behavior is reducing the availability of visual stimuli potentially eliciting aggressions. In this study, we investigated the expression of agonistic behavior by growing pigs and the resulting accumulation of skin lesions over a period of 14 days following the formation of new social groups, which occurred in a condition of darkness maintained for 48 h. Compared to a simulated natural photoperiod (12 h light/day), darkness significantly reduced the number of skin lesions on the mid- and rear thirds of pigs' body ($p \leq 0.01$). A lack of corresponding decrease in frequency and duration of agonistic interactions suggests that darkness acts by decreasing the efficacy, not the expression, of aggressions. Furthermore, the location of lesions mostly affected by darkness indicates that the latter mostly acted by reducing the possibility of pigs to convey damage to a fleeing conspecific, rather than to one involved in a reciprocal fighting. The lighting regime provided did not affect growth performance traits of a 17-weeks feeding trial. The present results identify in the provision of darkness an easily applicable, and relatively inexpensive intervention, that leads to the reduction of skin lesions.

Keywords: aggression; agonistic behavior; darkness; light; mixing; photoperiod; pig; regrouping; skin lesions; *Sus scrofa*

1. Introduction

Growing pigs in commercial herds are usually subjected to mixing events with unrelated and unacquainted animals [1]. This management procedure may occur several times from birth to slaughter [2] and generally aims at balancing the body weight of pigs within pens, in order to increase uniformity and to control stocking density by adjusting the group size to the pen dimensions [3]. Following regrouping, agonistic behavior may be intense, primarily serving to establish a new relative social ranking, thereby reducing future needs of disputes among animals [4]. Agonistic behavior can lead to fights, which result in skin lesions (SL), frequently used as a practical indicator of the extent and the severity of post-mixing aggressive behavior [5], as well as increased risk of lameness and of infections due to immunosuppressive effects [6]. Apart from the negative effects on animal welfare, the regrouping of unfamiliar pigs may also cause detrimental economic effects, negatively affecting growth rate and meat quality [3].

Agonistic behavior aimed at establishing relative social ranking in wild boars and feral pigs rarely ends with severe aggressions (i.e., bites), thanks to greater freedom of movement due to space allowance and fighting tactics based on complex and gradual behaviors [1,7]. Starting with reciprocal visual and olfactory inspection and gentle nudging, the interactions may escalate up to full-blown fights depending on signals indicating opponents' intention to submit [8–11]. When the overt fight is started, the behavioral patterns mainly aim at minimizing the risk of being bitten and increasing the likeliness of biting. Accordingly, strategies at regrouping should reduce the number of interactions that escalate to aggressions or reduce the efficacy of aggressions in terms of reciprocal injuries. In this respect, several studies have investigated the efficacy of manipulating housing system, pen dimension, stocking density, and group size as methods to reduce aggressive consequences [1,3]. The introduction of environmental enrichment, which may increase the opportunity to carry out exploratory behavior and diverting pigs' attention from conspecifics, has been explored [12], though with controversial results [1]. Other studies focused on the possibility to manipulate access to olfactory stimuli involved in the escalation of interactions by exposing animals to a diverse class of chemicals capable of altering olfactory information [13,14]. Much less attention has been paid to the possibility of manipulating visual signals and lighting regime; that has proven to affect growth rate and meat and ham quality of heavy pigs [15] and may be implicated in the escalation of inter-pig interactions.

To our knowledge, the manipulation of visual signals was only implemented by grouping animals after sunset [16,17], taking advantage of the lower phase of the circadian rhythm in a pig's activity. In these conditions, the number of aggressions was reduced by about 50% in the 90 min following mixing, but this effect disappeared the following morning, resulting in a comparable number of SL after three days from regrouping. Although these results suggest that darkness only delays aggressions, the beneficial effects of reducing visual information at mixing might have been biased due to the duration of the treatment used. Indeed, the higher amount of fighting between pigs occurs in the first 24–48 h after regrouping [6], which suggests a possible advantage in applying darkness for longer than one night. Moreover, if darkness affects aggression by reducing availability of opponents' visual information, extending its period of application could reduce outcome of aggressions (i.e., reciprocal injuries), regardless of their occurrence.

The aim of the present study was to deepen our knowledge on the effects of darkness at regrouping on aggressive behavior and skin lesions of growing pigs in a commercial farming situation.

2. Materials and Methods

2.1. Animals, Housing, and Experimental Design

The pigs involved in the present study are part of a larger feeding trial carried out at the research farm of the DAFNAE Department of the University of Padova, Italy [18–20]. Pigs were reared in accordance with EU Directive (2008/120/EC), and experimental procedures were reviewed and approved by the Ethical Committee for the Care and Use of Experimental Animals of the University of Padova, in accordance with the Italian legislation (D.Lgs. 26/2014, transposition of the EU 2010/63/UE directive).

Data were collected on 100 pigs (skin lesion counts) and 48 pigs (behavior observations)—specifically, barrows and gilts belonging to four different genetic types used in Italy for the production of heavy pigs to provide dry-cured hams. The piglets, who were born within the same week, arrived at the research farm around 80 d old and with a body weight (BW) close to 38 kg. At arrival, and until the beginning of the study, pigs were kept in four pens, homogeneous for genetic type (12 or 13 pigs/pen, two pens for each genetic type) and fed the same commercial diets according to the same feeding regime until the twenty-second week of age (86.5 ± 6.5 kg BW). Pens were located in two rooms (four pens/room), managed with the same ambient conditions and with an identical arrangement of pens within each room. Each pen was 5.8 × 3.8 m, had a slatted floor, and was equipped with a single-space electronic feeder (Compident Pig–MLP; Schauer Agrotronic, Prambachkirchen, Austria). Readers are referred to Schiavon et al. [18] for further details regarding the characteristics of pigs, their diets, growth performance, and carcass traits.

At the beginning of the study, the pigs were mixed, with the formation of new social groups, housed in the eight pens described above. Each of the eight groups was composed of 12 or 13 individuals (stocking density ≥ 1.6 m²/pig). Groups were balanced for BW, genetic types (e.g., each pen containing three or four pigs per genetic type), and sex (six or seven gilts and barrows per pen, and one or two of each sex, for each genetic type).

During mixing procedures (Day 0) and for the subsequent 48 h, a lighting regimen of darkness was kept in one of the two rooms (Figure 1), thus affecting half of the pigs ($n = 50$) in the study; darkness was obtained by covering the windows, the only source of ambient light in the room, with a fourfold black plastic polypropylene sheets. Simulated natural photoperiod (12 h light/day) was reintroduced in this room at h 10:00 of Day 2 and maintained for the rest of the experiment; that ended after two weeks at Day 14. In the other room, a lighting regimen of 12 h light/day was kept for the entire duration of the experiment (windows were covered in this room as well to obtain precise control on the photoperiod). Apart from the lighting regimen in the first 48 h following mixing procedures, pigs of the two rooms were managed and fed in the same way.

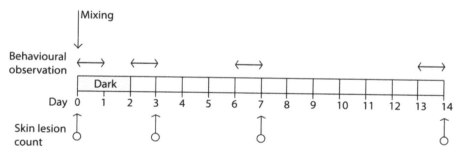

Figure 1. Schedule of skin lesion counting (on eight pens, $n = 100$ pigs) and behavior observations (on four pens, $n = 48$ pigs), relative to the day of mixing (Day 0); darkness was applied to half of the pens for the first 48 h after mixing (grey area).

2.2. Skin Lesion Counts

The total number of SL was recorded for each pig immediately before mixing (Day 0), after 72 h post-mixing (Day 3), 24 h after the natural photoperiod was reintroduced in the darkened room, and at Day 7 and Day 14 following regrouping (Figure 1). Lesions were recorded by direct observation of each pig, and it was performed independently by two trained observers who counted the total number of fresh lesions. A lesion was defined as a single and continuous scratch, regardless of severity, whereas freshness was judged on the basis of lesion color, usually red-pink, and development of scabbing [21,22]. Lesions were recorded independently on three different locations of the body: front (head, neck, shoulders, and front legs), middle (flanks and back), and the rear part of the animal (rump, hind legs, and tail), because the accumulation of skin lesions in different locations has been associated with different types of agonistic behavior [5,22].

2.3. Behavioral Observations

Infrared cameras, capable of recording in the dark, were installed overhead (Bullet IP cam, Y-cam Solutions Ltd., London, UK). Each camera framed the area occupied by one pen. A total of four cameras were installed, two for each room. Therefore, behavioral data were collected from a subsample of 48 animals, equally balanced between those subjected to darkness, and those kept in a 12 h photoperiod. Unfortunately, it was not possible to identify pigs of different genetic type or gender on videos, so these effects were not considered in the statistical models in which behavioral observations were analyzed.

To avoid interference due to the presence of operators performing the SL count, behavioral data were collected during the 24 h preceding each SL count. The only exception was represented by the behavioral data collected in the first 24 h following the regrouping of pigs, which occurred the day after the first (baseline) SL count. Collection of behavioral data was performed with the Observer software (ver. 12, Noldus Inc., Groeningen, the Netherdlands) on videos recorded on the following days of the trial (Figure 1):

- First session: from 10:00 a.m. (immediately after the end of mixing procedures) to 9:59 a.m., of Day 1;
- Second session: from 10:00 a.m. of Day 2 (immediately after reintroduction of the normal photoperiod in the pens that received the dark lighting regimen) to 9:59 a.m. of Day 3;
- Third session: from 10:00 a.m. of Day 6 to 9:59 a.m. of Day 7;
- Fourth session: from 10:00 a.m. of Day 13 to 9:59 a.m. of Day 14 (end of the trial).

Observations were performed in one interval of 10 min for each of the 24 h of observation days, resulting in a total of 24 intervals per day of observation and 96 intervals per pen for the whole study. During each observation interval, the expression of agonistic behavior by individual pigs was recorded with a focal animal, continuous sampling technique [23]. Agonistic behavior was defined as any interaction involving bites, attempts to bite, physical contact aimed at displacing, or putting off balance another pig (e.g., by pushing one's body against the other, or by putting one's muzzle under the body of the other pig). When such agonistic interaction lasted less than 1 s (i.e., one bite or one attempt to bite not followed by any other agonistic behavior), they were recorded as point events (AGO < 1 s). When the interactions lasted more than 1 s (AGO > 1 s), their duration was recorded, resulting in both number and duration of these interactions being used in statistical analysis.

Since the recording of agonistic behavior was performed for each pig in the pen, an interaction involving only two pigs would result in two recorded episodes of agonistic behavior of identical duration. For interactions involving more than two animals, as many episodes were recorded, as was the number of animals involved; the duration of such episodes, however, could be different since subjects could be involved for a different time in the same interaction (e.g., pig A starts an agonistic interaction with pig B, then pig C is involved along with A and B, then B stops interacting, leaving A and C to continue the interaction; in this case, three episodes of different duration would be recorded).

In addition to agonistic behavior, the number of animals in quadrupedal stance at the beginning of the 10 min observation interval was recorded as a measure of overall activity in the pen within the observation interval (STAND).

2.4. Performance Traits

In order to evaluate possible long-term effects of the darkness condition provided in the first 48 h following mixing, the main performance traits recorded for pigs in the feeding trial were taken into account. To this purpose, individual BW was collected at the start and at the end of the feeding trial for all the animals (100 pigs and eight pens), whereas individual feed intake (ADFI) was measured daily through the electronic feeder [18]. Data collected were used to compute individual average daily gain during the feeding trial (ADG), average individual daily feed intake, and individual feed efficiency, expressed as gain to feed ratio (G:F).

2.5. Editing and Statistical Analysis

Total SL count was computed for each pig by summing the SL recorded on the three different locations of the body. Behavioral observations were partitioned in two classes according to the daytime hours in which they occurred (DH: 08:00 to 19:59 h and 20:00 to 07:59 h), which also corresponded to the time at which lights were turned on/off, respectively, with the exception of the first 48 h in the pigs subjected to the dark lighting regimen. After a preliminary analysis aimed at examining their approximation to the normal distribution, data about the SL and the number of agonistic interactions were log transformed prior to statistical analysis.

Log of SL counts were analyzed according to a linear mixed model (SAS 9.4, SAS Institute, Cary, NC, USA) that included the fixed effects of sex (two levels), genetic types (four levels), lighting regime in the first 48 h following mixing (LR, two levels), days of the trial (DAY, four levels), operator (two levels), the DAY × LR interaction, and the random effects of pen within LR and of animal within genetic type and sex. Polynomial contrasts were estimated between the least square means of DAY to examine the response curve of each trait (linear, quadratic, and cubic components) with the advancing of time after mixing. Contrasts between least squares means of LR were estimated separately within each DAY for traits where the LR × DM interaction was significant ($p < 0.05$).

Data concerning the logarithm of the number of AGO < 1 s and AGO > 1 s, the total and mean duration of AGO > 1 s, and the incidence of STAND were analyzed according to a linear mixed model (SAS 9.4, SAS Institute, Cary, NC, USA) that included the fixed effects of LR, days from mixing (DM, four levels), daytime hours (DH, two levels) and the LR × DM and LR × DH interactions, and the random effects of hour of observation within DH and of pen within LR. Polynomial contrasts were estimated between the four least square means of DM to examine the response curve of each trait (linear, quadratic, and cubic components) with the advancing of time after mixing. Contrasts between least squares means of LR were estimated separately within each DH for traits where the LR × DH interaction was significant ($p < 0.05$).

Last, performance traits were analyzed according to a linear mixed model (SAS 9.4, SAS Institute, Cary, NC, USA) that included the fixed effects of sex (two levels), genetic types (four levels), diet (four levels), and LR, and the random effect of pen within LR and diet.

3. Results

3.1. General Statistics and Skin Lesions Count

Descriptive statistics of main performance traits recorded on pigs during the whole feeding trial, of SL counts, and of behavioral observation traits during the two weeks following pigs' regrouping are given in Table 1.

At the beginning of the feeding trial, when the pigs were moved to new pens and regrouped, the average BW of pigs approached 87 kg. At the end of the feeding trial, after around 17 weeks on feed, the BW of pigs averaged around 165 kg, which is the target weight for heavy pigs aimed to dry-cured ham production. The ADG was close to 0.66 kg/d and, given an ADFI around 2500 g/d from the start to the end of the trial, the average F:G ratio approached 3.85. The coefficient of variability was below 10% for all performance traits considered except for growth rate, which showed a coefficient of variation close to 14%.

At the fourteenth day following the regrouping procedure, an average total number of 5.24 skin lesions was recorded, with 56% of them being located in the front body area, whereas the middle and rear body area showed a similar SL count distribution. Variation in SL count was high for all the locations in the body.

Table 1. Descriptive statistics of main performance traits of growing pigs and of skin lesions count, number of agonistic interactions shorter and longer than 1 s (AGO > 1 s), total and mean duration of AGO > 1 s, and incidence of standing pigs on total number of pigs in the pen (STAND).

Item	No	Mean	SD	Min	Max
Main performance traits of pigs:					
Initial body weight, kg	100	86.5	6.9	66.4	103.7
Final body weight, kg	96	164.4	13.4	131.0	196.7
Average daily gain, kg/d	96	660	94	428	844
Average daily feed intake, g/d	96	2515	236	1696	2903
Feed to gain ratio	96	3.85	0.35	3.29	4.77
Counts of skin lesions assessed on:					
Front, no	798	2.98	3.58	0	29
Middle, no	798	1.21	2.01	0	17
Rear, no	798	1.04	1.54	0	12
Sum of skin lesions count, no	798	5.24	5.84	0	40
Agonistic interactions shorter than 1 s, no	383	1.78	3.42	0	26
Agonistic interactions longer than 1 s, no	383	2.59	5.16	0	38
Total duration of AGO > 1 s, s	114	56	99	2	649
Mean duration of AGO > 1 s, s	114	6.9	6.4	1	38
STAND, %	383	16.7	20.1	0	100

The average number of AGO > 1 s in the 10 min/h of observation interval approached 2.59, with an average mean duration close to 7 s, whereas on average, 17% of pigs in the pen were standing at the beginning of the 10 min of the observation interval. Additionally, for the behavioral observations, the variation observed was very large.

Average accumulation of SL in the two weeks following pigs regrouping was not influenced by the lighting regime adopted in the first 48 h from mixing (Table 2) independently from the body area. Conversely, the day of trial significantly influenced the distribution of SL irrespective of their position in the body ($p < 0.0001$). As a general trend, the change of log of SL with the advancing of days after regrouping followed a quadratic (SL evaluated in the flanks and back and total sum of SL counts) or cubic (SL evaluated in the front or in the rear part of the body) pattern. Namely, log of SL increased from the day of mixing (Day 0 was considered as a baseline reference for SL) until Day 3 (head, neck, shoulders, and front legs) or 7 from mixing (middle and rear part of the body and total sum of SL counts), whereas it decreased thereafter in all positions of the body.

Moreover, we found a significant ($p \leq 0.01$) LR × DAY interaction for all the SL counts except for those in the front body area; this suggests that the dynamic of SL accumulation was different according to the lighting regime provided to the pigs during the first 48 h since regrouping. Indeed, pigs kept in the dark room during the first 48 h since regrouping showed a similar pattern of variation since the day of mixing but lower SL accumulation 3 and 7 d following mixing, compared to those pigs provided with a 12 h photoperiod for the whole trial (Figure 2). Differences in SL accumulation between pigs of the two groups were no longer evident 14 d after mixing, with the only exception of skin lesions in the rear part of the body.

Table 2. Least squares means of logarithm of skin lesions count (SL) for lighting regimen during the first 48 h after mixing and days of trial.

Item	Body Location			Log of Sum of SL
	Front	Middle	Rear	
Lighting regimen (LR)				
0 h/d light	1.00	0.47	0.36	1.33
12 h/d light	1.18	0.61	0.67	1.63
SEM	0.10	0.09	0.10	0.14
p value	>0.10	>0.10	0.07	>0.10

Table 2. *Cont.*

Item	Body Location			Log of Sum of SL
	Front	Middle	Rear	
Days of trial (DAY)				
0	0.59	0.31	0.30	0.94
3	1.50	0.69	0.57	1.84
7	1.42	0.79	0.80	1.92
14	0.86	0.37	0.40	1.22
SEM	0.08	0.07	0.08	0.10
p value of effect	<0.0001	<0.0001	<0.0001	<0.0001
p value of contrasts:				
Linear	<0.0001	0.05	0.0002	<0.0001
Quadratic	<0.0001	<0.0001	<0.0001	<0.0001
Cubic	0.01	>0.10	<0.0001	>0.10
LR × DAY				
p value	>0.10	0.01	0.001	0.01

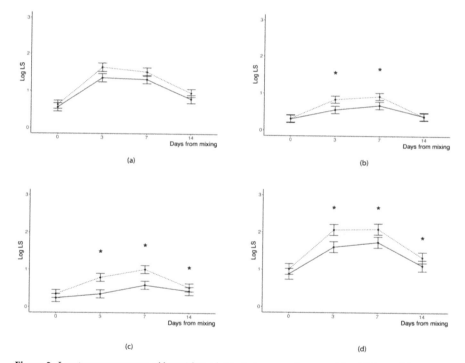

(a)   (b)

(c)   (d)

Figure 2. Least squares means of logarithm of skin lesions count assessed in: (**a**) front, (**b**) middle, and (**c**) rear position and of (**d**) logarithm of sum of counts at different days from mixing (Days Mix) for pigs kept in dark rooms (solid line) or with a 12 h photoperiod (dotted line) during the first 48 h after mixing (*$p < 0.05$ for difference between means of the two groups within any given day from mixing).

3.2. Behavioral Observations

Table 3 reports the least squares means of the agonistic behavior variables and of the overall activity, as a function of lighting regimen, days of trial, and daytime hours, as well as the LR × DM and LR × DH interactions on the same variables. No effect was found for the LR or its interaction with DAY on any of the agonistic behavioral variables or the overall activity.

Table 3. Least squares means of the number of agonistic interactions shorter (AGO < 1 s) and longer than 1 s (AGO > 1 s), of the total and mean duration of AGO > 1 s, and of the incidence of standing pigs on total number of pigs in the pen (STAND) for lighting regimen during the first 48 h after mixing, session of observation, and daytime hours [1].

Item	AGO < 1 s, log	AGO > 1 s, log	Duration of AGO > 1 s, s		STAND, %
			Total	Mean	
Lighting regimen (LR)					
0 h/d light	0.64	0.73	39	6	17.3
12 h/d light	0.57	0.64	41	5	16.2
SEM	0.14	0.14	20	2	2.6
p value	>0.10	>0.10	>0.10	>0.10	>0.10
Session of observation (DAY)					
First (day of trial 0 to 1)	0.70	0.88	103	9	20.3
Second (day of trial 2 to 3)	0.53	0.66	39	5	13.8
Third (day of trial 6 to 7)	0.54	0.60	4	5	15.9
Fourth (day of trial 13 to 14)	0.65	0.58	13	5	16.7
SEM	0.13	0.13	19	1	2.7
p value of effect	>0.10	0.06	<0.0001	0.007	0.05
p value of contrasts:					
Linear		0.01	<0.0001	0.01	>0.10
Quadratic		>0.10	0.02	0.07	0.03
Cubic		>0.10	>0.10	>0.10	>0.10
Daytime hours (DH)					
08:00 to 19:59 h	0.86	1.02	65	8	24.1
20:00 to 07:59 h	0.35	0.34	15	3	9.3
SEM	0.13	0.14	17	1	8.0
p value	0.001	<0.001	0.02	<0.001	<0.001
LR × DAY					
p value	>0.10	>0.10	>0.10	>0.10	>0.10
LR × DH					
p value	>0.10	0.07	>0.10	>0.10	>0.10

[1] Agonistic behavior and activity measured during the first 10 min of each hour.

There were more AGO < 1 during daytime than at night ($p = 0.001$); no change was observed in the number of such interactions as a function of DAY.

There were more agonistic interactions longer than 1 s during daytime than at night, and they were also longer, in terms of average as well as total duration. The mean and total duration of such interactions decreased with increasing days from mixing, and fewer of such interactions occurred as the days from mixing increased.

The incidence of standing pigs on total number of pigs in the pen was affected in a similar manner, with a higher overall activity during daytime than at night, and a decrease of overall activity as a function of days from mixing.

3.3. Performance Traits

As shown in Figure 3, the lighting regime during the first 48 h following regrouping did not affect growth performance traits of a 17-weeks feeding trial ($p > 0.10$). Pigs of two groups showed similar BW at the end of the feeding trial and comparable growth rate. As average feed intake was nearly identical in pigs provided with 48 h dark or normal photoperiod after mixing, the feed-to-gain ratios of the pigs of the two groups were also very similar.

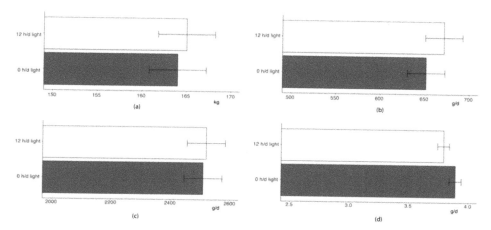

Figure 3. Least squares means of: (**a**) final BW, (**b**) overall average daily gain, (**c**) average daily feed intake, and (**d**) feed-to-gain ratio of pigs given 0 h (grey bar) or 12 h light daily (white bar) during the first 48 h after mixing (*p* value of the differences between means > 0.10).

4. Discussion

Agonistic behavior expressed when unfamiliar pigs are housed into newly formed social groups has been recognized as a one of the major welfare issues for pig husbandry [1]. Although aggression following mixing of growing or breeding pigs has been widely investigated in the last decades, mitigation strategies proposed seem scarcely implemented in commercial herds, so that the problem has not been reduced yet [3,4]. In the present study, we investigated if the provision of darkness in the 48 h after the formation of new social groups in growing pigs is effective in reducing the expression of agonistic behavior, and its outcome in terms of accumulated skin lesions.

Skin lesions are a useful and practical indicator of aggressive behavior and poor welfare, as their assessment requires little time, no specific equipment, and limited training [22]. Moreover, SL are a direct outcome of physical damages due to agonistic interactions, and their frequency and intensity can be related to the level of welfare impairment following regrouping.

In this study, a large variation in the total number of SL was found, similar to Turner et al. [5]. In agreement with the latter and other studies [5,9,24], lesions were mostly concentrated in frontal part of the body. Turner and collaborators [5] suggested that lesions in such region are the outcome of reciprocal active fighting, whereas those accumulated in the medium and rear part of the body are correlated to receiving aggression and retreating.

The accumulation of SL progressively increased over time, from the third to the seventh day of trial for front SL and middle, rear, and total ones, respectively. This pattern is generally consistent with data from the literature, although the schedule of SL evaluation after regrouping is variable. Turner and collaborators [5] observed an increase of SL 24 h post-mixing in the vast majority of pigs evaluated, with a greater increase for front SL compared to the rear body part. Similarly, Wurtz and collaborators [22] reported a steep increase of SL in all body locations 24 h following regrouping, whereas three weeks after regrouping SL decreased and accumulation was generally lower than that scored at regrouping. Stukenborg and collaborators [24] observed an increase in SL evaluated 48 h after regrouping on the front part of the body on the majority of pigs considered; conversely, no positive difference was found for over 60% and 70% of pigs in LS observed in the middle and rear regions, respectively, concluding that their contribution in the prediction of agonistic behavior seemed to be rather insignificant. Differences in the trend of variation of SL found in the present study could corroborate such conclusion, as front SL peaked 3 d after mixing, including the period when agonistic behavior is particularly intense, whereas SL judged at the medium and rear parts of the body peaked at later times.

Keeping pigs in the dark during the first 48 h since regrouping, compared to those provided with a 12 h photoperiod for the whole trial, did not affect the average accumulation of SL over the two weeks following regrouping or the pattern of variation of SL since the day of mixing; however, it significantly decreased the sum of SL and the accumulation of SL in the medium and rear part of the body in the first 7 d following regrouping, thus mitigating the negative effects of mixing unfamiliar pigs on skin integrity. Barnett and collaborators [16] observed a short-term decrease of aggression in pigs mixed 30 min after sunset compared to pigs mixed in the morning. However, the accumulation of SL three days post-mixing was similar between groups, suggesting that mixing after sunset simply delayed SL rather than really mitigating the effects of regrouping.

With regard to agonistic behavior, its expression was mostly affected by the time of day, with both duration and frequency of agonistic interactions being fourfold higher during daytime than nighttime. Our results are in agreement with previous studies reporting higher peaks in the expression of agonistic interactions in the middle of the day and lower peaks at night following a circadian rhythm [24]. In the present study, this pattern was clearly associated with the pigs' overall activity level, which was also, predictably, lower at night than during daytime. It is worth noting, however, that no difference in the effect of daytime on agonistic behavior or activity levels was found between the two experimental groups. Therefore, the provision of 48 h of darkness did not alter pigs' circadian rhythm, at least in terms of behavior. Although the timing by which photoperiod acts on agonistic behavior has not been investigated before, other physiological traits, such as melatonin concentrations, have been shown to closely follow abrupt changes in photoperiod; nonetheless, even melatonin secretion may take up to one week to fully entrain after a new photoperiod is instated [25]. Thus, our findings are well consistent with a lack of relevant effects in the provision of 48 h of darkness on circadian rhythm.

Agonistic behavior was also affected by the time elapsed from the day of mixing. The effect was clearly evident on the average and total duration of agonistic interaction, which decreased linearly (for average and total duration) or along a quadratic curve (average duration only), from Day 0 to the fourteenth day after mixing. Additionally, the number of agonistic interactions longer than 1 s decreased linearly with the advancing of days of trial, whereas no significant effect of day from mixing was observed on the number of short, instantaneous agonistic events. Therefore, although agonistic behaviors do not cease to occur, they appear to be solved significantly faster over time [26]. Therefore, our results confirm that aggressive behaviors aimed at re-establishing a social hierarchy in the new groups mostly occur during the first 48 h after mixing, as previously reported [6].

Previous studies suggested that impeding access to visual stimuli when groups of unacquainted pigs are newly formed may reduce the expression of agonistic behavior [16]. However, as the aggressions resume at the re-establishment of visibility (end of darkness period), this practice merely delayed the expression of this behavior [16]. In our experiment, the expression of agonistic behavior was not affected by the provision of 48 h of darkness, nor by its interaction with the time from mixing, indicating that agonistic interactions were concentrated during the first days after mixing, and progressively decreased over time, in both groups. This implies that there was no rebound in the frequency or duration of agonistic interactions in animals that had been kept in darkness once visibility was re-established. Our results are in contrast with those reported by Barnett et al. [16], who observed increased agonistic interactions between pigs being mixed before a 12 h (overnight) of darkness as the end of this period coincided with the peak of expression of agonistic behaviors within the group of pigs. On the contrary, in our study, this peak occurred while pigs were still kept in the dark, indicating that the provision of a 48-h period of darkness is sufficient to overcome such an acute agonistic phase; at the same time, the period is long enough to avoid relapses when visual stimuli are again made available. A further implication of the lack of differences between experimental groups in the expression of agonistic behavior over time is that the removal of visual stimuli of conspecifics does not seem to prevent pigs from engaging in agonistic interactions, nor to carry them on for as long as in plain visibility. Thus, at least in the conditions assessed by the present study, other sensory modalities seem sufficient to drive pigs' agonistic behavior. Again, this is in line with previous literature, showing not only a significant role of olfactory [27–30] and pheromonal perception [14,31,32] on agonistic behavior, but also that removal of visual stimuli (e.g., by temporarily blinding the animals, or by covering their heads with hoods) brings no alteration in pigs ability to form and maintain a hierarchy [33,34].

At first glance, the significant effect of the provision of darkness in the first days after regrouping on the accumulation of SL stands at odds with a lack of corresponding effects on the frequency and duration of agonistic behavior. On a closer look, however, the two findings are quite informative of the mechanism by which darkness affected pigs' agonistic behavior. While the lack of availability of visual stimuli did not seem to be a relevant factor in eliciting agonistic behavior, it did impact pigs' abilities to accurately aim at the opponent and inflict damage. It should be further noted that the difference in SL between experimental groups was limited to the mid- and rear body regions, rather than the frontal ones. As discussed above, the differential location of SL is thought to reflect a different role of the animal in the agonistic interaction [5]. In this sense, the lack of access to visual stimuli, rather than impacting the efficacy of close-contact, reciprocated fights, seems to have reduced the possibility of pigs to convey damage to a fleeing companion.

Last, managing photoperiod in the first 48 h following regrouping did not affect long-term performance of pigs. Indeed, pigs of the two groups evidenced comparable growth rate and feed efficiency and ended the 17 weeks of finishing at similar BW.

5. Conclusions

In this study, we showed that provision of 48 h of darkness in newly formed groups of fattening pigs significantly reduces the accumulation of skin lesions, particularly on the mid- and rear thirds of pigs' bodies. A lack of corresponding decrease in frequency and duration of agonistic interactions indicates that darkness acts by decreasing the efficacy of aggressions. Furthermore, the location of lesions mostly affected by darkness indicates that the effect was specific to aggressions towards a fleeing subject. The present findings have both theoretical and practical relevance. On the one hand, they shed light on the (limited) role of visual stimuli in eliciting agonistic behavior in pigs. They also provide suggestive evidence that an abrupt alteration of photoperiod does not bear a relevant impact on pig circadian rhythms, at least for what concerns overall activity levels and agonistic behavior. On the other hand, the results identify in the provision of darkness an easily applicable and relatively inexpensive intervention that leads to the reduction of one of the most problematic consequences of agonistic interactions, i.e., skin lesions. Certainly, some aspects will have to be addressed in further studies. For instance, it would be important to determine if the positive effects of darkness would also be observed in different categories of pigs than the ones assessed in this study (e.g., younger animals, intact males, pigs belonging to other genetic types). Moreover, it would be interesting to assess whether longer extension of the darkness period would exert more profound effects on the expression of agonistic interactions or their outcomes. However, considering the relatively quick effects that abrupt changes may have in the circadian rhythm in pigs, it is possible that longer exposures to darkness would have a larger effect, including possibly undesirable consequences on their welfare or growth.

Author Contributions: Conceptualization, L.M., L.G.; methodology, L.M., P.M., S.S., P.C., and L.G.; writing—original draft preparation, L.M., P.M., and L.G.; investigation, L.M., P.M., S.S., P.C., and L.G.; writing—review and editing, L.M., S.S., P.C., and L.G. All authors have read and agreed to the published version of the manuscript.

Funding: This research was funded and supported by Progetto AGER (Italy).

Acknowledgments: The authors greatly appreciate the technical assistance of Alberto Simonetto, Luca Carraro, Carlo Poltronieri, and Mirco Dalla Bona.

Conflicts of Interest: The authors declare no conflict of interest. The funders had no role in the design of the study; in the collection, analyses, or interpretation of data; in the writing of the manuscript, or in the decision to publish the results.

References

1. Marchant-Forde, J.; Marchant-Forde, R.M. Minimizing inter-pig aggression during mixing. *Pig News Inf.* **2005**, *26*, 63–71.
2. Camerlink, I.; Turner, S.P. Farmers' perception of aggression between growing pigs. *Appl. Anim. Behav. Sci.* **2017**, *192*, 42–47. [CrossRef]
3. Peden, R.S.E.; Turner, S.P.; Boyle, L.A.; Camerlink, I. The translation of animal welfare research into practice: The case of mixing aggression between pigs. *Appl. Anim. Behav. Sci.* **2018**, *204*, 1–9. [CrossRef]
4. Meese, G.B.; Ewbank, R. The establishment and nature of the dominance hierarchy in the domesticated pig. *Anim. Behav.* **1973**, *21*, 326–334. [CrossRef]
5. Turner, S.P.; Farnworth, M.J.; White, I.M.S.; Brotherstone, S.; Mendl, M.; Knap, P.; Penny, P.; Lawrence, A.B. The accumulation of skin lesions and their use as a predictor of individual aggressiveness in pigs. *Appl. Anim. Behav. Sci.* **2006**, *96*, 245–259. [CrossRef]
6. Ison, S.H.; Bates, R.O.; Ernst, C.W.; Steibel, J.P.; Siegford, J.M. Housing, ease of handling and minimising inter-pig aggression at mixing for nursery to finishing pigs as reported in a survey of North American pork producers. *Appl. Anim. Behav. Sci.* **2018**, *205*, 159–166. [CrossRef]
7. Gabor, T.M.; Hellgren, E.C.; Bussche, R.A.; Silvy, N.J. Demography, sociospatial behaviour and genetics of feral pigs (Sus scrofa) in a semi-arid environment. *J. Zool.* **1999**, *247*, 311–322. [CrossRef]
8. Jensen, P. An analysis of agonistic interaction patterns in group-housed dry sows—Aggression regulation through an "avoidance order". *Appl. Anim. Ethol.* **1982**, *9*, 47–61. [CrossRef]
9. McGlone, J.J. A Quantitative Ethogram of Aggressive and Submissive Behaviors in Recently Regrouped Pigs1. *J. Anim. Sci.* **1985**, *61*, 556–566. [CrossRef]
10. McGlone, J.J. Olfactory cues and pig agonistic behavior: Evidence for a submissive pheromone. *Physiol. Behav.* **1985**, *34*, 195–198. [CrossRef]
11. Camerlink, I.; Arnott, G.; Farish, M.; Turner, S.P. Complex contests and the influence of aggressiveness in pigs. *Anim. Behav.* **2016**, *121*, 71–78. [CrossRef]
12. Godyń, D.; Nowicki, J.; Herbut, P. Effects of Environmental Enrichment on Pig Welfare—A Review. *Animals* **2019**, *9*, 383. [CrossRef] [PubMed]
13. Barnett, J.L.; Cronin, G.M.; McCallum, T.H.; Newman, E.A. Effects of "chemical intervention" techniques on aggression and injuries when grouping unfamiliar adult pigs. *Appl. Anim. Behav. Sci.* **1993**, *36*, 135–148. [CrossRef]
14. Guy, J.H.; Burns, S.E.; Barker, J.M.; Edwards, S.A. Reducing post-mixing aggression and skin lesions in weaned pigs by application of a synthetic maternal pheromone. *Anim. Welf.* **2009**, *18*, 249–255.
15. Martelli, G.; Nannoni, E.; Grandi, M.; Bonaldo, A.; Zaghini, G.; Vitali, M.; Biagi, G.; Sardi, L. Growth parameters, behavior, and meat and ham quality of heavy pigs subjected to photoperiods of different duration. *J. Anim. Sci.* **2015**, *93*, 758–766. [CrossRef]
16. Barnett, J.L.; Cronin, G.M.; McCallum, T.H.; Newman, E.A.; Hennessy, D.P. Effects of grouping unfamiliar adult pigs after dark, after treatment with amperozide and by using pens with stalls, on aggression, skin lesions and plasma cortisol concentrations. *Appl. Anim. Behav. Sci.* **1996**, *50*, 121–133. [CrossRef]
17. Barnett, J.L.; Cronin, G.M.; McCallum, T.H.; Newman, E.A. Effects of food and time of day on aggression when grouping unfamiliar adult pigs. *Appl. Anim. Behav. Sci.* **1994**, *39*, 339–347. [CrossRef]
18. Schiavon, S.; Carraro, L.; Dalla Bona, M.; Cesaro, G.; Carnier, P.; Tagliapietra, F.; Sturaro, E.; Galassi, G.; Malagutti, L.; Trevisi, E.; et al. Growth performance, and carcass and raw ham quality of crossbred heavy pigs from four genetic groups fed low protein diets for dry-cured ham production. *Anim. Feed Sci. Technol.* **2015**, *208*, 170–181. [CrossRef]
19. Carcò, G.; Dalla Bona, M.; Carraro, L.; Latorre, M.A.; Fondevila, M.; Gallo, L.; Schiavon, S. Influence of mild feed restriction and mild reduction in dietary amino acid content on feeding behaviour of group-housed growing pigs. *Appl. Anim. Behav. Sci.* **2018**, *198*, 27–35. [CrossRef]
20. Carcò, G.; Schiavon, S.; Casiraghi, E.; Grassi, S.; Sturaro, E.; Dalla Bona, M.; Novelli, E.; Gallo, L. Influence of dietary protein content on the chemico-physical profile of dry-cured hams produced by pigs of two breeds. *Sci. Rep.* **2019**, *9*, 1–12. [CrossRef]

21. Turner, S.P.; Roehe, R.; Mekkawy, W.; Farnworth, M.J.; Knap, P.W.; Lawrence, A.B. Bayesian analysis of genetic associations of skin lesions and behavioural traits to identify genetic components of individual aggressiveness in pigs. *Behav. Genet.* **2008**, *38*, 67–75. [CrossRef] [PubMed]

22. Wurtz, K.E.; Siegford, J.M.; Bates, R.O.; Ernst, C.W.; Steibel, J.P. Estimation of genetic parameters for lesion scores and growth traits in group-housed pigs1. *J. Anim. Sci.* **2017**, *95*, 4310–4317. [CrossRef] [PubMed]

23. Martin, P.; Bateson, P. Recording Methods. In *Measuring Behaviour*; Cambridge University Press: Cambridge, UK, 1993.

24. Stukenborg, A.; Traulsen, I.; Puppe, B.; Presuhn, U.; Krieter, J. Agonistic behaviour after mixing in pigs under commercial farm conditions. *Appl. Anim. Behav. Sci.* **2011**, *129*, 28–35. [CrossRef]

25. Tast, A.; Love, R.J.; Evans, G.; Telsfer, S.; Giles, R.; Nicholls, P.; Voultsios, A.; Kennaway, D.J. The pattern of melatonin secretion is rhythmic in the domestic pig and responds rapidly to changes in daylength. *J. Pineal Res.* **2001**, *31*, 294–300. [CrossRef] [PubMed]

26. Arey, D.S.; Edwards, S.A. Factors influencing aggression between sows after mixing and the consequences for welfare and production. *Livest. Prod. Sci.* **1998**, *56*, 61–70. [CrossRef]

27. Meese, G.B.; Baldwin, B.A. The effects of ablation of the olfactory bulbs on aggressive behaviour in pigs. *Appl. Anim. Ethol.* **1975**, *1*, 251–262. [CrossRef]

28. McGlone, J.J. Olfactory signals that modulate pig aggressive and submissive behavior. *Soc. Stress Domest. Anim.* **1990**, 86–109.

29. Fuentes, M.; Otal, J.; Hevia, M.L.; Quiles, A.; Fuentes, F.C. Effect of olfactory stimulation during suckling on agonistic behavior in weaned pigs. *J. Swine Heal. Prod.* **2012**, *20*, 25–33.

30. Nowicki, J.; Swierkosz, S.; Tuz, R.; Schwarz, T. The influence of aromatized environmental enrichment objects with changeable aromas on the behaviour of weaned piglets. *Vet. Arh.* **2015**, *85*, 425–435.

31. Plush, K.; Hughes, P.; Herde, P.; van Wettere, W. A synthetic olfactory agonist reduces aggression when sows are mixed into small groups. *Appl. Anim. Behav. Sci.* **2016**, *185*, 45–51. [CrossRef]

32. McGlone, J.J.; Anderson, D.L. Synthetic maternal pheromone stimulates feeding behavior and weight gain in weaned pigs1. *J. Anim. Sci.* **2002**, *80*, 3179–3183. [CrossRef] [PubMed]

33. Ewbank, R.; Meese, G.B.; Cox, J.E. Individual recognition and the dominance hierarchy in the domesticated pig. The role of sight. *Anim. Behav.* **1974**, *22*, 473–480. [CrossRef]

34. Büttner, K.; Czycholl, I.; Mees, K.; Krieter, J. Temporal development of agonistic interactions as well as dominance indices and centrality parameters in pigs after mixing. *Appl. Anim. Behav. Sci.* **2020**, *222*, 104913. [CrossRef]

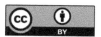

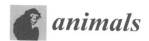

Article

Views of Farmers and Industrial Entrepreneurs on the Iberian Pig Quality Standard: An In-Depth Interview Research Study

Alberto Ortiz [1], Natalia Carrillo [2], Ahmed Elghannam [3], Miguel Escribano [2] and Paula Gaspar [2,*]

1   Meat Quality Area, Center for Scientific and Technological Research of Extremadura (CICYTEX-La Orden), Junta de Extremadura, 06187 Guadajira, Badajoz, Spain; alberto.ortiz@juntaex.es
2   Department of Animal Production and Food Science, School of Agricultural Engineering, University of Extremadura, Avda. Adolfo Suarez, s/n, 06007 Badajoz, Spain; ncarrillh@alumnos.unex.es (N.C.); mescriba@unex.es (M.E.)
3   Department of Economics, School of Agricultural Engineering, University of Extremadura, Avda. Adolfo Suarez, s/n, 06007 Badajoz, Spain; ahmedelghannam66@gmail.com
*   Correspondence: pgaspar@unex.es; Tel.: +34-924286200 (ext. 86264)

Received: 4 September 2020; Accepted: 26 September 2020; Published: 30 September 2020

Simple Summary: This paper aims to assess the main opinions of farmers and industrial entrepreneurs on the implementation of the current Spanish Iberian Pig Quality Standards regulation as well as on the processing technologies of Iberian cured products. The study is based on a qualitative research process through in-depth interviews, and has allowed the identification of aspects that can be improved both at the level of the Iberian meat industry and in the administrative processes in the view of the main actors of the Iberian pork sector in Spain. The aspects of the Quality Standard related to the protection of the base of the Iberian breed, the conditions of production in the traditional system (the montanera), as well as the ripening time of the products were mostly supported by the farmers and industrial entrepreneurs. However, they showed certain inconformity with the requirements established by the Quality Standard for other production systems such as the non-free-range fodder-fed and free-range fodder-fed, therefore they demanded changes in these aspects.

Abstract: Since 2014, the Quality Standard for Iberian meat, leg ham, shoulder ham and dry-cured loin has regulated production factors and processes involved in the raw material and manufactured products from Iberian pigs, the most important pig breed in both population size and economic importance of the southwest Iberian Peninsula. Regarding the changes to the Quality Standard that industrial entrepreneurs and farmers are currently demanding, a qualitative research study has been developed through 14 in-depth interviews with the purpose of understanding the perception of Iberian pig farmers and industrial entrepreneurs of the requirements of the currently-effective Quality Standard, as well as the conditions under which this is being applied. The results showed a consensus amongst the majority of the participants in aspects such as the maintenance of the breed base as 100% Iberian for reproductive females, weight and age requirements at the time of slaughter for the montanera category and the manufacturing lengths for dry-cured products. On the other hand, there were discrepancies between the requirements defined by the Quality Standard and those requested by the respondents for the non-free-range fodder-fed and free-range fodder-fed categories, with the industrial entrepreneurs and farmers being inclined towards the reduction in the age of slaughter of the former and the distinction in the production conditions of the latter.

Keywords: Iberian pork; quality standard; qualitative analysis; in-depth interviews

1. Introduction

Pork meat consumption represents a major part of the diet of the European countries, with pork being the most consumed and preferred meat, before chicken and beef [1]. In recent years there has been an increasing demand of meat products deriving from autochthonous breeds that are reared in extensive systems, which is potentially due to a positive perception of society as to their contribution in the preservation of the environment [2], animal welfare [3], as well as the perceived high quality of the derivative products [4].

This is the case of the Iberian pork, the most important pig breed in both population size and economic importance of the southwest Iberian Peninsula [5]. High acceptance and demand of Iberian products have enabled the development of the industry involved, which still has major problems to deal with, such as the great variability of factors associated with the various stages of the production chain, giving rise to a diversity of production models and therefore differences in the final quality of the products. These factors include the genetic background of animal [6], the production system, the feed provided to the animal, especially during the final finishing stage [7]. Additionally, animal age and weight at the beginning of the finishing stage [8] and at the time of slaughter [9,10] are factors to consider in the quality of the products derived. Further, this variability to which the Iberian pork products are subjected makes it difficult for the detection of any fraudulent activity that may take place within the industry [11].

The first Spanish Iberian Quality Standard [12] emerged in 2001 within this context with the main purpose of guaranteeing and defining the quality traits and control process, regulating Iberian pig production factors and the commercialization of their derived dry-cured products. Its subsequent amendment in 2007 [13] extended its scope of application to pork cuts that are commercialized as fresh meat. The current Spanish Iberian Quality Standard—known as the Quality Standard for Iberian meat, leg ham, shoulder ham and seasoned pork loin—came into force in 2014 [14] (hereinafter, QS) as an attempt to clarify and provide transparency to the industry, as well as providing a simpler perception of the market products and their various agreed quality standards grouping them under a new labeling system. Thus, four commercial categories (labels) were defined: the Black label (100% Iberian breed acorn-fed pigs), Red label (at least 50% Iberian breed acorn-fed pigs), Green label (at least 50% Iberian breed pigs, reared in pastures (dehesas) and fed on fodder and grass) and White label (at least 50% Iberian breed pigs, reared in confinement and fed only on fodder (Table 1).

Thus, the commercialization of the products under the aforementioned labels requires an effort by farmers, industrial entrepreneurs and traceability and control systems. This in turn means an increase in the production costs, which at times is not compensated by the selling price, given that all this effort to improve the industry is not always perceived and translated in the consumer purchasing decisions [15].

Several years since the implementation of the current QS, there is certain degree of disagreement amongst the involved stakeholders, i.e., farmers and industrial entrepreneurs, with regards to some of the requirements set out in the QS for the various categories, specifically in relation to production factor in the farm, certification process and technological processing of the products. Amongst others, one of the factors raising most of the interest and controversy within the production aspects is the age of slaughter of animals, which is determined according to production system (montanera, free-range fodder-fed and non-free-range fodder-fed) and, disregarding the animal Iberian breed percentage. Although traditionally, a long production cycle has been the preferred option for the Iberian breed in order to obtain high-quality products [8], the improvement in the production parameters deriving from the use of the Duroc breed [6]—authorized by the current quality standard—could generate a misalignment between the QS's required age of slaughter and the farmers' interests, who broadly use this breed in order to increase productivity, reduce production cycles and therefore costs. Nevertheless, in spite of the relevance of the age of slaughter [16], as far as we are concerned, there are no studies that explore the recommended age in association to genetics, and there are only few studies that assess its influence on the quality of the meat derivatives [8], [17] and therefore that may combine the demands and interests of farmers and consumers alike. On the other hand, there is a clear lack of definition of the feeding and rearing system used for pigs under the Green label category (free-range fodder-fed animals), a fact that has even led to this category being excluded from sensorial studies on account of the lack of uniformity of its production aspects [18].

Table 1. Requirements for the production aspects of the various categories of Iberian products and manufacture minimum times according to the current Quality Standard (QS).

Production Aspects	Commercial Label			
	Black Label	**Red Label**	**Green Label**	**White Label**
Breed (100%, 75% and 50% Iberian) provided that the female is 100% Iberian breed and the male is Duroc breed, both registered in a genealogic tree	100%	75%, 50%	100%, 75%, 50%	100%, 75%, 50%
Management system (the animals can be reared under various levels of intensiveness)	Extensive		Semi-intensive	Intensive
	(0.25–1.25 animals/ha) subject to the wooded area available and the availability of acorns		At least 100 square metres/animal when the live weight exceeds 110 kg	At least 2 square metres/animal when the live weight exceeds 110 kg
Weight and minimum weight gain during the finishing stage	46 kg for over 60 days		At least 60 days prior to slaughter	
Minimum age at slaughter	14 months		12 months	10 months
Feed allowed during the finishing stage for each category	Feed based only on acorn, grass and other natural resources found during *Montanera* in the *dehesa*		Feed based on fodder made of cereal and legumes with the possibility for the animals to either fully or partially rearing in *Montanera*	Fodder made of cereal and legumes
Carcass minimum weight	115 kg, except for 100% Iberian animals, which will be 108 kg			
Product	**Leg Ham**		**Shoulder Ham**	**Loin**
Minimum time of manufacture of the products	W < 7 Kg 600 days, W ≥ 7 Kg 730 days		365 days (regardless of weight)	70 days (regardless of weight)

W: weight; Own source based on the current QS [14].

Additionally, the current QS does not contemplate any measures to help overcome the seasonality to which Iberian products are subjected—especially montanera Iberian dry-cured loins, which are launched to the market in the summer months with lesser demand, and considering that the period of greatest consumption of this type of products is from November to December (because of Christmas season), there is a gap between industry and consumer demand. In order to overcome this situation, industrial entrepreneurs use practices such as freezing the raw material prior to its technological process of curing, but the lack of European Regulations for the freezing of animal products [19], together with scarce scientific literature [20,21], has led to a situation of uncertainty regarding how this practice may affect the quality of the end product, which in turn has made it difficult to regulate and control it at the industrial level.

Given the above concerns and the over four years since the implementation of the QS, it is vital to assess the current QS, as well as any improvement proposals made by the stakeholders, and thus contribute to form a bases for a decision tool that may focus on these specific industry and administrative issues.

In this context our purpose was to understand the main views of farmers and industrial entrepreneurs on the application of the current QS for the Iberian product through an in-depth interview qualitative research study, in order to identify the limitations and opportunities for the commercialization of Iberian products in the current environment.

2. Materials and Methods

This research study has been based on a qualitative method throughout in-depth interviews on account of its exploratory nature and because of the high level of controversy amongst the various stakeholders involved in this industry. The research team selected a widely-recognized semi-structured model that is largely used in these types of research studies [22]. Two versions of the interview script were designed and adapted to the purposes of the study, one per type of stakeholder (farmers and industrial entrepreneurs). Figure 1 presents the full methodological process followed for the research study.

2.1. Data Collection

For the purposes of this research study, all the interviews were face to face interviews carried out at the workplace of the respondents. The final sample was selected following a convenience sampling process, which is a non-probability type of sampling that is broadly used in qualitative research [23,24]. For this piece of research, the respondent selection process was progressive, as interviews were conducted at the same time as the respondents were classified by characteristics. Subsequently, from the information obtained, new farmers and industrial entrepreneurs with different characteristics from the ones that had already been interviewed were sought. This particular selection process was adopted with the purpose of covering the various types of businesses in terms of size (small, medium and large), categories (or labels) of products sold (Black, Red, Green and White label) and production type; both in the case of farmers (closed cycle, only montanera/fodder, other integrations) and industrial entrepreneurs (dry-cured products, fresh products, both) and finally, the various market plans for the products (local, national or international).

Subsequently, a telephone conversation was held with the selected respondents, where the purpose of the research study was explained, and they were asked cooperation in the conduction of the semi-structured interviews. Additionally, they were assured that the data provided would be confidential in compliance with the Spanish Data Protection Act. Fourteen in-depth interviews were conducted in total, seven of which were conducted with farmers and the other seven with industrial entrepreneurs. This number of interviews was in line with that of other qualitative research studies carried out using semi-structured interviews [25]. All the participants were asked for their consent to be audio recorded during the interviews and they all accepted. The average length of each interview was approximately 120 min.

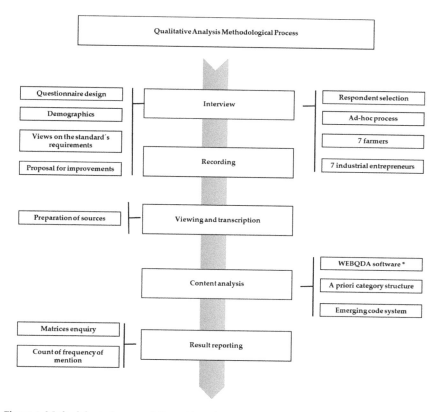

Figure 1. Methodological process followed in order to carry out the in-depth interviews. * WebQDA Software V 3.1. is a qualitative data software analysis. It allows editing, viewing, linking and organizing different sources as text documents or audio files. It can create categories, codes, manage, filter, search and question the data in order to answer the questions that emerge in the research. WebQDA Software has been developed by the partnership Universidade de Aveiro; CIDTFF; Esfera Crítica and Ludomedia (https://www.webqda.net/).

2.2. Interview Script Design

The interviews were structured in five sections designed to meet the purposes of the research study. As Table 2 shows, the interviews included similar questions for farmers and industrial entrepreneurs, although in some cases there were specific questions for each group.

2.3. Data Analysis

Once the interviews had been conducted, the recordings were transcribed and the information collected was analyzed by means of a Content Analysis methodology [26]. Content analysis is method attempting to obtain valid and applicable inferences from the texts with the purpose of reducing the original material [27]. The webQDA software (v. 3.1, Ludomedia, Oliveira de Azeméis, Portugal) was used for the purpose of this analysis, establishing a tree structure with a priori categories and an "emerging" code system linked to each category. Building a priori categories consists of establishing a preliminary hierarchical system prior to reading the documents, which for the purposes of this research study was predetermined by the items included in the semi-structured interview. Coding is a systematic way of developing and refining the data interpretation. The coding process includes the collection and analysis of all the data relating to subjects, ideas, concepts, interpretations and propositions [28]. Specifically, emerging coding is characterized by being inductive or open with codes being generated as the information is processed, in a way that as the data are being read or interpreted, new amendments emerge. Subsequently, the frequency of mention of each opinion was obtained from the views of each respondent that were coherent with the ideas or concepts contained in each code with respect to the total of responses, converted to a percentage [29].

Table 2. Script of the interviews conducted with farmers and industrial entrepreneurs.

Interview Design	Farmers	Industrial Entrepreneurs
Demographics	Information on the age, sex, education level, job title and experience in the position	
Type of farm/industry	Business activity (farming, industrial or both), number of employees and their distribution in the various departments, production type under the QS, commercialisation channels and sales	
	N° of pigs sold per category	Main product type sold (fresh, cured)
	Animal breed base	Brands under which the products are commercialised
		Countries for export, if any
Views on the various aspects of the Quality Standard (RD 4/2014)	Views on the requirements of the QS in terms of breed base, feeding type, weight gain at the finishing stage and weight/age at time of slaughter	
	Views on the certification process for farms and industrial businesses	
		Manufacturing time for products according to the QS
Views on production seasonality and Iberian product demand	-	Strategies used to correct discontinuity of demand of Iberian products
		Freezing of the fine cuts prior to the curing process. Impact on the final quality of the
	-	product and production costs. Need to specify such practice on the label
Proposals for improvement	Applicable measures aimed at improving the identified deficiencies or others not referred to previously. Individuals responsible for their implementation.	

QS: Quality Standard.

3. Results

The results are presented according to the a priori categories established in the methodological process. These are a total of eight categories of which the first four are categories related to the requirements of the QS at the farms, the next two have to do with the administrative aspects that the QS also establishes, such as certification and inspection processes as well as product labeling. The last two categories refer to aspects related to the processing of the products by the manufacturers.

3.1. Farmers and Industrial Entrepreneur Views on the Requirements of the Quality Standard for Farms

3.1.1. Requirements in Terms of the Breed Base of the Reproductive Animals

With the purpose of protecting the genetic value of the Iberian breed, the QS establishes that all females must be 100% Iberian breed. These can be used for the Iberian female x Duroc male cross-breeding, whereas the Duroc breed is reserved for the male line, provided always that both are registered in the herd book. In Figure 2 we can see how in their majority, both farmers and industrial entrepreneurs who are asked about this, are inclined towards the protection and preservation of a 100% Iberian female, with 63.6% and 56.3% in frequency of mention, respectively.

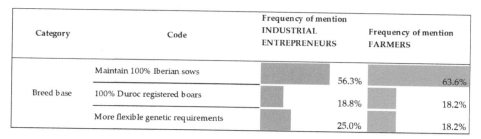

Figure 2. Industrial entrepreneur/farmer views on the requirements of the QS in terms of breed base. (Scale: frequency of mention of each opinion. Percentage is based on responses in the given code out of all responses to equal 100%).

The following were some of the literal comments made by the respondents:

"This has been one of the major contributions of the QS to the industry because it has maintained production at the same time as preserving the pure Iberian female".

"It is great for the Standard to protect the Iberian female because, otherwise, this would all get out of hand".

Another idea that was contributed during the interviews by industrial entrepreneurs and farmers was the need to guarantee the breed purity of Duroc boars in the farms where they decide to have cross-bred animal products, with over 18% in the frequency of mention both by farmers and industrial entrepreneurs.

Lastly, some views were in favor of making the genetic requirements more flexible (Figure 2), mainly amongst the industrial entrepreneurs (25.0% of frequency of mention), in a way that the QS would allow animals whose characteristics were compatible with the breed standards, even when they were not registered in the herd books. This goes against the currently effective regulations which are supported by Iberian Breed Association [14].

3.1.2. Requirements in Terms of Minimum-Weight Gain at the Finishing Stage and Minimum Carcass Weight

According to the current QS, the average weight of the animal lot at the beginning of the montanera stage (Black and Red labels) must be between 92 and 115 kg, gaining a minimum of 46 Kg during at least 60 days. In the case of animals produced under the free-range fodder-fed and non-free-range fodder-fed categories (Green and White labels, respectively), the QS does not establish the weight gain applicable during the finishing stage. As a common feature for all categories, the carcass weight must be greater than 115 kg in cross-breeds (Iberian x Duroc), and 108 kg in pure Iberian animals.

Almost half of respondents when asked for this requirement, both from the farm and the industrial backgrounds, were of the opinion that the weight gain and weight at slaughter were adequate (in order to achieve the minimum carcass weight) in all categories (42.9% and 44.4% in frequency of mention, respectively) (Figure 3). Examples of comments in this line are:

"With regards to weight, I think it is important to maintain the limits established by the QS, because a pig that does not reach the adequate weight will not prove an adequate carcass later on".

Nevertheless, some interviewed farmers would agree to not establishing minimum-weight gains for animals reared under the montanera system (Black and Red labels) (21.4% of frequency of mention).

On the other hand, a large proportion of farmers, and especially industrial entrepreneurs, (35.7% and 44.4%, respectively) pointed out that the issue might not be so much in the minimum carcass weights required by the QS (108 to 115 kg) but in the minimum age of slaughter, which was inferred from the interviews through comments such as the following:

"I think it is OK, although the industry complains about it being a bit high and with a little less weight they would have better selling hams, especially because the new Duroc hams have caused the ham meat yield to increase and, back then, when the Standard was published in 2014, it was assumed that a 115 kg carcass would yield 7–8 kg hams, which are easy to sell. They are now finding this is not the case, the average weight per ham is 8.5 to 8.6 kg which is way higher than the expected average".

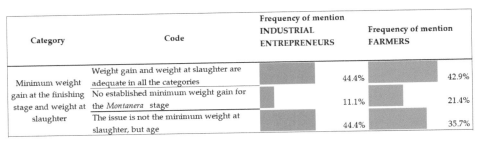

Category	Code	Frequency of mention INDUSTRIAL ENTREPRENEURS	Frequency of mention FARMERS
Minimum weight gain at the finishing stage and weight at slaughter	Weight gain and weight at slaughter are adequate in all the categories	44.4%	42.9%
	No established minimum weight gain for the *Montanera* stage	11.1%	21.4%
	The issue is not the minimum weight at slaughter, but age	44.4%	35.7%

Figure 3. Industrial entrepreneur/farmer views on the requirements of the QS (Quality Standard) in terms of weight gain at the finishing stage and minimum weight at slaughter. (Scale: frequency of mention of each opinion. Percentage is based on responses in the given code out of all responses to equal 100%).

3.1.3. Requirements in Terms of Feeding at the Finishing Stage

The QS establishes that pigs reared under the montanera system (Black and Red labels) must be only fed on natural resources (acorns and grass); free-range fodder-fed pigs (Green label) must feed on fodder made of cereal and legumes, without prejudice to the use they may make of the natural resources, and that non-free-range fodder-fed animals (White label) are fed only on fodder. Figure 4 collects the respondents' main views on the aspects set out by the QS in terms of the feeding at the finishing stage.

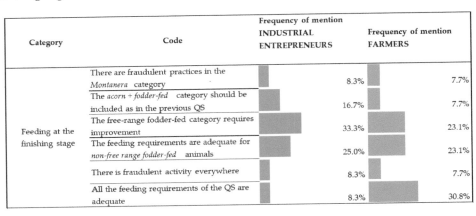

Category	Code	Frequency of mention INDUSTRIAL ENTREPRENEURS	Frequency of mention FARMERS
Feeding at the finishing stage	There are fraudulent practices in the *Montanera* category	8.3%	7.7%
	The *acorn + fodder-fed* category should be included as in the previous QS	16.7%	7.7%
	The free-range fodder-fed category requires improvement	33.3%	23.1%
	The feeding requirements are adequate for *non-free range fodder-fed* animals	25.0%	23.1%
	There is fraudulent activity everywhere	8.3%	7.7%
	All the feeding requirements of the QS are adequate	8.3%	30.8%

Figure 4. Industrial entrepreneur/farmer views on the QS (Quality Standard) feeding requirements. (Scale: frequency of mention of each opinion. Percentage is based on responses in the given code out of all responses to equal 100%).

The perception that "there are fraudulent practices with animals reared in the montanera production system" represented 8.3% and 7.7%, in frequency of mention by industrial entrepreneurs and farmers, respectively. On the other hand, there were some which were in favor of "including again the free-range acorn + fodder-fed animal category that was contemplated in the previous QS" (16.7% and 7.7% of frequency of mention by industrial entrepreneurs and farmers, respectively).

With regards to the animal feeding requirements for free-range fodder-fed animals (Green label), most of the views of the industrial entrepreneurs and farmers, with 33.3% and 23.1% in frequency of mention, respectively, concluded that it was necessary to improve the current QS requirements.

Participants generally showed a consensus with the requirements of the QS in terms of feeding in the non-free-range fodder-fed category (White label).

Lastly, in spite of not being a majoritarian view, some participants expressed the idea that there are generally fraudulent practices in the industry in terms of the feeding at the finishing stage (coded as "There is fraudulent activity everywhere"; Figure 4), which attempts to classify animals fed on fodder as montanera animals.

3.1.4. Requirements in Terms of the Minimum Age for Slaughter

For each of the production systems set out in the QS, a series of requirements is established for minimum age of slaughter: for pigs reared under the montanera system (Black and Red labels), the minimum age for slaughter is 14 months and for free-range fodder-fed (Green label) and non-free-range fodder-fed (White label) the age is 12 and 10 months, respectively.

A percentage of industrial entrepreneurs and farmers (30.0% and 45.5% in frequency of mention, respectively) were supportive of a reduction in the age of slaughter by two months for non-free-range fodder-fed pigs (White label), going from 10 to 8 months (Figure 5). Some examples of these comments were:

"The fair thing to do would be to adjust the age of the animal in order to obtain a product that is more adapted to the market and able to make it stable".

"Thanks to the existing technological advances, pigs cannot be slaughtered at the age of 10 months, which would not comply with the requirements of the market; this is where by trying to improve the pig or other parameters, we may forget that the purpose is to sell it in a market demanding an 8-month-old pig, not because it is 8 months old, but because this is the age at which it can be sold into the market; the consumer does not want a ham that weights more than 7 kg".

"The age of slaughter should be earlier for non-free-range fodder-fed animals at least by two months".

"The genetics of pigs have been improved and currently 8-month-old pigs or younger would be ready for slaughter".

Category	Code	Frequency of mention INDUSTRIAL ENTREPRENEURS		Frequency of mention FARMERS	
Minimum age for slaughter	Reduction of the minimum age for *non-free range fodder-fed* category by two months		30.0%		45.5%
	Adequate only for the *Montanera* category		25.0%		18.2%
	Adequate for the *Montanera* and the *free-range fodder-fed* categories		15.0%		18.2%
	The minimum age of slaughter is adequate for all categories		25.0%		18.2%

Figure 5. Industrial entrepreneur/farmer views on the QS (Quality Standard) requirements for age of slaughter (Scale: frequency of mention of each opinion. Percentage is based on responses in the given code out of all responses to equal 100%).

In the case of animals that are fed under the montanera system, industry entrepreneurs and farmers thought—with 25.0% and 18.2% of frequency of mention, respectively—that the currently-established age of slaughter is adequate. Amongst their statements, the following can be highlighted:

"Animals like those my father used to rear, montanera all his life. If I tell him that the current minimum is 14 months old, he will laugh at me, because that is so little time, if you think of the time an animal with good qualities and traits needs to fully rear".

Finally, other farmers and industrial entrepreneurs also expressed their views on keeping the age of slaughter proposed by the QS for the various production systems as they thought they were adequate (montanera, free-range fodder-fed and non-free-range fodder-fed), with 18.2% and 25% in frequency of mention, respectively.

3.2. Farmer and Industrial Entrepreneur Views on the Certification Processes and the Product Labeling

3.2.1. Views on the Certification/Inspection Process

The certification and inspection processes are key for Iberian pigs and their meat products, as they are the tool that guarantees they comply with the QS both at the production stage in the fields and the manufacturing and commercialization stages. In this regard, various matters were dealt with during the interviews, with the results being shown in Figure 6.

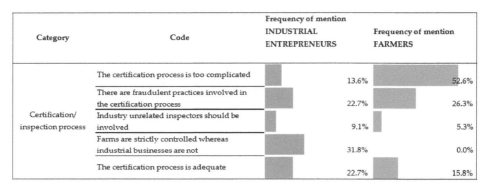

Figure 6. Industrial entrepreneur/farmer views on the requirements of the QS (Quality Standard) in terms of certification/inspection. (Scale: frequency of mention of each opinion. Percentage is based on responses in the given code out of all responses to equal 100%).

Notably, the participating farmers (52.6% in frequency of mention) complained about the excessive control measures they are required to submit their practices, especially at production level, with the purpose of ensuring the quality of the inspections, as well as the amount of documents that they need to provide in order to prove their situation.

3.2.2. Views on the Labeling Process

In terms of the labeling of the Iberian pork products, the majority of the industrial entrepreneurs mentioned the excessive importance that the QS places on the font size and type to be used, which was considered irrelevant by the above in contrast with more important aspects, such as the information that is provided to the consumer.

The participants thought it was much more important to mention the animal's breed purity (whether it is pure or a cross-breed with Duroc), the production system (extensive or in confinement) and even indicating the age at which it was slaughtered.

On the other hand, they also felt that it would be important to select the key words to be used on each label depending on the type of animal (words such as Iberian, black leg, free-range fodder-fed, etc.).

3.3. Industrial Entrepreneur Views on the Processing of the Products by the Manufacturers

3.3.1. Views on the Freezing Process of Raw Materials

Part of industrial entrepreneurs saw freezing as a feasible solution to manage the excess product in the industry and to adapt it to market demand, with 19.2% mentions. On the other hand, with the same frequency of mention, industrial entrepreneurs pointed that freezing was a solution for importing and exporting products since the useful life of fresh meat is quite limited. However, the participants pointed out that consideration must be given to the alterations the product might suffer in terms of quality. Thus, the same proportion of respondents indicated that freezing affects the quality of the products as those stating that it does not (15.4%).

On the other hand, the seasonality to which the Iberian products are subject, especially those deriving from pigs reared under the montanera system (Black and Red label), makes it necessary for this industry to innovate in order to adapt production to consumer demand. A potential solution would be freezing the hams raw material prior to their curing process as mentioned by the industrial entrepreneurs in this research study with 11.5% frequency of mention (Figure 7).

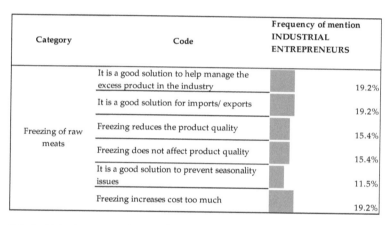

Category	Code	Frequency of mention INDUSTRIAL ENTREPRENEURS	
Freezing of raw meats	It is a good solution to help manage the excess product in the industry		19.2%
	It is a good solution for imports/ exports		19.2%
	Freezing reduces the product quality		15.4%
	Freezing does not affect product quality		15.4%
	It is a good solution to prevent seasonality issues		11.5%
	Freezing increases cost too much		19.2%

Figure 7. Industrial entrepreneur views on the requirements of the QS (Quality Standard) in terms of product freezing. (Scale: frequency of mention of each opinion. Percentage is based on responses in the given code out of all responses to equal 100%).

On the other hand, other opinions were related with the idea that freezing the product increases the costs.

Some contributed the above opinions with statements such as:

"The freezing process clearly increases the cost of the product, which does necessarily translate into an increase in the final product".

"Freezing the hams is a solution that would help optimize the facilities of this industry".

"Slaughtering and acorn-fed animals have a seasonal component to them, and Christmas is when most of the acorn-fed product is sold. For example, loin is always frozen in preparation for the Christmas demand".

3.3.2. Views on the Minimum Obligatory Maturity Time

An aspect that is defined by the standard is the minimum manufacturing times, which range from 600 to 730 days for leg hams, 365 days for shoulder hams and 70 for dry-cured loins. It is important to point out that these timings are minimums, and the final maturity period can be much longer, depending on the manufacturing method used in the industry. In this regard, Figure 8 portrays the views of respondents on these maturity times.

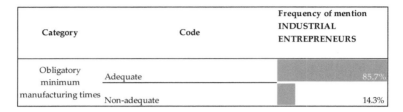

Figure 8. Industrial entrepreneurs' views on the requirements of the QS (Quality Standard) in terms of the maturity times. (Scale: frequency of mention of each opinion. Percentage is based on responses in the given code out of all responses to equal 100%).

As Figure 8 shows, with over 85% in frequency of mention, industrial entrepreneurs stated that the maturity times for Iberian products—leg hams, shoulder hams and dry-cured loins—were adequate.

"The acorn-fed product fully complies with it under the traditional system and in the case of the free-range fodder-fed product, it must comply too, as it is the case of a greased animal. If anyone were able to put it out earlier in the market by artificial means, they will do it, but . . . to what extent should we tell them: put it out now! One thing is clear: quality takes time and the standard is the reference stating the times in order to prevent us from going the fastest way possible".

4. Discussion

The regulation of the breed base of reproductive animals was certainly the main motivating aspect for the implementation of the first QS in 2001 [12] and this has been maintained through to the current QS [14]. Both sectors, farmers and industrial entrepreneurs, were of the opinion that this requirement has given rise to a positive increase in the number of Iberian animals [30], thus preventing the loss of purity of the Iberian breed against the cross with Duroc, as was the case before the application of the first Iberian QS [11,31]. On the other hand, the main reasons for the need to guarantee the breed purity of Duroc boars may be associated with characteristics of the Duroc breed itself, such as an improvement in the production parameters, prolificacy, higher energy efficiency, lean meat yield and growth ratio of the cross-bred animals, which are consistent with the scientific literature [6]. In spite of this requirement being effective since the QS was published in 2001, it became more demanding with the application of a new inspection protocol in 2017 [32]. This gave rise to an increase in the demand of registered pure Duroc boars and a price increase [33].

With respect to the minimum-weight gain at the finishing stage and minimum carcass weight, the fact that some responders, mainly farmers, considered not to establish a minimum-weight gain during montanera could be explained due to years of bad weather resulting in lack of natural resources (acorns and grass), and therefore inability to reach the minimum weight gain threshold required—46 kg—on only natural resources. On the other hand, the large proportion of respondents that indicated that the minimum age of slaughter was the main issue to solve, instead of the minimum-weight gain during the finishing stage, could be attributed to financial terms. Thus, most of the animals currently being slaughtered in Spain are those yielding White and Red label products, being 80% and 14%, respectively, of the total slaughtered animals [34], which are therefore Iberian-Duroc crossed animals. Since the QS establishes the age at slaughter for each category, regardless of the breed purity, the greater growth speed of Iberian × Duroc crossed animals [6] could lead to animals reaching the age of slaughter required by the QS with heavier weights to those the farmer deems optimum to render the most profit [35]. On the other hand, industrial entrepreneurs are faced with the difficulty of processing hams from animals which are overweight, especially leg hams above 8 Kg, which forces the increase of curing and stocking times, as well as the commercializing of products that are not in line with the current trends and habits of consumption [36].

Regarding to the requirements in terms of feeding at the finishing stage it should be highlighted that respondents think it is not well defined for free-range fodder-fed animals (Green label). This may be due to the lack of specific criteria to differentiate the degree of intensiveness in which the animals are reared (animals per hectare), as well as the percentage of feed the animal has eaten from natural resources in the dehesa and from fodder. This situation gives rise to a lack of an adequate distinction within the free-range fodder-fed category that is translatable into a differentiated type and therefore into the price of the derived products, thus acting in detriment of the profitability threshold of the extensive producer. In this sense, the scientific literature we find on the relevance of the production factors [15] or the influence of the various QS Iberian packaged products [18] on consumer preference have omitted the Green label as a commercial category due to the lack of uniformity of the farming conditions and therefore the high degree of heterogeneity of the end product.

With respect to the requirements in terms of the minimum age for slaughter, the relative high portion of respondents who agreed with the adequacy of the slaughtering age established by the QS for montanera animals could be explained by the greater presence of 100% Iberian animals in the montanera production system (Black label), which, according to the existing scientific literature, grow and mature slowly and have low meat yield [16], which indicates the requirement for them to have a longer production cycle in order to obtain quality products. In this line, there are studies which analyzed the traits of the carcass and the meat quality of pure Iberian pigs by age, concluding that the animals being introduced to the montanera rearing system at a younger age might not be mature enough to make the most of it [17], and could led to poorer growth rate, as well as carcass quality and fat traits [8]. As far as we are aware, there are no studies on the impact of the age of slaughter on cross-breed pigs reared under the montanera system (Red label). The free-range fodder-fed animal (Green label), however, has a more complex context, due to the great variability of the production factors. On the one hand, extensive farmers state these animals are very similar to the pigs reared under the montanera system and therefore, the age at slaughter is adequate. On the other hand, intensive farmers state that the age of slaughter should be reduced or maintained due to its similarities with the non-free-range fodder-fed animals (White label). Contrarily, most of the industrial entrepreneurs and farmers agreed with a reduction in the age of slaughter by two months for non-free-range fodder-fed pigs (White label), maybe because animals reared under this category come from Iberian × Duroc crossed animals and therefore, they grow faster and yield more meat [6] in comparison to the pure Iberian breed, and they could reach the optimum weight for slaughter at a younger age.

Moving to certification processes and the product labeling, the high frequency of mentions reporting the too complicated certification process by farmers could be explained by overlap between the various institutions carrying out inspections and the certifying companies in the first place, and then the Autonomous Communities Authorities and Interprofessional Iberian Pig Association (ASICI, in its Spanish abbreviation), which leads to a general sense of irritation in the industry [37]. To overcome this situation, farmers and industrial entrepreneurs suggested that inspections could be conducted by independent experts unrelated to the farming industry, but with sufficient knowledge and skills to perform the job, since the main purpose of this is to prevent industry fraud.

On the other hand, the importance given by respondents to mention the animal's breed purity in product's labeling may be due to the fact that participants understood that breed is a quality indicator for the consumer, in spite of the fact that various studies may not support the same position, demonstrating that consumer places much more importance on the type of feed than the breed [38] and concluding, additionally, that consumers cannot distinguish—from the sensorial point of view—between dry-cured products coming from pure Iberian pigs or crossed with Duroc, when the feed is the same [15].

In regard to the views on the freezing process of raw materials, there was no consensus about its impact on quality. In this line, no detriment in quality has been reported in Iberian pork meat after a year and a half frozen [39]. On the other hand, freezing raw material from pigs under montanera system could help to overcome the seasonality to which these products are subjected. However, this practice is not contemplated by the current QS [14] nor by the European standards dealing with freezing animal meats [19]. As far as we are concerned, there are few research studies relating to the freezing of meats prior to their curing process and mostly carried out on leg ham from commercial pigs [40,41]. Few studies deal with such topic in leg hams from Iberian pigs [42–44], and that analyze its effects on Iberian loins [21], so further studies being required in order to assess the effects of freezing on the final product as well as consumer acceptance.

Lastly, where a consensus was observed was in the fact that freezing the product increases the costs. In the first place, because a frozen product translates into money that is not circulating and, in the second place, because the maintenance of the freezing process implies a relevant cost for any industry.

With respect to the views on the minimum obligatory maturity time, the general agreement about the manufacturing length follow the lines of the scientific literature. Research studies concluded [45] that consumers prefer leg hams that have a long process to mature, as they positively associate this fact with an improvement in texture, flavor and aroma. We can conclude that maturity time is a parameter that does not give rise to much dispute, as the nature itself of the production process defines minimum times that must be observed.

5. Conclusions

A qualitative research study involving the use of in-depth interviews allowed the stakeholders to identify key aspects for future potential modifications in the current Iberian QS. Our findings showed industrial entrepreneurs and farmers were of the same opinion in aspects of the QS that have a significant impact on the profitability, the production yield and the quality of the end product. There was general consensus in terms of the preservation of the Iberian breed for sows, the elimination of the minimum weigh gains in animals under the montanera system as well as establishing an additional difference within the free-range fodder-fed category. Additionally, the participants shared the view that the age of slaughter established by the QS for non-free-range-fodder-fed animals is too high, which leads to a detriment in the commercial value of derivatives due to excessive weight.

On the other hand, this research study highlighted the dissatisfaction of the participants with the excessive bureaucracy required for the commercialization of products under the current QS. This aspect could potentially pose a risk for the industry, as farmers may be inclined to abandon their activities given the highly atomized environment with a lack of qualified personnel that characterizes the Iberian sector.

With regards to technological processing, the participants thought freezing was an adequate solution in order to manage the balance between production and demand, which was particularly relevant for the animals reared under the montanera system. They believe that any future amendments to the QS should take the regulation of such practice into account.

Author Contributions: Conceptualization, P.G.; data curation, A.O. and N.C.; formal analysis, N.C.; funding acquisition, P.G.; investigation, A.O. and P.G.; methodology, A.O.; project administration, P.G.; supervision, P.G.; validation, M.E.; writing—original draft, A.O., N.C. and A.E.; writing—review and editing, A.O., M.E. and P.G. All authors have read and agreed to the published version of the manuscript.

Funding: This research was supported by the RTA2015-00002-C04-03 "Effect of different production system and technology processing of meat from Iberian pigs" project funding by INIA-AEI Spanish organization and FEDER funds. Alberto Ortiz thanks the Government of Extremadura and the European Social Fund for the pre-doctoral grant (PD16057).

Acknowledgments: The authors would like to acknowledge the time and availability provided by the farmers and industrial entrepreneurs dedicated to carry on the interviews.

Conflicts of Interest: The authors declare no conflict of interest.

References

1. European Commission: Directorate-General for Agriculture and Rural Development. *Prospects for Agricultural Markets and Income in the EU 2011–2020*; Directorate-General for Agriculture and Rural Development: Brussels, Belgium, 2012.
2. Trícia, A.N.; Monteiro, R.; Wilfart, E.; Utzeri, V.J.; Luka, N.B.; Tomazin, U.; Nanni Costa, L.; Candek-Potokar, M.; Fontanesi, L.; Garcia-Launay, F. Environmental impacts of pig production systems using European local breeds: The contribution of carbon sequestration and emissions from grazing. *J. Clean. Prod.* **2019**, *237*, 117843. [CrossRef]
3. Temple, D.; Manteca, X.; Velarde, A.; Dalmau, A. Assessment of animal welfare through behavioural parameters in Iberian pigs in intensive and extensive conditions. *Appl. Anim. Behav. Sci.* **2011**, 29–39. [CrossRef]
4. Pugliese, C.; Sirtori, F. Quality of meat and meat products produced from southern European pig breeds. *Meat Sci.* **2102**, *93*, 511–518. [CrossRef] [PubMed]
5. Serra, X.; Gil, F.; Pérez-Enciso, M.; Oliver, M.A.; Vázquez, J.M.; Gispert, M.; Díaz, I.; Moreno, F.; Latorre, R.; Noguera, J.L. A comparison of carcass, meat quality and histochemical characteristics of Iberian (Guadyerbas line) and Landrace pigs. *Livest. Prod. Sci.* **1998**, *56*, 215–223. [CrossRef]
6. Ramírez, R.; Cava, R. The crossbreeding of different Duroc lines with the Iberian pig affects colour and oxidative stability of meat during storage. *Meat Sci.* **2007**, *77*, 339–347. [CrossRef] [PubMed]
7. Tejerina, D.; García-Torres, S.; Cabeza De Vaca, M.; Vázquez, F.M.; Cava, R. Effect of production system on physical-chemical, antioxidant and fatty acids composition of Longissimus dorsi and Serratus ventralis muscles from Iberian pig. *Food Chem.* **2012**, *133*, 293–299. [CrossRef]
8. Daza, A.; Lopez-Bote, C.J.; Olivares, A.; Menoyo, D.; Ruiz, J. Age at the beginning of the fattening period of Iberian pigs under free-range conditions affects growth, carcass characteristics and the fatty acid profile of lipids. *Anim. Feed Sci. Technol.* **2007**, *139*, 81–91. [CrossRef]
9. Bahelka, I.; Hanusová, E.; Peškovičová, D.; Demo, P. The effect of sex and slaughter weight on intramuscular fat content and its relationship to carcass traits of pigs. *Czech. J. Anim. Sci.* **2007**, 122–129. [CrossRef]
10. Candek-Potokar, M.; Ilender, B.; Lefaucheur, L.; Bonneauc, M. Effects of Age and/or Weight at Slaughter on Longissimus dorsi Muscle: Biochemical Traits and Sensory Quality in Pigs. *Meat Sci.* **1998**, *48*, 287–300. [CrossRef]
11. Espárrago, F.; Cabeza de Vaca, F.; Molina, R. Censos y precios de porcino ibérico 1986–1999. *Solo Cerdo Ibérico* **2001**, *2*, 113–122.
12. Spanish Ministry of the Presidency. *Real Decreto 1083/2001, por el que se Aprueba la Norma de Calidad para el Jamón Ibérico, Paleta Ibérica y Caña de lomo Ibérico Elaborados en España*; Spanish Ministry of the Presidency: Madrid, Spain, 2001.
13. Spanish Ministry of Agriculture, Fisheries and Food. *Real Decreto 1469/2007, Por el que se Aprueba la Norma de Calidad Para la Carne, el Jamón, la Paleta y la Caña de lomo Ibéricos*; Spanish Ministry of Agriculture, Fisheries and Food: Madrid, Spain, 2007.
14. Spanish Ministry of Agriculture, Food and Environment. *Real Decreto 4/2014 Por el que se Aprueba la Norma de Calidad para la Carne, el Jamón, la Paleta y la Caña de Lomo Ibérico*; Spanish Ministry of Agriculture, Food and Environment: Madrid, Spain, 2014.
15. Díaz-Caro, C.; García-Torres, S.; Elghannam, A.; Tejerina, D.; Mesias, F.J.; Ortiz, A. Is production system a relevant attribute in consumers' food preferences? The case of Iberian dry-cured ham in Spain. *Meat Sci.* **2019**, *158*. [CrossRef] [PubMed]
16. Bonneau, M.; Lebret, B. Production systems and influence on eating quality of pork. *Meat Sci.* **2010**, *84*, 293–300. [CrossRef] [PubMed]
17. Mayoral, A.I.; Dorado, M.; Guillén, M.T.; Robina, A.; Vivo, J.M.; Vázquez, C.; Ruiz, J. Development of meat and carcass quality characteristics in Iberian pigs reared outdoors. *Meat Sci.* **1999**, 315–324. [CrossRef]
18. Ortiz, A.; Tejerina, D.; Díaz-Caro, C.; Elghannam, A.; García-Torres, S.; Mesías, F.J.; Trujillo, J.; Crespo-Cebada, E. Is packaging affecting consumers' preferences for meat products? A study of modified atmosphere packaging and vacuum packaging in Iberian dry-cured ham. *J. Sens. Stud.* **2020**. [CrossRef]

19. European Union Regulation N° 16/2012 Concerning Requirements for Frozen Food of Animal Origin Intended for Human Consumption. 2012. Available online: https://eur-lex.europa.eu/eli/reg/2012/16/oj. (accessed on 30 April 2020).

20. Abellán, A.; Salazar, E.; Vázquez, J.; Cayuela, J.M.; Tejada, L. Changes in proteolysis during the dry-cured processing of refrigerated and frozen loin. *LWT* **2018**, *96*, 507–512. [CrossRef]

21. Lorido, L.; Ventanas, S.; Akcan, T.; Estévez, M. Effect of protein oxidation on the impaired quality of dry-cured loins produced from frozen pork meat. *Food Chem.* **2016**, *196*, 1310–1314. [CrossRef]

22. McEachern, M.G.; Seaman, C. Consumer perceptions of meat production: Enhancing the competitiveness of British agriculture by understanding communication with the consumer. *Br. Food J.* **2005**, *107*, 572–593. [CrossRef]

23. Mesias, F.J.; Pulido, F.; Escribano, M.; Gaspar, P.; Pulido, A.F.; Escribano, A.; Rodríguez_ledesma, A. Evaluation of new packaging formats for dry-cured meat products using conjoint analysis: An application to dry-cured iberian ham. *J. Sens. Stud.* **2013**, *28*, 238–247. [CrossRef]

24. Kinnear, T.; Taylor, J. *Investigacion de Mercados: Un Enfoque Aplicado*; McGraw-Hill: Santafé de Bogotá, Colombia, 1998.

25. Gatley, A.; Caraher, M.; Lang, T. A qualitative, cross cultural examination of attitudes and behaviour in relation to cooking habits in France and Britain. *Appetite* **2014**, *75*, 71–81. [CrossRef]

26. Stewart, D.; Shamdasani, P.; Rook, D. *Focus Groups*, 2nd ed.; Applied Social Research Methods Series; SAGE Publications, Inc.: Thousand Oaks, CA, USA, 2007; Volume 20.

27. Flick, U. *An Introduction to Qualitative Research*, 4th ed.; Sage Publications Lt.: Thousand Oaks, CA, USA, 2009.

28. Taylor, S.J.; Bogdan, R. Introducción a los métodos cualitativos. *Paidós* **1986**, *37*, 1-342.

29. Neri de Souza, F.; Costa, A.P.; Moreira, A. Análise de Dados Qualitativos Suportada pelo Software WebQDA. In Proceedings of the VII Conferência Internacional de TIC na Educação: Perspetivas de Inovação, Braga, Portugal, 12–13 May 2011.

30. Ministry of Agriculture, Fisheries and Food. Sistema Nacional de Información de Razas ARCA. Explotación de datos Censales. Available online: https://www.mapa.gob.es/es/ganaderia/temas/default.aspx (accessed on 30 April 2020).

31. Vargas Giraldo, J.; Aparicio Tovar, M. Análisis de la evolución de los censos y sistemas de producción del cerdo ibérico. *Rev. Española Estud. Agrosociales y Pesq.* **2001**, *193*, 87–118.

32. Spanish Ministry of Agriculture, Food and Environment. Norma de Calidad del Ibérico (RD 4/2014). Protocolos de Actuación. 2017. Available online: https://www.mapa.gob.es/es/alimentacion/temas/control-calidad/protocolodeinspeccionrevision18122018version2rev1_tcm30-500158.pdf (accessed on 29 September 2020).

33. Vinagre, C. Los Cochinos de Raza Duroc Siguen de Moda. *Periodico Hoy.* 2020. Available online: https://www.hoy.es/extremadura/cochinos-raza-duroc-20200118001044-ntvo.html (accessed on 29 September 2020).

34. Higuera, M.A. El Sector Porcino Español. In *El Sector Porcino. De la Incertidumbre al Liderazgo*; Díaz Yubero, M.A., Ed.; Cajamar Caja Rural: Almería, Spain, 2018; pp. 95–108. Available online: https://www.publicacionescajamar.es/publicacionescajamar/public/pdf/series-tematicas/informes-coyuntura-monografias/el-sector-porcino-de-la-incertidumbre.pdf (accessed on 29 September 2020).

35. Muñoz, A. Bases para la gestión de explotaciones de porcino ibérico. In *Porcino Ibérico: Aspectos Claves*; Buxade, C., Daza, A., Eds.; Mundi Prensa: Madrid, Spain, 2001; pp. 665–687.

36. Parra, V.; Viguera, J.; Sánchez, J.; Peinado, J.; Espárrago, F.; Gutiérrez, J.L.; Andrés, A.I. Effect of exposure to light on physico-chemical quality attributes of sliced dry-cured Iberian ham under different packaging system. *Meat Sci.* **2012**, *90*, 236–243. [CrossRef] [PubMed]

37. Resano, H.; Sanjuán, A.I.; Albisu, L.M. Consumers' acceptability of cured ham in Spain and the influence of information. *Food Qual. Prefer.* **2007**, *18*, 1064–1076. [CrossRef]

38. Hallenstvedt, E.; Øverland, M.; Rehnberg, A.; Kjos, N.P.; Thomassen, M. Sensory quality of short- and long-term frozen stored pork products. Influence of diets varying in polyunsaturated fatty acid (PUFA) content and iodine value. *Meat Sci.* **2012**, *90*, 244–251. [CrossRef]

39. Martín, M.J. Aptitud de Distintos Sistemas de Conservación para la Prolongación de la vida útil de Carne Fresca de Cerdo Ibérico para el Consumo Directo y de Productos Derivados. Ph.D. Thesis, University of Extremadura, Badajoz, Spain, 2013.

40. Bañón, S.; Cayuela, J.M.; Granados, M.V.; Garrido, M.D. Pre-cure freezing affects proteolysis in dry-cured hams. *Meat Sci.* **1999**, *51*, 11–16. [CrossRef]

41. Flores, M.; Soler, C.; Aristoy, M.; Toldrá, F. Effect of brine thawing/salting for time reduction in Spanish dry-cured ham manufacturing on proteolysisand liplysis during salting and post-salting periods. *Eur. J. Food Res. Technol.* **2006**, *222*, 509–515. [CrossRef]

42. Pérez-Palacios, T.; Ruiz, J.; Martín, D.; Barat, J.M.; Antequera, T. Pre-cure freezing effect on physicochemical, texture and sensory characteristics of Iberian ham. *Food Sci. Technol. Int.* **2011**, *17*, 127–133. [CrossRef]

43. Pérez-Palacios, T.; Ruiz, J.; Barat, J.M.; Aristoy, M.C.; Antequera, T. Influence of pre-cure freezing of Iberian ham on proteolytic changes throughout the ripening process. *Meat Sci.* **2010**, *85*, 121–126. [CrossRef]

44. Pérez-Palacios, T.; Ruiz, J.; Grau, R.; Flores, M.; Antequera, T. Influence of pre-cure freezing of Iberian hams on lipolytic changes and lipid oxidation. *Int. J. Food Sci. Technol.* **2009**, *44*, 2287–2295. [CrossRef]

45. Flores, M.; Ingram, D.A.; Bett, K.L.; Toldrá, F.; Spanier, A.M. Sensory characteristics of Spanish 'Serrano' dry-cured ham. *J. Sens. Stud.* **1997**, *12*, 169–179. [CrossRef]

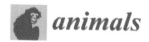

Article

Free-Range and Low-Protein Concentrated Diets in Iberian Pigs: Effect on Plasma Insulin and Leptin Concentration, Lipogenic Enzyme Activity, and Fatty Acid Composition of Adipose Tissue

Juan F. Tejeda [1,2,*], Alejandro Hernández-Matamoros [1] and Elena González [2,3]

[1] Food Science and Technology, Escuela de Ingenierías Agrarias, Universidad de Extremadura, Avda. Adolfo Suárez s/n, 06007 Badajoz, Spain; alejandro@nutricionespecial.com

[2] Research University Institute of Agricultural Resources (INURA), Avda. de Elvas s/n, Campus Universitario, 06006 Badajoz, Spain; malena@unex.es

[3] Animal Production, Escuela de Ingenierías Agrarias, Universidad de Extremadura, Avda. Adolfo Suárez, 06007 Badajoz, Spain

* Correspondence: jftejeda@unex.es; Tel.: +34-924-289-300

Received: 10 September 2020; Accepted: 16 October 2020; Published: 19 October 2020

Simple Summary: Recently, it has been shown that reducing dietary crude-protein levels during the final fattening period prior to slaughter is a suitable strategy to increase intramuscular fat content in Iberian pig meat, without affecting pig growth. Investigating the effect of a low-protein diet on the metabolism, development, and composition of the adipose tissue of Iberian pigs, and the obese porcine breed, was the objective of this study. Three groups of pigs fed under free-range conditions and in confinement with concentrated diets with low- and standard-protein contents were studied. All three groups exhibited the same backfat thickness at the end of the fattening period. The level of hormones and activities of enzymes related to adipogenic metabolism were affected by diet, with differences between free-range and intensive feeding systems. Therefore, we suggest that feeding Iberian pigs on low-protein diets did not result in fatter carcasses, and is thus a useful strategy to improve Iberian pig meat quality.

Abstract: The purpose of this study was to investigate the effect of diets with different protein contents on carcass traits, plasma hormone concentration, lipogenic enzyme activities, and fatty acid (FA) composition in the adipose tissue of Iberian pigs. Twenty-four castrated male Iberian pigs (eight per feeding diet) were fed under free-range conditions with acorns and grass (FR), and in confinement with concentrated diets with standard (SP) and low-protein contents (LP) from 116.0 to 174.2 kg live weight. Backfat thickness was not affected by diet. The plasma leptin concentration was higher ($p < 0.001$) in the FR group than in the LP and SP groups, while insulin concentration was higher in the SP group than in the LP and FR groups. The lipogenic enzyme activities of glucose-6-phosphate dehydrogenase, malic enzyme, and glycerol-3-phosphate dehydrogenase were lower in the FR group compared to the LP and SP pigs. The activities of these enzymes were adipose-tissue-specific. No differences were found in FA composition of adipose tissue between the SP and LP groups, while the FR pigs had lower proportions of saturated FA and higher proportions of monounsaturated and polyunsaturated FA than the SP and LP pigs. In conclusion, feeding low-protein diets in Iberian pigs does not seem to affect adipose carcass traits, strengthening previous findings that indicate that this is a good strategy to improve meat and dry-cured product quality.

Keywords: Iberian pig; extensive system; low-protein diet; adipose tissue; plasma hormones; lipogenic enzymes; fatty acids

1. Introduction

The high level of crude protein in pig diets, usually formulated to provide the requirements for certain essential amino acids, leads to an excess of other essential amino acids [1] and excretion of excess nitrogen [2], resulting in a lower efficiency of nitrogen utilization, and also protein fermentation in the hindgut, which can damage the gut health [3]. Moreover, in the last years, there has been increased interest in reducing ammonia emissions from pig farms due to their negative impact on the environment and on human health [4]. Therefore, feeding pigs on low-protein diets is a tool not only to reduce feed costs, nitrogen excretion, and gut health, but also could contribute to improving meat quality without affecting pig production performance. In this sense, several studies have been carried out to explore the effect of different nutritional strategies, based on reducing crude-protein content [5–10], essential amino acids levels, such as lysine [11–15], or both of these [16] in the diet, on growth performance, carcass composition, and meat quality of pigs. It is well known that a high amount of intramuscular fat (IMF) is one the most relevant aspects of meat quality [17], and although low-fat pork could be interesting for reducing caloric intake in humans, an IMF level below 2.5% is related to lower sensory meat quality [18]. In a recent paper, we evidenced that reduced dietary crude-protein levels during the final fattening period prior to slaughter in intensive conditions, as occur in free-range pigs reared with natural resources (acorns and grass) in the south-west Iberian Peninsula, is a suitable strategy to increase IMF content in Iberian pig meat, without affecting the pig growth [19]. The Iberian pig is an autochthonous breed characterized by its low potential for lean tissue deposition and its high tendency to accumulate fat [20], as a consequence of an excessive and continuous intake, since their sensation of satiety is altered [21]. Therefore, it is of great importance to understand how a low-protein diet affects the biochemical mechanisms related to the production and development of adipose tissue. In this sense, some authors have reported that protein-deficient diets increased backfat thickness [5,22] or modified monounsaturated fatty acids (MUFA) biosynthesis in muscle, by increasing the activity and protein expression of stearoyl-CoA desaturase [23]. Katsumata et al. [11] reported an increase in m(messenger)RNA abundance of PPARG (the nuclear hormone receptor involved in adipocyte gene expression and differentiation) in the *longissimus* muscle. However, the effects of this type of diet on biochemical mechanisms are different in muscle and subcutaneous backfat-adipose tissue [23]. In this context, it is very interesting to determine the effect of the reduction in the protein content in the pig diet, not only on muscle tissue, but also on the metabolism, development, and composition of the adipose tissue, mainly on the backfat, especially in the case of fatty pigs, as is the case with the Iberian pig. The present study is, to our knowledge, the first report to look at the hormone profile and lipogenic enzyme activity of the Iberian pig fed in free-range conditions compared with pigs fed intensively on concentrate diets. With this background, we hypothesized that exploring the effect of dietary protein deficiency on metabolic changes, studying plasma hormones and lipogenic enzyme activity, and the fatty acid composition of different adipose tissues from Iberian pigs fed in free-range and intensive conditions could help better understand the findings previously reported [19] on the effect of this feeding strategy on Iberian pig productive performances and meat quality.

2. Materials and Methods

2.1. Animals, Experimental Design, and Diets

The experimental design carried out in this study was described in detail in a previous paper [19]. Briefly, 24 castrated male Iberian pigs of the Retinto variety were selected at a 116.0 ± 5.9 kg live weight and an age of 425 days, and randomly divided into 3 groups according to the rearing system during the fattening period. Eight pigs were fattened in the traditional extensive rearing system based on local resources (acorn and grass) in a large enclosure (FR). The others were fed on two different concentrate diets: 1 group of 8 pigs was fed on a standard protein diet (SP) and the other on a low-protein diet (LP); both groups were fed in confinement. Diet composition, including daily feed intake of acorn, grass, and concentrates; handling; and carcass sampling were detailed in the above-mentioned study by

Tejeda et al. [19]. In brief, pigs were fattened for 45–57 days (45.4, 46.3, and 56.8 days for LP, SP, and FR pigs, respectively) in order to reach a similar slaughter weight (174.2 ± 6.1 kg live weight), and daily feed intakes were of 5161 and 5088 g DM/pig in LP and SP pigs; while in FR pigs estimated daily feed intakes were of 3600 and 655 g DM/pig for acorn pulp and grass, respectively. The backfat thickness of pigs was measured using a hand-held ultrasonic device (Aquila vet, Esaote Pie Medical, Genoa, Italy), equipped with an ultrasonic linear probe (3.5 Mhz and 18 cm long) with a silicone acoustic loin adapter, by placing the probe perpendicular to the loin at the level of the last rib. The captured images were processed using the AutoCAD® 2008 software (AutoDESK®, Inc., San Rafael, CA, USA) to determine total backfat thickness and the thickness of the 3 layers that can be differentiated into subcutaneous fat [24] at 10 cm from the dorsal midline. These 3 layers will be referred to as SC1, SC2, and SC3, for each of the outer, middle, and inner layers, respectively, in the following text. Pigs were restrained in a crate during ultrasound scanning to restrict movement and maintain a standing posture and were ultrasonically scanned the on the first and the last day (24 h before slaughter) of the fattening period. The backfat thickness increase was calculated as the difference between the 2 ultrasonic measurements, and divided by the total number of days in fattening period, and multiplied by 10 (backfat thickness increasing every 10 days). Feed was withheld from animals for 12 h before slaughter. FR pigs were locked in a pen and fed with acorns collected from the same place where they usually ate, until the pre-slaughter fasting. Pigs were slaughtered by electrical stunning and killed by exsanguination. Then, they were scalded, skinned, eviscerated, and split down both sides of the vertebral column according to the standard commercial procedures of the Iberian pig industry. Hot carcass weights without pelvic renal fat were recorded and used to calculate carcass yield. Samples of perirenal fat (PE), backfat, at the level of the tailbone (TB), and samples from SC1, SC2, and SC3 layers of backfat at the level of the last rib were collected for lipid analysis, frozen in liquid nitrogen, and stored at −80 °C until analysis. Blood samples were collected during postmortem exsanguinations and were immediately stored at 4 °C in tubes with heparin to prevent clotting, until arrival at the laboratory. In the laboratory, blood samples were centrifuged at 5000× g for 10 min, and plasma was collected and stored at −80 °C until analysis. Hams and shoulders were removed from the carcasses, weighed 2 h postmortem, and trimmed 24 h later according to the approved procedure for the production of Iberian ham; they were weighed again to calculate trimmed yields.

2.2. Analyses

2.2.1. Assessment of Plasma Hormone Concentrations

The circulating leptin and insulin concentrations were measured using the radioimmunoassay (RIA) kits Multi-Species Leptin RIA Kit (cat. no. XL-85K, Merck Millipore, Darmstadt, Germany) and Porcine Insulin RIA Kit (cat. no. PI-12K, Merck Millipore, Darmstadt, Germany), respectively. The leptin and insulin assays were performed according to the manufacturer's instructions, including standard and sample tubes. Briefly, for leptin determination, 300 μL of assay buffer, 100 μL of standards, and 100 μL of each sample were added to the respective tubes, followed by 100 μL of Multi Species Leptin antibody; they were then vortexed, covered, and incubated overnight at 4 °C. After incubation, 100 μL of 125I-Human Leptin was added and incubated overnight again at 4 °C. On the third day, 1.0 mL of cold (4 °C) precipitating reagent was added to the tubes, vortexed, and incubated for 20 min at 4 °C. After that, the tubes were centrifuged for 20 min at 2500× g, the supernatant was decanted and counted in a gamma counter (model 5500; Beckman Instrument, Irvine, CA, USA) for 1 min. The analyses were carried out in duplicate, and the results were expressed as ng/mL human equivalent of leptin. For insulin determination, after adding the assay buffer (300 μL), standards (100 μL), and samples (100 μL) to the tubes, 100 μL of 125I-Insulin and 100 μL of Porcine Insulin antibody were added. After mixing, this was incubated for 24 h at 4 °C. On the second day, 1.0 mL of cold (4 °C) precipitating reagent was added to the tubes and re-incubated for 20 min at 4 °C. Finally, the tubes were centrifuged (20 min at 2500× g) and the supernatant was decanted and counted in the gamma counter for 1 min.

The analyses were carried out in duplicate, and the results were expressed as µU/mL of porcine insulin. In both the leptin and insulin assays, the difference between the duplicate results of a sample was <10% coefficient of variation, and the sensitivity was <1 ng/mL and <2 µU/mL, respectively.

2.2.2. Assessment of Lipogenic Enzyme Activity

The activities of 4 lipogenic enzymes, glucose-6-phosphate dehydrogenase (G6PDH) (EC 1.1.1.49) [25], malic enzyme (ME) (EC 1.1.1.40) [26], glycerol-3-phosphate dehydrogenase (G3PDH) (EC 1.1.1.8) [27], and fatty acid synthetase (FAS) (EC 2.3.1.85) [28] were assessed on subcutaneous (TB, SC1, SC2, and SC3) and perirenal adipose tissue homogenates. The analytical procedure followed was: 0.7 g of adipose tissue, previously frozen at −80 °C, was homogenized in 4 mL of STEG ice-cold buffer (containing 300 mM saccharose, 30 mM trizma base, 1 mM EDTA and 1 mM glutatión, at pH = 7.4) using an Omni-Mixer homogenizer (OMNI Int., Waterbury, CT, USA) at 50,000 rpm for 3 cycles of 10 s each. The homogenate was filtered (20 µm pore size filter) and centrifuged at 4000× g for 10 min at 4 °C in an Eppendorf Centrifuge 5810R (Eppendorf, Hamburg, Germany). The supernatant fraction was re-filtered (0.45 µm pore size filter) and re-centrifuged at 14,000× g for 10 min at 4 °C. Then, the resulting supernatant (cytoplasmic soluble fraction) was collected, filtered (0.45 µm pore size cellulose filter), and stored at −80 °C for further analyses. The G6DPH, ME, G3PDH, and FAS activities were assessed at 37 °C by absorbance at 340 nm using a spectrophometer (Fluostar Optima, BMG Labtech, Aylesbury, UK). One unit of activity was defined as the amount of enzyme that increases (for ME and G6PDH) or decreases (for FAS and G3PDH) the presence of 1 nmol of nicotinamide adenine dinucleotide phosphate (NADPH) (NADH for G3PDH) per minute and per gram of fresh tissue. The amount of substrate was adjusted so that the reactions were linear over time during the assay period.

2.2.3. Fatty Acid Composition

Fatty acid compositions of backfat and perirenal fat samples were determined, after lipid extraction in a microwave oven [29], by acidic trans-esterification with 0.1 N sodium metal and 5% sulphuric acid in methanol [30]. The fatty acid methyl esters were analyzed using a Hewlett-Packard HP-4890 Series II gas chromatograph (Hewlett-Packard, Palo Alto, CA, USA) equipped with a split/splitless injector and a flame ionization detector (FID). The derivatives were separated on a capillary column (HP-INNOWax 30 m long, 0.25 mm id, 0.25 µm film thickness; Hewlett-Packard, Palo Alto, CA, USA) containing a polar stationary phase (polyethylene glycol). The oven temperature was held at 260 °C for 25 min. The injector and detector temperatures were held at 320 °C. The carrier gas was nitrogen at 1.8 mL/min. The methyl esters were identified by comparing their retention times with those of the reference standard mixtures (Sigma Chemical Co., St. Louis, MO, USA). The results were labeled as a percentage of the total fatty acids present, considering a total of 15 fatty acids.

2.3. Statistical Analysis

The mean and the standard error of the mean were used for the descriptive data analysis. The pig was used as the experimental unit. One-way ANOVA was used to determine the effect of dietary treatment on carcass traits and plasma hormone concentrations. The effect on lipogenic enzyme activities and fatty acid compositions of the backfat and perirenal fat, and their interaction, was carried out by Factorial (3 diet × 5 adipose tissue) ANOVA procedure. Tukey's test was applied to compare the means of each group. The General Linear Model procedure of the SPSS package (SPSS for Windows Ver. 19.0; SPSS Inc., Chicago, IL, USA, 2004) was used. Differences between means were significant for $p < 0.05$.

3. Results

3.1. Carcass Measurements and Plasma Hormones

The results from the trimmed ham and shoulder, and backfat traits and from the plasma hormone concentration are shown in Table 1. According to the data published by the authors in a previous paper [19], the trimming, carried out according to the procedure approved for the production of Iberian ham, leads to a reduction in the weight of the ham and shoulder by 21% and 30%, respectively. The effect of the feeding system was only significant ($p < 0.05$) for trimmed shoulder yield, with the SP group showing higher scores than the FR and LP groups. Backfat thickness, at the level of the last rib, varied between 58.0 and 62.8 mm, without significant differences between the different feeding systems. With respect to the thickness increase in the three backfat layers studied, it was observed that the middle layer (SC2) showed the highest increase during the pig fattening period, followed by the inner layer (SC3), and finally the outer one (SC1). However, no significant differences were observed related to diet in terms of increasing thickness of any of the three layers studied. Regarding hormone concentrations, leptin contents varied widely, with significantly higher levels ($p = 0.001$) in the FR group than in the LP group; the SP pigs showed the lowest concentration. In contrast, plasma insulin concentration was higher ($p = 0.007$) in the SP group than in the LP group, with the FR animals showing intermediate levels.

Table 1. Carcass traits and plasma hormone concentrations from Iberian pigs fed with the experimental diets.

Items	FR	LP	SP	SEM	*p*-Value
Carcass traits					
Trimmed ham weight (kg)	11.4	11.4	11.6	0.10	0.772
Trimmed shoulder weight (kg)	7.4	7.5	7.9	0.10	0.068
Trimmed ham yield (%)	16.6	16.6	17.1	0.18	0.415
Trimmed shoulder yield (%)	10.8 [a]	10.8 [a]	11.7 [b]	0.16	0.024
Backfat thickness (last rib) (mm) [1]	62.8	62.6	58.0	1.86	0.490
Backfat thickness increasing (mm) [2]					
SC1	0.7	0.4	0.5	0.05	0.129
SC2	2.1	2.6	2.8	0.25	0.577
SC3	1.6	2.0	2.2	0.18	0.358
Hormone concentration					
Leptin (ng/mL)	30.3 [a]	21.2 [b]	13.9 [b]	1.97	0.001
Insulin (µU/mL)	10.4 [a,b]	7.9 [a]	11.8 [b]	0.55	0.007

[a,b] Values within a row with different superscripts differ significantly at $p < 0.05$. SEM, standard error of the mean. SC1, outer backfat layer. SC2, middle backfat layer. SC3, inner backfat layer. Diets: FR, Iberian pigs reared in free-range conditions; LP, Iberian pig fed on experimental low-protein diet; SP, Iberian pig fed on experimental standard protein diet. [1] Measurements were carried out ultrasonically, 24 h before slaughter, 10 cm from the dorsal midline at the level of the last rib. [2] Increase was calculated as the difference between the two measurements carried out ultrasonically on the first and the last day (24 h before slaughter) of the fattening period, and divided by the total number of days in this period and multiplied by 10 (backfat thickness increasing every 10 days).

3.2. Fat Biochemical Characteristics

The lipogenic enzyme activities of the four enzymes determined in the different diets and adipose tissues studied are shown in Table 2. The activities of the G6PDH and ME enzymes were similar (on average, 427 and 421 nmol NADPH/min/g of lipids, respectively), but higher than the G3PDH activity (189 nmol), with the FAS enzyme demonstrating the lowest activity (34 nmol). The activity of G6PDH, ME, and G3PDH was affected by the feeding treatment. The FR diet displayed significantly lower activities of G6PDH (−25%, $p < 0.001$), ME (−34%, $p < 0.001$), and G3PDH (−35%, $p < 0.001$) compared to the LP and SP diets. The FAS activity was not affected by diet.

Table 2. Effect of diet and adipose tissue on the lipogenic enzyme activities of backfat and perirenal fat from Iberian pigs. Results are expressed in nmol of nicotinamide adenine dinucleotide phosphate (NADPH) produced (ME, G6PDH) or consumed (FAS), and NADH consumed (G3PDH) per min and per g lipids.

	Diet				Tissue				*p*-Value			
	FR	LP	SP	TB	SC1	SC2	SC3	PE	SEM	Diet	Tissue	Int.
G6PDH	352 [a]	456 [b]	472 [b]	497 [a]	484 [a,b]	438 [a,b]	423 [b]	297 [c]	12.9	0.000	0.000	0.851
ME	315 [a]	490 [b]	459 [b]	357 [a]	481 [b]	477 [b]	413 [a,b]	379 [a]	15.4	0.000	0.000	0.458
G3PDH	140 [a]	213 [b]	212 [b]	238 [a]	207 [a,b]	186 [b,c]	155 [c]	158 [c]	6.6	0.000	0.000	0.993
FAS	29	34	33	34	37	28	29	36	1.7	0.689	0.434	0.951

[a,b,c] Values within a row with different superscripts differ significantly at $p < 0.05$. SEM, standard error of the mean. Int., interaction Diet $\times$ Tissue. G6PDH, glucose-6-phosphate dehydrogenase; ME, malic enzyme; G3PDH, glycerol-3-phosphate dehydrogenase; FAS, fatty acid synthase. Diets: FR, Iberian pigs reared in free-range conditions; LP, Iberian pig fed on experimental low-protein diet; SP, Iberian pig fed on experimental standard protein diet. Tissues: TB, backfat, at the level of the tailbone; SC1, outer backfat layer; SC2, middle backfat layer; SC3, inner backfat layer; PE, perirenal fat.

For TB, backfat layers, and PE, significant differences were also detected in G6PDH, ME, and G3PDH enzyme activities. The FAS activity did not differ between the five different tissues studied. For G6PDH, TB exhibited the highest enzyme activity, followed by SC1 and SC2, SC3, and finally, PE. A similar trend was followed by G3PDH, with the highest levels being in TB and the lowest in PE and SC3; SC1 and SC2 showed intermediate levels. In contrast, ME showed lower enzyme activity in TB and PE than the SC layers. No interaction was observed between diet and tissue.

3.3. Fatty Acid Composition

The fatty acid composition of total subcutaneous fat at the level of the tail bone (TB), including the outer (SC1), middle (SC2), and inner (SC3) layers, and perirenal (PE) fat is presented in Table 3. Pigs reared in free-range conditions (FR) had significantly lower proportions ($p < 0.01$) of C16:0, C18:0, C20:0, and total saturated fatty acids (SFA) than pigs fed intensively with standard (SP) and low-protein diets (LP). In contrast, FR pigs showed higher ($p < 0.05$) percentages of C18:1 n-9, C18:2 n-6, C18:3 n-3, total monounsaturated (MUFA), and total polyunsaturated fatty acids (PUFA) than SP and LP pigs. However, no differences were found in any of the above-mentioned fatty acids between the SP and LP groups. With respect to the fatty acid composition of the different adipose tissues studied, the effect was significant in most of the fatty acids analyzed. Briefly, the fatty acid composition of total backfat at the level of the tail bone (TB) and the outer layer of subcutaneous fat (SC1) at level of the last rib were quite similar, but different to the SC2 and SC3 layers. Perirenal fat (PE) presented a different fatty acid composition, mainly SFA and MUFA, compared to the other fat tissues studied. The proportions of C18:1 n-9, C20:1 n-9, and total MUFA were higher in TB and SC1 than in SC2 and SC3, with PE showing the lowest percentages ($p < 0.001$). In contrast, total SFA, including C16:0 and C18:0, the two main saturated fatty acids, were lower in TB and SC1 compared to SC2 and SC3, with the highest proportions in PE ($p < 0.001$). Regarding PUFA, significant differences ($p < 0.05$) were observed between the different tissues studied, although they were less marked than those described in SFA and MUFA. No significant effect ($p > 0.05$) of interaction between the diet and adipose tissue was observed.

Table 3. Effect of diet and adipose tissue on fatty acid composition (%) of the backfat and perirenal fat from Iberian pigs.

	Diet			Tissue					SEM	p-Value		
	FR	LP	SP	TB	SC1	SC2	SC3	PE		Diet	Tissue	Int.
C14:0	1.21	1.21	1.18	1.21	1.21	1.20	1.16	1.21	0.010	0.335	0.402	0.082
C16:0	20.79 [a]	21.61 [b]	21.55 [b]	20.29 [a]	20.02 [a]	21.03 [b]	21.57 [b]	23.66 [c]	0.144	0.000	0.000	0.053
C16:1 n-7	2.04	2.14	2.22	2.22 [a]	2.34 [a]	2.26 [a]	2.03 [a,b]	1.81 [b]	0.039	0.116	0.000	0.635
C17:0	0.34 [a]	0.31 [b]	0.34 [a]	0.28 [a]	0.33 [a,b]	0.39 [b]	0.33 [a]	0.32 [a]	0.007	0.044	0.000	0.969
C17:1	0.34	0.32	0.35	0.33 [b]	0.38 [a,b]	0.41 [a]	0.33 [b]	0.24 [c]	0.008	0.273	0.000	0.993
C18:0	10.66 [a]	12.14 [b]	11.92 [b]	9.63 [a]	9.51 [a]	11.12 [b]	12.22 [c]	15.39 [d]	0.237	0.000	0.000	0.863
C18:1 n-9	51.10 [a]	49.88 [b]	49.99 [b]	53.04 [a]	52.72 [a]	50.07 [b]	50.31 [b]	45.49 [c]	0.293	0.003	0.000	0.880
C18:2 n-6	9.93 [a]	8.70 [b]	8.84 [b]	9.10 [a,b]	9.53 [a,b]	9.66 [b]	8.62 [a]	8.88 [a,b]	0.120	0.000	0.013	0.813
C18:3 n-3	0.80 [a]	0.71 [b]	0.71 [b]	0.69 [a,b]	0.74 [a,b,c]	0.80 [b,c]	0.66 [a]	0.81 [c]	0.014	0.012	0.002	0.999
C20:0	0.18 [a]	0.21 [a,b]	0.25 [b]	0.19	0.25	0.22	0.21	0.19	0.010	0.042	0.429	0.533
C20:1 n-9	1.47 [a]	1.67 [b]	1.58 [a,b]	1.82 [a]	1.70 [a,b]	1.60 [b]	1.55 [b]	1.19 [c]	0.028	0.001	0.000	0.342
C20:2 n-9	0.63	0.62	0.59	0.70 [a]	0.69 [a]	0.68 [a]	0.55 [b]	0.43 [c]	0.013	0.135	0.000	0.172
C20:3 n-6	0.10	0.09	0.10	0.09 [a,b]	0.11 [a]	0.11 [a]	0.09 [a]	0.07 [b]	0.002	0.314	0.000	0.446
C20:4 n-6	0.15	0.13	0.15	0.15 [a]	0.15 [a,b]	0.17 [b]	0.14 [a,b]	0.14 [a,b]	0.003	0.138	0.012	0.908
C20:3 n-3	0.26	0.26	0.25	0.27 [a,b]	0.31 [a]	0.30 [a]	0.23 [b]	0.16 [c]	0.007	0.759	0.000	0.474
SFA	33.18 [a]	35.47 [b]	35.23 [b]	31.60 [a]	31.32 [a]	33.95 [b]	35.48 [c]	40.78 [d]	0.368	0.000	0.000	0.583
MUFA	54.95 [a]	54.02 [b]	54.14 [b]	57.42 [a]	57.14 [a]	54.33 [b]	54.23 [b]	48.74 [c]	0.325	0.036	0.000	0.929
PUFA	11.86 [a]	10.51 [b]	10.63 [b]	10.97 [a,b,c]	11.53 [a,b]	11.72 [a]	10.29 [c]	10.49 [b,c]	0.146	0.000	0.002	0.856

[a,b,c] Values within a row with different superscripts differ significantly at *p* < 0.05. SEM, standard error of the mean. Int., interaction Diet × Tissue. SFA, total saturated fatty acids; MUFA, total monounsaturated fatty acids; PUFA, total polyunsaturated fatty acids. Diets: FR, Iberian pigs reared in free-range conditions; LP, Iberian pig fed on experimental low-protein diet; SP, Iberian pig fed on experimental standard protein diet. Tissues: TB: backfat, at the level of the tailbone; SC1, outer backfat layer; SC2, middle backfat layer; SC3, inner backfat layer; PE, perirenal fat. Results are expressed as means in percentage of a total of 15 fatty acids identified.

4. Discussion

The purpose of this study was to investigate the influence of a protein-restricted diet on the lipogenic response of the main fat depots of Iberian pigs carcasses, such as subcutaneous and perirenal fat [31]. Subcutaneous fat tissue in pigs consists of two or three layers (SC1, SC2, and SC3), depending on the carcass point [24], with differences in allometry coefficients and the composition between them [32], which suggests that it would be better to study the composition of individual fat layers as an indicator of carcass composition [33]. However, the Spanish Ministry of Agriculture, Fishery, and Food established a procedure to take backfat samples in Iberian pigs from the area of tail insertion in the coxal region of the carcass (TB), where no differentiation between the different layers is observed [34], in order to avoid the possible error that would be made if only one of the layers were sampled. Perirenal fat (PE) is a tissue that is found close to pig maturity [35], which probably could better reflect the diet composition at the end of the fattening period.

4.1. Carcass Traits

Trimmed shoulder yield was affected by Iberian pig diet, which implies a higher lean percentage in the SP trimmed shoulders than in the FR and LP trimmed shoulders, in agreement with the results observed previously in *longissimus thoracis* and *lumborum* muscle [19]. Trimming, the procedure that removes rind and external fat in the traditional V-shape, facilitates the salting phase and standardizes the subcutaneous fat thickness [36]. However, no significant effect of diet was observed as regards the final weight and yield of trimmed hams, in accordance with others studies carried out in Cinta Senese [10] and Large White × Landrace [7] pigs, respectively. This is important because ham is the main dry-cured product obtained from Iberian pigs, characterized by its high sensory quality and high price in the market [37]. In the same way, backfat thickness and backfat thickness increase were not affected by diet, showing that low-crude-protein diets did not result in fatter carcasses, in agreement with the data from previous studies in heavy [7,13] and lighter [8,38] pigs. Furthermore, other authors [32,39] reported that total backfat thickness and the different backfat layers thickness were no influenced by the feeding of Iberian pigs in extensive or intensive conditions. In the same way, these authors reported a slight increase over the finished fattening period in the external subcutaneous layer compared to the medium and internal ones, the medium layer representing nearly 60% of the total backfat [39]. A similar trend was observed by González et al. [40], who reported that the middle layer of backfat showed more growth than the inner layer, with the outer layer demonstrating the lowest fat thickness. In contrast, the increase in backfat thickness in pigs fed on low-protein diets has been previously reported [5]. These discrepancies between the published results could be related to the extent of crude-protein reduction in the diet, the amount of indispensable amino acids supplemented, and the net energy of the diet [7]. A great reduction in protein percentage, i.e., greater than about 3% below the control values, could significantly affect backfat thickness [8], since this diet protein reduction would cause levels of other important amino acids to be too low [41].

4.2. Plasma Hormones

Regarding the plasma hormone concentrations, significant differences in leptin and insulin contents were observed between the three diets studied. Iberian pigs fed on the SP diet had 55% and 35% less leptin content than the FR and LP groups, respectively. Leptin is a protein encoded by the gene responsible for obesity. The positive correlation between plasma leptin levels, pig fatness [21], and subcutaneous fat depth [42] is well documented, since this hormone is synthesized and secreted by adipocytes [43]. The effect of the dietary treatment of Iberian pigs on plasma leptin concentration has been reported by several authors [14,21]. To our knowledge, no studies have been previously carried out to determine plasma leptin levels in Iberian pigs fed in free-range conditions, according to the traditional system known as *montanera*, with acorns and pasture, which is recognized as a poor natural source of protein [44]. Therefore, there are no studies that compare the free-range and the intensive feeding systems. However, differences in the plasma leptin levels of Iberian pigs fed intensively with crude-protein diets or lys-deficient diets have been previously evidenced [14], with the pigs with greater relative weights of fatty components (backfat, belly, kidney fat, and mesenteric fat) [14] and intramuscular fat [15] demonstrating higher hormone levels. Nevertheless, these authors revealed only slight differences in subcutaneous fat depth measured at the first and last rib and last lumbar vertebra [15], in agreement with our results, where no differences in backfat thickness between the three feeding systems studied were detected. Furthermore, in accordance with the study carried out previously in our lab, Iberian pigs fed according to the FR system, with higher plasma leptin concentrations, exhibited greater intramuscular fat content compared to pigs fed on diets with higher protein contents (SP) [19].

Plasma insulin concentration was also influenced by diet, with SP pigs demonstrating higher levels than FR and LP pigs ($p < 0.01$). Some studies reported that the reduction in the crude-protein [45] or lysine [46] content in the pig diets resulted in a decrease in plasma insulin levels, which is in agreement with our results. The difference between diets in plasma insulin concentration, in spite of a higher intake of carbohydrates in LP compared to SP pigs, could be attributable to the higher protein content in SP diet, since the ingestion of protein elicits a rise in insulin in non-ruminants [47]. On the contrary, other studies reported no difference in the plasma insulin concentration of pigs fed different levels of protein [21,48]. These differences could be explained by the level of protein or lysine reduction in diets. Therefore, as suggested by Fernández-Figares et al. [21], apparently only severe protein restriction is able to elicit changes in the hormonal profile of pigs. The lipogenic action of insulin on adipose tissue is well documented [49]. The lack of differences in backfat thickness between Iberian pigs fed on the three diet treatments in our study could indicate that the lipogenic effect of insulin, as occurs with lipogenic enzyme activities [23], could be expressed less readily in subcutaneous fat than in muscle.

4.3. Effect of Diet and Adipose Tissue on Lipogenic Enzyme Activity

Lipogenic pathways could play a determining role in the amount of lipid deposited in tissues [15], because more than 80% of the total fatty acid deposition in pig tissues is attributed to de novo synthesis [50]. To further investigate adipogenesis and metabolism in different carcass adipose tissues, such as backfat—total (TB) and the SC1, SC2, and SC3 layers—and perirenal (PE) fat in

Iberian pigs fattened in free-range and in intensive conditions, with different protein contents in their diets, the activity of four lipogenic enzymes (G6PDH, ME, G3PDH, and FAS) was analyzed. These enzymes play an important role in lipid metabolism: G6PDH and ME are involved in reduced nicotinamide adenine dinucleotide phosphate (NADPH) supply for de novo fatty acid synthesis; G3PDH produces glicerol-3-phosphate, involved in triglyceride synthesis, from the glucose; and FAS catalyzes the palmitate synthesis pathway from malonil-CoA and is therefore also involved in de novo fatty acid synthesis.

Differences in lipogenic enzyme activity between lean and fatty pig breeds during the fattening period have been pointed out by several authors [51,52], which lead to a more intense lipid metabolism [15] and greater capacity for tissue lipid synthesis in fatty pigs, such as Iberian pigs, as compared to conventional pigs [53]. The effect of animal tissue, muscle, and adipose tissue on lipogenic enzyme activity is also well known [13,23], which would suggest different regulatory lipid metabolism mechanisms for subcutaneous and intramuscular fat [15]. Finally, feeding regimes involving dietary crude protein [22,23] or lysine [13,15] restriction can also affect the lipogenic enzyme activity in pigs, although this effect is closely related to the fatty tissue studied, as mentioned above. The results of lipogenic enzyme activity in adipose tissues between diet regimes in our study showed a significant difference between Iberian pigs fed on natural resources in free-range conditions (FR), with lower G6PDH, ME, and G3PDH activities, compared to pigs fed intensively on concentrates (LP and SP). A possible explanation for this difference between the FR group and intensive fed pigs could be the very high amount of feed consumed by the SP and LP pigs (see Tejeda et al. [19]), which results in high-energy intake, leading to an increase in fat synthesis and consequently an increase in lipogenic enzyme activity. However, no differences in backfat thickness measured at the end of the fattening period were detected, probably because the FR pigs exhibited a lower average daily intake and needed more days to reach slaughtering weight compared to the LP and SP pigs (56.8 vs. 45.4 and 46.3 days, respectively) [19]. In contrast, the present results evidenced that diet protein restriction in Iberian pigs fed intensively with standard (SP) and low-protein concentrates (LP) had no effect on backfat and perirenal fat lipogenic enzyme activity, which is in agreement with previous studies carried out with protein [51] or lysine [11] deficient diets, both in Iberian and lean pigs, which could help explain the absence of differences in the carcass traits of the pigs, specifically the backfat thickness and thickness increase in the three backfat layers studied. The differences in the enzymatic activity of lipogenic enzymes between subcutaneous fat and muscle, as suggested by Palma Granados et al. [15], could be the cause of the significant effect of low-protein diet on IMF content in Iberian pigs previously reported in our lab [19], and by other authors [54], compared to the absence of effect on subcutaneous or perirenal fat. Nevertheless, it would be interesting to study further the lipogenic enzyme activity in Iberian pig muscles to find more evidence of the effect of low-protein diets on carcass and meat quality.

With respect to the effect of adipose tissue on the lipogenic enzyme activity, our results show differences between backfat (TB, SC1, SC2, and SC3) and PE fat from Iberian pigs, with the metabolic enzyme activity being less intense in global terms in PE compared to subcutaneous fat. These results confirm the effect of tissue on lipogenic enzyme activity as studies comparing muscle and subcutaneous tissues demonstrated [13,15,23]. This fact could help explain the significantly different enzyme activity described in our study in PE with respect to TB, SC1, SC2, and SC3, since PE is a tissue that develops at a later age compared to other fat depots [35].

4.4. Effect of Diet and Adipose Tissue on Fatty Acid Composition

The fatty acid composition of pig tissues can be altered by several factors, such as genotype, sex, age, slaughter weight, and environmental temperature, with the diet being the main factor through which this fatty acid profile can be modified [54,55]. In the present study, no effect was observed regarding protein restriction in the diet in the different adipose tissues studied. In agreement with our results, Daza et al. [56] reported that a low-crude-protein diet had no effect on the major fatty acid proportions of the total subcutaneous fat. In addition, partially agreeing with our results, Aquilani et al. [10] did not detect any effect as regards crude-protein restriction on the backfat inner layer from Cinta Senese pigs, corresponding to the middle layer in our study. However, this was opposite to the findings of most studies, which reported dietary crude-protein reduction having a significant effect on the fatty acid composition of subcutaneous [23,38] and intramuscular [38] fat from finishing lean pigs, as well as in Iberian piglets growing from 10 to 25 kg in body weight and fed on low-lysine diets [14,15]. All these studies have an increase in SFA and MUFA, and a reduction in PUFA in pigs fed on low-protein compared to standard-protein diets in common, which could indicate an activation of lipogenic enzymes at the adipose or muscular tissue [57], and consequently, the increase in de novo fatty acid synthesis and stearoyl-CoA desaturase activity [23]. In this regard, it has been pointed out that these discrepancies in the results described in the literature could be related to the level of dietary protein reduction [38], in addition to genetic factors and the slaughter age of the pigs in the different studies [14,15,38]. The increase in de novo synthesis in pigs fed on the LP diet compared to those fed the SP diet could be diminished as a result of the high proportion of oleic acid (about 72%) in the concentrated feed used in our study. Moreover, it is important to highlight again that the Iberian pig is a rustic fatty pig slaughtered at high weights, which could also contribute to the lack of effect related to diet protein level on fatty acid composition of the different fatty tissues studied. The dietary effect detected in the current study was associated with free-range rearing vs. feeding in intensive conditions, since FR pigs exhibited lower C16:0, C18:0, C20:0, and SFA, and higher C18:1, C18:2, C18:3, MUFA, and PUFA in adipose tissues compared to LP and SP pigs. An explanation for these results could be related to the composition of natural resources (acorn and grass) consumed by pigs during the fattening period [19,58,59].

Regarding the effect of carcass fat tissue on the fatty acid composition, our results are in accordance with those previously reported [60] for Iberian pigs, with differences between the three subcutaneous layers studied, with the outer layer (SC1) showing the highest proportions of MUFA, mainly C18:1 n-9, and PUFA, mainly C18:2 n-6 and C18:3 n-3, and the lowest of SFA, mainly C16:0 and C18:0. The same trend was observed in Cinta Senese pigs, an obese genotype characterized by great lipogenic potential [10], similar to the Iberian pig, although these authors only studied two subcutaneous fat layers. These differences in the fatty acid composition could be attributed to variations in lipogenic enzyme activity in the different fat depots. The hierarchy observed in the G3PDH activity, with higher values in the outer compared to the inner layers, and the observed decreasing tendency in G6PDH and ME activities in the outer, middle, and inner backfat layers (SC1, SC2, and SC3, respectively) and in PE tissue in our study, evidenced the tissue-specific lipogenic enzyme activity.

5. Conclusions

Under the experimental conditions of our study, which was carried out on Iberian pigs, a fatty, rustic breed, slaughtered at an advanced age and weight, dietary crude-protein restriction during the final fattening period prior to slaughter did not affect the carcass fatness or the enzyme activity and fatty acid composition of fatty tissues. This fact provides relevant details regarding the usefulness of feeding Iberian pigs with LP diets in intensive conditions to improve meat quality. On the other hand, our results showed that the free-range feeding system, characterized by a low-crude-protein content, increased the plasma leptin content, but had no effect on carcass fatness traits, supporting the described leptin resistance of the Iberian pig. The extensive feeding system, which implies a slower pig growth, and consequently, a longer fattening period in order to reach the final fattening weight as compared to intensive feeding system, decreased the lipogenic enzyme activity and modified the fatty acid composition of fatty tissues. Additionally, the present results confirm that lipogenic metabolic pathways are adipose tissue-specific, with the different adipose tissues being affected by the feeding system.

Author Contributions: Conceptualization, J.F.T. and E.G.; methodology, J.F.T., E.G., and A.H.-M.; data analysis, E.G.; animal management, E.G. and A.H.-M.; writing—original draft preparation, J.F.T., E.G., and A.H.-M.;

writing—review, J.F.T., E.G. and A.H.-M.; writing—editing, J.F.T.; project administration and funding acquisition, J.F.T. and E.G. All authors have read and agreed to the published version of the manuscript.

Funding: The research was funded by the regional government of Extremadura and the European Social Fund (Research Project PRI08B091). A. Hernández-Matamoros wants to thank the regional government of Extremadura for his pre-doctoral grant.

Acknowledgments: The authors gratefully acknowledge María Angeles Tormo (Deparment of Physiology, Medical School, University of Extremadura, Badajoz, Spain) for their technical assistance in hormone determinations, and José Antonio Mendizabal (IS-FOOD Institute; ETS Ingenieros Agrónomos, Departamento de Agronomía, Biotecnología y Alimentación, Universidad Pública de Navarra, Pamplona, Spain) for its contribution to the development of the technique for determining enzyme activity in our laboratory. Thanks also are given to M. Paniagua and the workers of Valdesequera farm (CICYTEX-Agricultural Research Center Finca La Orden-Valdesequera, Junta de Extremadura) for their technical assistance in animal management.

Conflicts of Interest: The authors declare no conflict of interest. The funders had no role in the design of the study; in the collection, analyses, or interpretation of data; in the writing of the manuscript, or in the decision to publish the results.

References

1. Wang, Y.; Zhou, J.; Wang, G.; Cai, S.; Zeng, X.; Qiao, S. Advances in low-protein diets for swine. *J. Anim. Sci. Biotechnol.* **2018**, *9*, 1–14. [CrossRef]
2. Prandini, A.; Sigolo, S.; Morlacchini, M.; Grilli, E.; Fiorentini, L. Microencapsulated lysine and low-protein diets: Effects on performance, carcass characteristics and nitrogen excretion in heavy growing-finishing pigs. *J. Anim. Sci.* **2013**, *91*, 4226–4234. [CrossRef] [PubMed]
3. Rist, V.T.S.; Weiss, E.; Eklund, M.; Mosenthin, R. Impact of dietary protein on microbiota composition and activity in the gastrointestinal tract of piglets in relation to gut health: A review. *Animal* **2013**, *7*, 1067–1078. [CrossRef] [PubMed]
4. Portejoie, S.; Martinez, J.; Landmann, G. Ammonia of farm origin: Impact on human and animal health and on the natural habitat. *Prod. Anim.* **2002**, *15*, 151–160.
5. Ruusunen, M.; Partanen, K.; Pösö, R.; Puolanne, E. The effect of dietary protein supply on carcass composition, size of organs, muscle properties and meat quality of pigs. *Livest. Sci.* **2007**, *107*, 170–181. [CrossRef]
6. Barea, R.; Nieto, R.; Aguilera, J.F. Effects of the dietary protein content and the feeding level on protein and energy metabolism in Iberian pigs growing from 50 to 100 kg body weight. *Animal* **2007**, *1*, 357–365. [CrossRef]
7. Galassi, G.; Colombini, S.; Malagutti, L.; Crovetto, G.M.; Rapetti, L. Effects of high fibre and low protein diets on performance, digestibility, nitrogen excretion and ammonia emission in the heavy pig. *Anim. Feed Sci. Technol.* **2010**, *161*, 140–148. [CrossRef]
8. Wood, J.D.; Lambe, N.R.; Walling, G.A.; Whitney, H.; Jagger, S.; Fullarton, P.J.; Bayntun, J.; Hallett, K.; Bünger, L.; Bünger, L. Effects of low protein diets on pigs with a lean genotype. 1. Carcass composition measured by dissection and muscle fatty acid composition. *Meat Sci.* **2013**, *95*, 123–128. [CrossRef]
9. Monteiro, A.N.T.R.; Bertol, T.M.; Oliveira, P.A.V.D.; Dourmad, J.; Coldebella, A. The impact of feeding growing- finishing pigs with reduced dietary protein levels on performance, carcass traits, meat quality and environmental impacts. *Livest. Sci.* **2017**, *198*, 162–169. [CrossRef]
10. Aquilani, C.; Sirtori, F.; Franci, O.; Acciaioli, A.; Bozzi, R.; Pezzati, A.; Pugliese, C. Effects of protein restriction on performances and meat quality of cinta senese pig reared in an organic system. *Animals* **2019**, *9*, 310. [CrossRef] [PubMed]
11. Katsumata, M.; Kobayashi, S.-I.; Matsumoto, M.; Tsuneishi, E.; Kaji, Y. Reduced intake of dietary lysine promotes accumulation of intramuscular fat in the Longissimus dorsi muscles of finishing gilts. *Anim. Sci. J.* **2005**, *76*, 237–244. [CrossRef]
12. Katsumata, M.; Kyoya, T.; Ishida, A.; Ohtsuka, M.; Nakashima, K. Dose-dependent response of intramuscular fat accumulation in longissimus dorsi muscle of finishing pigs to dietary lysine levels. *Livest. Sci.* **2012**, *149*, 41–45. [CrossRef]
13. Madeira, M.S.; Costa, P.; Alfaia, C.M.; Lopes, P.A.; Bessa, R.J.B.; Lemos, J.P.C.; Prates, J.A.M. The increased intramuscular fat promoted by dietary lysine restriction in lean but not in fatty pig genotypes improves pork sensory attributes. *J. Anim. Sci.* **2013**, *91*, 3177–3187. [CrossRef] [PubMed]

14. Palma-Granados, P.; Haro, A.; Seiquer, I.; Lara, L.; Aguilera, J.F.; Nieto, R. Similar effects of lysine deficiency in muscle biochemical characteristics of fatty and lean piglets. *J. Anim. Sci.* **2017**, *95*, 3025–3036. [CrossRef] [PubMed]

15. Palma-Granados, P.; Seiquer, I.; Benítez, R.; Óvilo, C.; Nieto, R. Effects of lysine deficiency on carcass composition and activity and gene expression of lipogenic enzymes in muscles and backfat adipose tissue of fatty and lean piglets. *Animal* **2019**, *13*, 2406–2418. [CrossRef] [PubMed]

16. Ruiz-Ascacibar, I.; Stoll, P.; Kreuzer, M.; Boillat, V.; Spring, P.; Bee, G. Impact of amino acid and CP restriction from 20 to 140 kg BW on performance and dynamics in empty body protein and lipid deposition of entire male, castrated and female pigs. *Animal* **2017**, *11*, 394–404. [CrossRef] [PubMed]

17. Wood, J.D.; Enser, M.; Fisher, A.V.; Nute, G.R.; Sheard, P.R.; Richardson, R.I.; Hughes, S.I.; Whittington, F.M. Fat deposition, fatty acid composition and meat quality: A review. *Meat Sci.* **2008**, *78*, 343–358. [CrossRef]

18. Fernandez, X.; Monin, G.; Talmant, A.; Mourot, J.; Lebret, B. Influence of intramuscular fat content on the quality of pig meat—1. Composition of the lipid fraction and sensory characteristics of m. longissimus lumborum. *Meat Sci.* **1999**, *53*, 59–65. [CrossRef]

19. Tejeda, J.F.; Hernández-Matamoros, A.; Paniagua, M.; González, E. Effect of free-range and low-protein concentrated diets on growth performance, carcass traits, and meat composition of iberian pig. *Animals* **2020**, *10*, 273. [CrossRef]

20. Nieto, R.; Miranda, A.; García, M.A.; Aguilera, J.F. The effect of dietary protein content and feeding level on the rate of protein deposition and energy utilization in growing Iberian pigs from 15 to 50kg body weight. *Br. J. Nutr.* **2002**, *88*, 39–49. [CrossRef]

21. Fernández-Fígares, I.; Lachica, M.; Nieto, R.; Rivera-Ferre, M.G.; Aguilera, J.F. Serum profile of metabolites and hormones in obese (Iberian) and lean (Landrace) growing gilts fed balanced or lysine deficient diets. *Livest. Sci.* **2007**, *110*, 73–81. [CrossRef]

22. Gondret, F.; Lebret, B. Feeding intensity and dietary protein level affect adipocyte cellularity and lipogenic capacity of muscle homogenates in growing pigs, without modification of the expression of sterol regulatory element binding protein. *J. Anim. Sci.* **2002**, *80*, 3184–3193. [CrossRef] [PubMed]

23. Doran, O.; Moule, S.K.; Teye, G.A.; Whittington, F.M.; Hallett, K.G.; Wood, J.D. A reduced protein diet induces stearoyl-CoA desaturase protein expression in pig muscle but not in subcutaneous adipose tissue: Relationship with intramuscular lipid formation. *Br. J. Nutr.* **2006**, *95*, 609–617. [CrossRef] [PubMed]

24. Fortin, A. Development of backfat and individual fat layers in the pig and its relationship with carcass lean. *Meat Sci.* **1986**, *18*, 255–270. [CrossRef]

25. Glock, B.G.E.; Mclean, P. Further Studies on the Properties and Assay of Glucose 6-Phosphate Dehydrogenase and 6-Phosphogluconate Dehydrogenase of Rat Liver. *Biochem. J.* **1953**, *55*, 400–408. [CrossRef] [PubMed]

26. Ochoa, S. "Malic"-enzyme. *Methods Enzymol.* **1955**, *1*, 739–753. [CrossRef]

27. Wise, L.S.; Green, H. Participation of One Isozyme Cytosolic Glycerophosphate Dehydrogenase in the Adipose Conversion of 3T3 Cells. *J. Biol. Chem.* **1979**, *254*, 273–275. [PubMed]

28. Halestrap, A.P.; Denton, R.M. Insulin and the regulation of adipose-tissue acetyl-coenzyme A carboxylase. *Biochem. J.* **1973**, *132*, 509–517. [CrossRef] [PubMed]

29. De Pedro, E.; Casillas, M.; Miranda, C.M. Microwave oven application in the extraction of fat from the subcutaneous tissue of Iberian pig ham. *Meat Sci.* **1997**, *45*, 45–51. [CrossRef]

30. Sandler, S.R.; Karo, W. *Sourcebook of Advanced Organic Laboratory Preparations*; Academic Press: Cambridge, MA, USA, 1992; ISBN 0126185069. [CrossRef]

31. García-Valverde, R.; Barea, R.; Lara, L.; Nieto, R.; Aguilera, J.F. The effects of feeding level upon protein and fat deposition in Iberian heavy pigs. *Livest. Sci.* **2008**, *114*, 263–273. [CrossRef]

32. Almeida, J.M.; Bressan, M.C.; Amaral, A.J.; Bettencourt, C.; Santos-Silva, J.; Moreira, O.; Gama, L.T. Body weight and ultrasound measurements over the finishing period in Iberian and F1 Large White × Landrace pigs raised intensively or in free-range conditions. *Livest. Sci.* **2019**, *229*, 170–178. [CrossRef]

33. McEvoy, F.J.; Strathe, A.B.; Madsen, M.T.; Svalastoga, E. Changes in the relative thickness of individual subcutaneous adipose tissue layers in growing pigs. *Acta Vet. Scand.* **2007**, *49*, 1–7. [CrossRef] [PubMed]

34. Ayuso, D.; González, A.; Hernández, F.; Corral, J.M.; Izquierdo, M. Prediction of carcass composition, ham and foreleg weights, and lean meat yields of Iberian pigs using ultrasound measurements in live animals. *J. Anim. Sci.* **2013**, *91*, 1884–1892. [CrossRef]

35. Wood, J.D.; Buxton, P.J.; Whittington, F.M.; Enser, M. The chemical composition of fat tissues in the pig: Effects of castration and feeding treatment. *Livest. Prod. Sci.* **1986**, *15*, 73–82. [CrossRef]

36. Arnau, J. Principales problemas tecnológicos en la elaboración del jamón curado. In Proceedings of the 44th International Congress of Meat Science, ICOMST, Barcelona, Spain, 30 August–4 September 1998; pp. 72–86.

37. Ventanas, S.; Ventanas, J.; Ruiz, J.; Estévez, M. Iberian pigs for the development of high-quality cured products. *Recent Res. Devel. Agric. Food Chem.* **2005**, *6*, 1–27.

38. Tous, N.; Lizardo, R.; Vilà, B.; Gispert, M.; Font-i-Furnols, M.; Esteve-Garcia, E. Effect of reducing dietary protein and lysine on growth performance, carcass characteristics, intramuscular fat, and fatty acid profile of finishing barrows. *J. Anim. Sci.* **2014**, *92*, 129–140. [CrossRef] [PubMed]

39. Ayuso, D.; González, A.; Hernández, F.; Peña, F.; Izquierdo, M. Effect of sex and final fattening on ultrasound and carcass traits in Iberian pigs. *Meat Sci.* **2014**, *96*, 562–567. [CrossRef] [PubMed]

40. González, A.; Ayuso, D.; Peña, F.; Martínez, A.L.; Izquierdo, M. Effects of gender and diet on back fat and loin area ultrasound measurements during the growth and final stage of fattening in Iberian pigs. *Arch. Anim. Breed.* **2017**, *60*, 213–223. [CrossRef]

41. Tuitoek, K.; Young, L.G.; De Lange, C.F.M.; Kerr, B.J. The Effect of Reducing Excess Dietary Amino Acids on Growing-Finishing Pig Performance: An Evaluation of the Ideal Protein Concept. *J. Anim. Sci.* **1997**, *75*, 1575–1583. [CrossRef]

42. Deng, D.; Li, A.K.; Chu, W.Y.; Huang, R.L.; Li, T.J.; Kong, X.F.; Liu, Z.J.; Wu, G.Y.; Zhang, Y.M.; Yin, Y.L. Growth performance and metabolic responses in barrows fed low-protein diets supplemented with essential amino acids. *Livest. Sci.* **2007**, *109*, 224–227. [CrossRef]

43. Zhang, Y.; Proenca, R.; Maffei, M.; Barone, M.; Leopold, L.; Friedman, J.M. Positional cloning of the mouse obese gene and its human homologue. *Nature* **1994**, *372*, 425–432. [CrossRef] [PubMed]

44. García-Valverde, R.; Nieto, R.; Lachica, M.; Aguilera, J.F. Effects of herbage ingestion on the digestion site and nitrogen balance in heavy Iberian pigs fed on an acorn-based diet. *Livest. Sci.* **2007**, *112*, 63–77. [CrossRef]

45. Mejia-Guadarrama, C.A.; Pasquier, A.; Dourmad, J.Y.; Prunier, A.; Quesnel, H. Protein (lysine) restriction in primiparous lactating sows: Effects on metabolic state, somatotropic axis, and reproductive performance after weaning. *J. Anim. Sci.* **2002**, *80*, 3286–3300. [CrossRef]

46. Ren, J.B.; Zhao, G.Y.; Li, Y.X.; Meng, Q.X. Influence of dietary lysine level on whole-body protein turnover, plasma IGF-I, GH and insulin concentration in growing pigs. *Livest. Sci.* **2007**, *110*, 126–132. [CrossRef]

47. Unger, R.H. Alpha- and beta-cell interrelationships in health and disease. *Metabolism* **1974**, *23*, 581–593. [CrossRef]

48. Farmer, C.; Petitclerc, D.; Sorensen, M.T.; Vignola, M.; Dourmad, J.Y. Impacts of dietary protein level and feed restriction during prepuberty on mammogenesis in gilts. *J. Anim. Sci.* **2004**, *82*, 2343–2351. [CrossRef]

49. Poretsky, L.; Cataldo, N.A.; Rosenwaks, Z.; Giudice, L. The insulin-related ovarian regulatory system in health and disease. *Endocr. Rev.* **1999**, *20*, 535–582. [CrossRef] [PubMed]

50. Kloareg, M.; Noblet, J.; van Milgen, J. Deposition of dietary fatty acids, de novo synthesis and anatomical partitioning of fatty acids in finishing pigs. *Br. J. Nutr.* **2007**, *97*, 35–44. [CrossRef] [PubMed]

51. Morales, J.; Pérez, J.F.; Baucells, M.D.; Mourot, J.; Gasa, J. Comparative digestibility and lipogenic activity in Landrace and Iberian finishing pigs fed ad libitum corn- and corn-sorghum-acorn-based diets. *Livest. Prod. Sci.* **2002**, *77*, 195–205. [CrossRef]

52. Benítez, R.; Fernández, A.; Isabel, B.; Núñez, Y.; De Mercado, E.; Gómez-Izquierdo, E.; García-Casco, J.; López-Bote, C.; Óvilo, C. Modulatory effects of breed, feeding status, and diet on adipogenic, lipogenic, and lipolytic gene expression in growing iberian and duroc pigs. *Int. J. Mol. Sci.* **2018**, *19*, 22. [CrossRef]

53. Nieto, R.; Lara, L.; Barea, R.; García-Valverde, R.; Conde-Aguilera, J.A.; Aguilera, J.F. Growth of body components and carcass composition of Iberian pigs of 10 to 150 kg body weight as affected by the level of feeding and dietary protein concentration. *J. Anim. Sci.* **2013**, *91*, 4197–4207. [CrossRef] [PubMed]

54. Lebret, B. Effects of feeding and rearing systems on growth, carcass composition and meat quality in pigs. *Animal* **2008**, *2*, 1548–1558. [CrossRef] [PubMed]

55. Wood, J.D.; Nute, G.R.; Richardson, R.I.; Whittington, F.M.; Southwood, O.; Plastow, G.; Mansbridge, R.; Da Costa, N.; Chang, K.C. Effects of breed, diet and muscle on fat deposition and eating quality in pigs. *Meat Sci.* **2004**, *67*, 651–667. [CrossRef] [PubMed]

56. Daza, A.; Latorre, M.A.; Olivares, A.; Amazán, D.; López Bote, C.J. Effect of replacement of a conventional diet by granulated barley during finishing period on growth performance and carcass and meat characteristics in 130-kg gilts. *Livest. Sci.* **2012**, *148*, 196–200. [CrossRef]

57. Gerfault, V.; Louveau, I.; Mourot, J.; Le Dividich, J. Lipogenic enzyme activities in subcutaneous adipose tissue and skeletal muscle from neonatal pigs consuming maternal or formula milk. *Reprod. Nutr. Dev.* **2000**, *40*, 103–112. [CrossRef]

58. Tejeda, J.F.; Gandemer, G.; Antequera, T.; Viau, M.; García, C. Lipid traits of muscles as related to genotype and fattening diet in Iberian pigs: Total intramuscular lipids and triacylglycerols. *Meat Sci.* **2002**, *60*, 357–363. [CrossRef]

59. Pérez-Palacios, T.; Ruiz, J.; Tejeda, J.F.; Antequera, T. Subcutaneous and intramuscular lipid traits as tools for classifying Iberian pigs as a function of their feeding background. *Meat Sci.* **2009**, *81*, 632–640. [CrossRef]

60. Daza, A.; Menoyo, D.; López Bote, C.J. Carcass traits and fatty acid composition of subcutaneous, intramuscular and liver fat from iberian pigs fed in confinement only with acorns or a formulated diet. *Food Sci. Technol. Int.* **2009**, *15*, 563–569. [CrossRef]

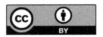

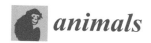

Article

Pre-Slaughter Sources of Fresh Meat Quality Variation: The Case of Heavy Pigs Intended for Protected Designation of Origin Products

Luca Sardi [1], Alessandro Gastaldo [2], Marzia Borciani [3], Andrea Bertolini [2], Valeria Musi [3], Anna Garavaldi [3], Giovanna Martelli [1,*], Damiano Cavallini [1] and Eleonora Nannoni [1]

1   Department of Veterinary Medical Sciences, University of Bologna, Via Tolara di Sopra 50,
    40064 Ozzano Emilia (BO), Italy; luca.sardi@unibo.it (L.S.); damiano.cavallini@unibo.it (D.C.);
    eleonora.nannoni2@unibo.it (E.N.)
2   Foundation C.R.P.A. (Research Centre on Animal Production) Studies and Researches,
    Viale Timavo 43/2, 42121 Reggio Emilia, Italy; a.gastaldo@crpa.it (A.G.); a.bertolini@crpa.it (A.B.)
3   C.R.P.A. (Research Centre on Animal Production), Viale Timavo 43/2, 42121 Reggio Emilia, Italy;
    m.borciani@crpa.it (M.B.); v.musi@crpa.it (V.M.); a.garavaldi@crpa.it (A.G.)
*   Correspondence: giovanna.martelli@unibo.it

Received: 29 October 2020; Accepted: 9 December 2020; Published: 14 December 2020

Simple Summary: This study aimed at investigating which pre-slaughter parameters determine variations in the quality of the loin derived from pigs intended for Italian PDO (Protected Designation of Origin) products. Data were collected on 44 commercial shipments of Italian heavy pigs. Meat quality parameters (pH, color lightness, drip loss, cooking loss, and shear force) identified two clusters: 'Higher Quality' (HQ) and 'Lower Quality' (LQ). The parameters which differed more widely between the two clusters were journey duration, ambient temperature, distance traveled and irregular behaviors (slipping, falling, and overlapping) at unloading. Among the pre slaughter parameters which negatively affect pork quality, consideration should be given to ambient temperatures above 22 °C, distance traveled above 26 km, travel duration between 38 and 66 min, and more than 5.9% of animals showing irregular behaviors at unloading. Journeys involving one or more of these risk factors may require additional attention in terms of animal welfare in order to obtain meat suitable for high-quality productions.

Abstract: This study focused on loin quality in Italian heavy pigs intended for the production of PDOs (Protected Designation of Origin) products, and investigated the pre-slaughter factors which negatively affect the quality of fresh meat. Data were collected on 44 shipments (loads) of pigs. Shipments were carried out under commercial conditions. Several pre-slaughter parameters were recorded within the entire process (on-farm, during transport, and at the slaughterhouse). On a subset of pigs (10 animals from every load, N = 440), serum cortisol and creatine kinase were measured and loin samples were analyzed for pH, instrumental color, drip loss, cooking loss, shear force, and sensory quality. Cluster analysis of the instrumentally-assessed meat quality parameters allowed the categorization of the shipments into two clusters: lower quality (LQ) and higher quality (HQ). Our results showed that the factors with significant differences between the two clusters were journey duration, ambient temperature, distance traveled, and irregular behaviors (slipping, falling, and overlapping) at unloading (all greater in LQ, $p < 0.05$). The pre-slaughter conditions associated with lower loin quality were ambient temperatures above 22 °C, distance traveled above 26 km, travel duration between 38–66 min, more than 5.9% of animals showing irregular behaviors at unloading.

Keywords: animal welfare; transport; stress; pigs; meat quality

1. Introduction

Animal welfare and meat quality in relation to road transportation have received much attention in terms of experimental research, but the effects of road transportation on animal welfare are difficult to monitor and validate under practical conditions, because of the numerous situations and variables which can change during the process (e.g., road condition, driver experience, animal handling, microclimate, etc.) [1]. Besides, according to a recent review [2] the literature currently available on pig transportation mostly focuses on pigs weighing between 100 and 135 kg, and little information is available on heavier pigs, which may react differently to transportation stressors. Besides the case of Italy, where pigs are traditionally transported and slaughtered at a minimum age of 9 months and at the average body weight (BW) of 160 kg ± 10% for the production of typical PDO (Protected Designation of Origin) products (such as Parma Ham, Salame Brianza, Coppa Piacentina, etc.) [3], other European and worldwide countries have been increasing pigs' slaughtering BW over the past decade. This increase is driven by both the dilution of fixed production cost over more weight per pig and the improvement of genetic selection of lean-type pigs [4]. Several studies evaluated the effects of greater slaughter weights on profitability, carcass quality, primal cuts yield, and pork quality (e.g., [5–10]); however, only in a few studies the slaughter weight considerably exceeded 125 kg [5,10]. This framework results in a pronounced lack of knowledge concerning the quality of the fresh meat of heavy pigs, and in particular on how pork quality of this productive category may be affected by pre-slaughter stressors under conventional conditions. Additionally, according to a recent review, the quality of dry-cured hams, which are the most valuable products, greatly depends on raw material properties (e.g., meat physicochemical properties such as pH and water holding capacity) and intrinsic properties of the muscle (moisture, fat, and enzyme activities), all of which are influenced by various ante-mortem factors [11]. The few available studies on pre-slaughter handling of Italian heavy pigs highlighted that animal losses increase when animals are kept in lairage overnight at the plant [12]. This effect, however, was observed to vary largely, depending on the characteristics and management of the lairage area at the slaughterhouse (i.e., presence of large open windows, stocking density in the lairage pens, and the use of cooling devices such as sprinklers) [13]. When heavy pigs are subjected to pre-slaughter handling and short transportation, the parameters found to have a negative impact on blood stress indicators were the following: high average speed of the vehicle during transport, low welfare index at slaughter, low TSWI (overall transport and slaughter welfare index), greater distance traveled, and greater percentage of irregular behaviors (slips, falls, and overlaps) during unloading [14]. However, in the mentioned studies, the consequences of different pre-slaughter handling on meat quality have not been evaluated [12,13], or have produced results inconsistent with the level of stress experienced by the animals (evaluated in terms of blood indicators) [14].

The aim of the present paper, which is part of a wider research project [14], was to fill this lack of knowledge by investigating the relationships between a some pre-slaughtering parameters (measured upon departure, during transport, and at slaughter) and loin quality, to identify which pre-slaughtering have the largest impact on pork quality. Within the framework of a typical pork production mainly focused on cured products, the identification and control of the parameters that have a positive effect on meat cuts to be consumed fresh can help reduce food wastage and promote higher standards of animal welfare.

2. Materials and Methods

2.1. Ethical Statement

The experiment did not include any invasive procedure in vivo, therefore no specific authorization by the institutional ethical committee was required (Directive 2010/63/EU [15]). Rearing, transport, and slaughtering were carried out in commercial farms/trucks/plants and according to the EU legislation (Directive 2008/120/EC [16], Council Regulation-EC-no. 1/2005 [17], and Council Regulation-EC-no. 1099/2009 [18]).

2.2. Experimental Design and Data Collection

Data were collected by monitoring 44 shipments of Italian heavy pigs. As per common commercial practice, animals were raised and transported in mixed-sex groups (gilts and barrows). Shipments originated from 11 randomly-selected commercial farms located in Northern Italy (Emilia Romagna region), with each farm providing 4 loads of pigs (2 during the warm and 2 during the cold season). All animals involved in the study were commercial hybrids suitable for the production of Parma hams according to the production rules [3]. Loads varied between a minimum of 59 and a maximum of 145 pigs (average: 118). Descriptive statistics of the transports analyzed in the present study can be found in Sardi et al. [14]. All animals were transported to the same commercial slaughter plant, where they were electrically stunned and then immediately exsanguinated. For each of the shipments, the experimental protocol included: (a) the assessment of several pre-slaughtered parameters; (b) the collection of blood samples from a subset of pigs, for the evaluation of stress biomarkers; and (c) the collection of meat samples from the same subset of animals, for meat quality and sensory evaluations. The methods by which these data/samples were collected and analyzed are fully described in a previous paper [14] and will be briefly outlined in this section.

2.2.1. Pre-Slaughter Parameters Checklists and Scores/Indexes Calculation

For every shipment (or load) of pigs (N = 44), several pre-slaughter parameters were assessed by filling three checklists: one upon departure from the farm, one during transport, and one at slaughter. All observations were carried out by the same two trained assessors, who worked together. Data were then submitted to a calculation system which allowed the calculation of (1) a farm (on departure) score; (2) a transport score; (3) a slaughter score, and (4) an overall TSWI (Transport and Slaughter Welfare Index). Additional information on the assessment method, together with a full list of the parameters assessed and how they were scored can be found in Barbari et al. [19] and in Sardi et al. [14]. Briefly, the characteristics of the indexes/scores can be summarized as follows:

- On departure (from the farm) checklist. The parameters assessed were: loading duration, path from the pen to the truck (length, width, design, flooring, presence of internal and external corridors, ramps, loading facilities), time taken to move the pigs, handling (tools used and mode of use), irregular behaviors during handling (pigs slipping, falling, overlapping). The integration of observations made according to this checklist resulted in an 'on-departure score', whose values could range from the lowest theoretical value of −30.5 points (pts) for the minimum possible welfare level to the highest theoretical value of 15.5 pts for the maximum possible welfare level.

- Transport checklist. The parameters assessed were: distance and duration of the journey, space allowance per pig, presence and number of drinkers, cooling systems, other characteristics of the lorry (possibility to inspect animals and take care of them, internal illumination, floor type and condition, presence or absence of bedding). The integration of the observations made according to this checklist resulted in a 'transport score' whose values could range from the lowest theoretical value of −18.0 pts for the minimum possible welfare level to the highest value of 9.5 pts for the maximum possible welfare level.

- Slaughter checklist. The parameters assessed were: unloading duration, path from the truck to the lairage pen and from the lairage pen to the stunning area (flooring, passages, presence of one-way gates), handling (tools used and mode of use), irregular behaviors during handling (pigs slipping, falling, overlapping), lairage pens characteristics (stocking density, ventilation, illumination, thermal insulation, conditions of floors and surfaces, type of pens, presence of mobile partitions, drinkers, cooling systems), stunning area characteristics (partitions, gates, devices, stunning method, stun-to-stick interval, procedures for the use and to check the efficiency of the stunning system, emergency stunning procedures, training of the personnel involved). The integration of the observations made according to this checklist resulted in a 'slaughter score', which could range from the lowest theoretical value of −41.5 pts for the minimum possible welfare level to the highest theoretical value of 50.5 pts for the maximum possible welfare level.

- TSWI: The Transport and Slaughter Welfare Index summarizes the welfare experienced by the animals during the entire pre-slaughter period (from when they are taken from their pen at the farm until when they are slaughtered). The TSWI integrated the three previously calculated scores and its theoretical values could range from a minimum of −90.0 pts for the lowest possible welfare level to a maximum of 75.5 for the highest possible welfare level.

2.2.2. Blood Sampling and Analysis

Blood samples were collected at exsanguination from 10 randomly-selected animals from each of the 44 loads (N = 440). Blood was refrigerated and transferred to the laboratory of the Department of Veterinary Medicine of the University of Bologna (Italy), where plasma was immediately separated and stored at −20 °C, pending subsequent analysis for cortisol, creatine kinase, and aldolase. Cortisol was used in this study as an indicator of acute pre-slaughter stress (e.g., during handling, transport, and/or restraint) [20]. Creatine kinase (CK) was chosen as a subacute indicator of intense physical activity (due for example to exhaustion, loading, or harsh handling) and as a biomarker of overall welfare during transport [21]. Blood CK concentration rises up to a peak approximately 6 h after muscle damage and returns to basal levels between 8 h and 48 h [22,23]. Aldolase is a less-studied, possible long-term indicator of muscle damage. Its blood concentration peaks after at least 48–72 h from the damage [24] and its activity has been correlated to meat quality traits such as pH and myofibrillar protein solubility [25]. Aldolase has been used in human medicine as a more accurate and objective indicator of muscle damage than CK due to its lower inter-individual variability [24]. In the present paper, cortisol concentration (which will be expressed as ng/mL) was measured using a radioimmunological assay technique [26], whereas creatine kinase and aldolase concentrations in plasma (which will both be expressed as U/L) were measured using two commercially available kits based on a colorimetric method with subsequent spectrophotometric UV readings (CK Nac Liquid and Aldolase, Sentinel Diagnostics, Milano, Italy).

2.2.3. Meat Sampling and Meat Quality Assessment

The meat parameters were measured on the longissimus thoracis and lumborum (LTL) muscle of the same animals from which the blood samples were collected (10 animals per shipment, N = 440). At the slaughter plant, carcass lean content was measured using a Fat-o-Meater (F-o-M SFK, Copenhagen, DK), and pH at 45 min (pH 45) was measured in the LTL muscle (at the second/third last rib level) using a portable pH meter equipped with a glass spear tip electrode and a temperature compensation probe (model 250A—Orion Research, Boston, MA, USA). Two portions of the LTL muscle were collected from each carcass, refrigerated and transferred to the laboratory for the assessment of instrumental color, pH at 24 h post mortem (pH 24), Drip Loss, Cooking Loss, and Warner–Bratzler Shear Force (WBSF). Measurements of pH were carried out by means of the same portable pH meter described above. Color was measured according to the CIE Lab (lightness index L*, green/red index a*, blue/yellow index b*) color space system [27] using a Minolta Chromameter set with D65 illuminant (model CR-400—Konica Minolta optics INC., Tokyo, Japan). Drip Loss, Cooking Loss (water bath cooking until core temperature reached 75 °C), and WBSF were assessed subsequently on the same meat sample according to the methods described previously by Honikel [28] and also reported by Sardi et al. [14].

The second muscle portion was transferred to the laboratories at the Research Centre on Animal Production (Reggio Emilia, Italy). Here samples were vacuum-packed and stored at −20 °C pending sensory analysis, which was carried out within a month by a panel of trained experts, according to the method described by Della Casa et al. [29]. The sensory analysis included a visual assessment on raw samples (lean color and marbling) and a subsequent evaluation of the cooked sample (initial tenderness, chewing tenderness, juiciness, final residue, chewiness, aroma intensity, buttery aroma, and off-flavors).

Photographic scales were provided for the assessment of lean color (0 = light pink, reference sample chicken breast; 10 = brown, reference samples horse steak after a few days) and marbling (0 = absent or low, on one side of the slice; 10 = high on all sides of the slice) [29]. All other factors were evaluated using a structured continuous scale with values ranging between 1 and 10 (1 = sensation absent, 10 = sensation of the greatest intensity).

2.3. Statistical Analysis

Statistical analysis was carried out using the software JMP v15.1 (SAS Institute Inc., Cary, NC, USA). Meat quality parameters (pH45, pH24, L*, Drip Loss, Cooking loss and WBSF) within the corresponding shipment were used in a k-means cluster analysis to differentiate clusters of animals based on their instrumentally-assessed meat quality. Three different models (with two, three, and four clusters) were tested and compared for their cubic clustering criterion (CCC) values. The two-cluster model was chosen, based on its greater fit statistics (CCC values of −1.4887, −3.1458, and −4.7393 for the two-, three-, and four-cluster model, respectively). The two-cluster model allowed the identification of two groups, including 34 and 10 shipments (clusters characteristics will be described more in detail in Section 3.1). For numerical variables, a linear mixed-model procedure was used to identify statistical differences between the two clusters in the pre-slaughter measures (including measures taken on departure, during transport, and at slaughter). Each shipment from the farm of origin was considered as an experimental unit and used as a random variable for all analyses. For blood parameters and meat quality, each shipment was used as the experimental unit, and the 10 measures for each shipment were considered as repeated measures with an autoregressive covariance structure (AR1). The cluster grouping was used as a fixed effect within the model. Means were separated based on least-square mean, and all pairwise multiple comparisons were carried out using Tukey post-hoc test. For categorical variables, a nominal logistic model with the chi-square likelihood ratio test was carried out. A p-value ≤ 0.10 was considered as a tendency, a $p \leq 0.05$ was considered statistically significant.

A random K-fold (5-fold) neural network model was also run to recognize underlying relationships between the meat quality clusters and the pre-slaughter variables. In the training set, the R-square statistic and the RMSE (root-mean-square error) were 0.9307 and 0.1469, respectively. In the validation set, the R-square statistics and the RMSE were 0.9032 and 0.1703, respectively. A ROC (receiver operating characteristic) curve procedure was used to identify thresholds, sensitivity, and specificity of a list of individual pre-slaughter variables.

3. Results and Discussion

3.1. Clusters Based on Meat Parameters

Meat quality parameters (pH45, pH24, L*, Drip Loss, Cooking Loss and WBSF) allowed the separation of the shipments in two clusters (which are graphically shown in Figure 2). Cluster 1 (red color) included 34 shipments (N = 340 meat samples), and cluster 2 (green color) included 10 shipments (N = 100 meat samples). The average value of the main instrumental meat quality parameters for the two clusters and the statistical differences between clusters are summarized in Table 1.

Concerning the parameters used for clusterization, Cluster 1 included shipments with animals having significantly greater ($p < 0.0001$) average pH45′ and pH24 h, as well as significantly lower ($p < 0.0001$) L* and Drip Loss values than Cluster 2. Cooking Loss tended to be lower ($p = 0.064$) in Cluster 1 than in Cluster 2. For these reasons, Cluster 1 and Cluster 2 were renamed Higher Meat Quality (HQ), and Lower Meat Quality (LQ), respectively. Shear force (WBSF) was significantly greater in HQ than in LQ cluster ($p < 0.0001$). Significant differences were observed also in a*, b*, and Chroma values, which were all greater in Cluster 2 (LQ). Carcass lean content was similar between clusters.

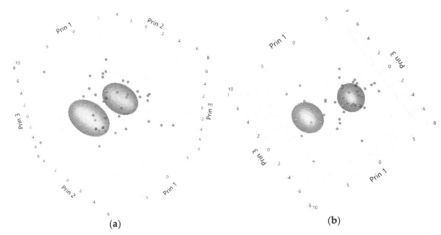

(a)   (b)

Figure 1. Three-dimensional representation of the shipments clustered according to meat quality parameters (pH 45, pH 24, L*, Drip Loss, Cooking Loss and WBSF) and seen from different angles (a) and (b). Each dot on the graph represents a shipment. Cluster 1 (red color, 34 shipments), Cluster 2 (green color, 10 shipments). The colored area represents the area around the cluster centroid.

Table 1. Summary of the meat quality characteristics of the two clusters. Variables in italics were used for data clusterization.

Parameter, U.M. [3]	Cluster 1 (HQ [1]) (N = 340 Pigs)		Cluster 2 (LQ [2]) (N = 100 Pigs)		*p*-Value
	Estimate	SE [4]	Estimate	SE [4]	-
pH 45	6.06	0.02	5.80	0.04	<0.0001
pH 24	5.54	0.006	5.43	0.01	<0.0001
*L**	46.6	0.5	53.0	0.9	<0.0001
Drip Loss, %	0.98	0.04	1.47	0.08	<0.0001
Cooking loss, %	25,8	0.6	28.1	1.0	0.0643
WBSF [5], kg/cm²	4.0	0.1	3.4	0.2	0.0054
F-o-M [6]	48.6	0.2	48.3	0.4	0.3413
a*	3.9	0.2	4.7	0.3	0.0491
b*	4.6	0.2	5.9	0.3	0.0002
Hue [7]	0.89	0.01	0.91	0.02	0.382
Chroma [8]	6.2	0.2	7.7	0.4	0.0016

[1] Higher Quality; [2] Lower Quality; [3] Unit of Measurement; [4] Standard Error; [5] Warner–Bratzler Shear Force; [6] Carcass lean content was measured using a Fat-o-Meater; [7] Hue = $\sqrt{(a^{*2} + b^{*2})}$; [8] Chroma = arctan(b*/a*).

Overall, the meat quality profile of Cluster 1 (HQ) indicates more favorable characteristics, due to the more limited rate and extent of pH decline, leading to a lower degree of protein denaturation and disintegration of cellular structures [30], resulting also in greater water holding capacity (WHC) both during conservation at +4 °C (drip loss) and during cooking (cooking loss). The combination of a high protein denaturation degree and a low WHC usually results in light meat color, due to greater light-scattering properties of the shrunk proteins, as it also happens in meat with the PSE (pale, soft, and exudative) defect [31]. Accordingly, greater L* values were observed in Cluster 2 (LQ), compared to Cluster 1 (HQ). The main characteristics of the LQ meat are compatible with the PSE definition, including also the consistency of meat assessed on the cooked samples, which was softer (lower WBSF values) in the LQ than in the HQ cluster. While several studies observed a reduced tenderness of PSE meat [32], our results seem to agree with Tornberg, who hypothesized that, when meat is cooked at temperatures above 60 °C, the WBSF decreases as the degree of contraction of the fibers increases [33].

This would imply that cooking PSE meat, which has a greater degree of longitudinal contraction, would result in a greater tenderness (i.e., a lower WBSF). It is, however, noteworthy that the drip loss observed in heavy pigs meat (being it either normal or similar to PSE) is usually considerably lower than what observed in lighter animals (e.g., [34,35]), probably due to the different age and weight at slaughter, reflecting on the moisture content of the carcass (and meat) [36].

Statistically significant differences between clusters were observed also with respect to the instrumentally-assessed meat color, with LQ cluster having greater redness index (a* value) and yellowness index (b* value), and an overall greater chroma value than HQ ($p < 0.05$ for the three variables). Such small differences in color, likely not detectable by the human eye, probably indicate that the meat belonging to the LQ cluster may fall within the case of untypical deviations like RSE (reddish-pink, soft, exudative), which can be defined as a mild occurrence of PSE [30,35].

3.2. Differences in Transport Variables, Blood Parameters, and Sensory Meat Quality between Clusters

Table 2 shows the linear mixed model applied to some of the pre-slaughter variables measured in the TSWI checklists.

Table 2. Results of the linear mixed-model procedure to identify statistical differences between the two clusters in the measured transport and slaughter variables.

Number of Shipments	HQ [1]		LQ [2]		
	34		10		
Variable	Estimate	SE [3]	Estimate	SE	p-Value
Loading duration, min	47.7	3.7	43.9	6.9	0.6469
Pigs loaded per hour, n	170	11	170	20	0.9870
Irregular behaviors (slipping, falling, overlapping) at loading, %	17.3	1.9	21.0	3.4	0.3362
Waiting time at the farm (before departure), min	14.3	0.8	11.5	1.5	0.1173
Journey duration, min	33.8	3.1	48.6	5.7	0.0277
Ambient temperature, °C	15.3	1.4	21.9	2.6	0.0291
Distance traveled, km	23.3	1.8	36.1	3.3	0.0014
Average vehicle speed during transport, km/h	72.0	2.8	77.7	5.2	0.3433
Waiting time at the slaughterhouse (before unloading), min	20.4	2.5	24.2	4.7	0.4796
Total journey duration (from loading to unloading), min	133.4	5.6	143.7	10.4	0.3906
Total waiting time on the truck (farm + slaughterhouse), min	34.7	2.8	35.7	5.2	0.8672
Unloading duration, min	17.4	0.9	15.5	1.6	0.3209
Pigs unloaded per hour, n	427	22	452	40	0.5919
Irregular behaviors (slipping, falling, overlapping) at unloading, %	4.82	0.58	7.77	1.06	0.0192
Total irregular behaviors (slipping, falling, overlapping), %	22.1	2.1	28.8	3.8	0.1243
Lairage duration (from unloading to stunning), min	576	89	528	164	0.7986
Transport + lairage duration, min	710	90	672	165	0.8423
Stable (unmixed) groups, odds ratio	0.59	0.39	0.70	0.39	0.5183
On-departure (at farm) score, pts	1.66	0.29	2.05	0.55	0.5391
Transport score, pts	3.10	0.28	3.90	0.51	0.1798
Slaughter score, pts	27.97	0.39	28.45	0.73	0.5645
TSWI [4] (farm + transport + slaughter), pts	32.73	0.59	34.40	1.09	0.1875

[1] Higher quality; [2] Lower quality; [3] Standard error; [4] Transport and Slaughter Welfare Index.

According to our model, some of the pre-slaughter parameters statistically differed between the two clusters. In particular, the variables journey duration, ambient temperature, distance traveled, and irregular behaviors (total of slipping, falling, and overlapping) observed at unloading were all significantly greater ($p < 0.05$) in the LQ than in the HQ cluster. The other variables and the calculated scores/indexes (on-departure score, transport score, slaughter score, and TSWI) did not significantly differ between clusters.

Despite the statistically significant differences found between the two clusters, it can be observed that some variables, such as transport duration and distance traveled, indicate that on average both groups of animals were transported for a short time and over small distances (for journey duration: average 37.2, SD 18.8, minimum 18, maximum 90 min; for distance traveled: average 26.2, SD 11.6, minimum 11, maximum 59 km, data shown in [14]). Short travel duration is common for Italian heavy pigs, and previous research indicated that between one half and 90% of these animals are transported for less than 2 h [12,13]. In the present study, however, differences in meat quality were observed despite the short average transportation time, with relatively greater transportation times and greater distances traveled negatively affecting meat quality. This result is in partial disagreement with the findings on lighter pigs of Warriss et al. [37], who compared two relatively short travel durations (1 h vs. 4 h) and found no major effects on meat quality. This may indicate that the meat quality of heavy pigs is more subjected to alterations even during short time transportations. It is, however, worth observing that, under some circumstances, short time (1 h) transportation has been deemed to be more stressful than longer ones (3 h) because, if conditions on the truck are good, during the journey animals can recover from the stress suffered at loading [38]. In our case, this may indicate that the transport conditions were quite good regardless of the cluster, and this is confirmed by the transport score value, which was similar between the clusters (3.10 vs. 3.90) and fell in the moderate-to-high welfare range. In fact, as shown in the Materials and Methods section, transport score ranges from −18 pts for the lowest welfare level possible to 9.5 pts for the highest welfare level; therefore, values of about 3–4 pts collocate the transport in the top 25% of the assessment checklist, indicating that most of the required parameters illustrated in Sardi et al. ([14]) were met.

The differences observed concerning ambient temperature are in agreement with the literature. It is well known that acute heat stress before slaughter stimulates muscle glycogenolysis and can therefore lead to low WHC and to PSE meat [39]. Accordingly, a study on lighter pigs (127 kg BW) showed that transports carried out during summer resulted in paler meat color (i.e., in greater L* value) than during winter [40]. Čobanović et al. [34] observed the lowest pH and the highest thawing loss, L* and b* values, and occurrence of PSE meat in pigs (110 kg BW) transported during summer.

To the best of our knowledge, no study specifically investigated the relationship between irregular behaviors and meat quality, although it has been observed that harsh handling or bad facility design (resulting in more slips, falls, and overlaps), especially at loading, is correlated with more intense stress response and reduced pork quality [41,42]. This may warrant the need for future studies on behavior during unloading.

Table 3 shows the results of the linear mixed model applied to the blood parameters and to the sensory meat quality traits. Our results show no substantial difference between clusters in stress and muscle damage parameters (cortisol, CK, and aldolase). This seems to confirm the poor-to-moderate relationship between physiological response to pre-slaughter stress and meat quality which has been previously observed in other studies (e.g., [43,44]).

As concerns sensory parameters, from a general standpoint, it can also be observed that several variables, despite not showing statistically significant differences, were in general agreement with the higher vs. lower meat quality characteristics observed in the two clusters (i.e., numerically greater marbling score, initial tenderness, chewing tenderness, juiciness, chewiness, and aroma intensity in the HQ cluster). Conversely, significant differences were observed in some sensory traits, with LQ cluster having a lower (i.e., paler) color score, and a greater final residue and buttery aroma scores. Color and final residue are in agreement with the instrumentally-measured meat characteristics described above (L* and WHC, respectively), whereas the differences in the buttery aroma are harder to explain, especially considering the almost identical marbling score and carcass lean meat content between the two clusters. It should, however, be mentioned that—despite being significant—the difference observed in the buttery aroma was detected by a panel of trained experts and amounted to 0.3 points out of a 10-point sensory scale, therefore it may not be easily perceived by the average consumer. The same observation can also be made for the differences detected in visually assessed color.

Table 3. Results of the linear mixed-model procedure to identify statistical differences between the two clusters in the measured blood parameters and sensory attributes of meat. Back-transformed data are presented between square brackets.

Number of Samples	HQ [1]		LQ [2]		
	340		100		
Variable	Estimate	SE [3]	Estimate	SE	*p*-Value
log Cortisol, ng/mL	1.033 [10.79]	0.030	1.040 [10.96]	0.054	0.9176
log CK [4], U/L	3.291 [1954]	0.014	3.263 [1832]	0.026	0.3623
log Aldolase, U/L	1.647 [44.36]	0.027	1.618 [41.50]	0.049	0.605
Color score	4.72	0.06	4.45	0.09	0.0126
Marbling score	4.96	0.11	4.89	0.17	0.7300
Initial tenderness	5.52	0.11	5.27	0.18	0.2676
Chewing tenderness	5.07	0.11	4.80	0.18	0.2282
Juiciness	3.88	0.13	3.76	0.21	0.6127
Final residue	2.90	0.05	3.16	0.07	0.0076
Chewiness	5.43	0.09	5.31	0.14	0.4788
Aroma intensity	5.38	0.12	5.27	0.18	0.5929
Buttery aroma	2.81	0.06	3.08	0.10	0.0318
Off-flavors	2.28	0.05	2.31	0.08	0.7858

[1] Higher quality, [2] Lower quality; [3] Standard error [4] Creatine kinase.

3.3. Results of the Neural Network Model to Identify Possible Thresholds for Meat Quality Variation in the Pre-Slaughtering Variables

As concerns the neural network analysis, the high R-Square statistic for the validation set (above 0.9) indicates that the model is predicting well on data not used to train it, and also indicates a good capability of the model to describe a phenomenon. Figure 2 shows the profile graphs resulting from the neural network model for each of the pre-slaughter variables presented in Table 2, to visually understand how the variables affect the predicted meat quality clusterization. For completeness, all variables considered are presented in Figure 2 and briefly described in the next paragraph, but only those significantly differing between the meat quality clusters will be discussed in detail. To improve readability, the caption below each graph indicates the variable plotted on the x-axis. Each graph indicates how the probability of the transport to be classified as either HQ or LQ changes as the pre-slaughter variable indicated on the horizontal axis varies.

This paragraph provides a general description of the results of the neural network shown in Figure 2. Some of the variables (loading duration, number of pigs loaded per hour, total journey duration, total waiting time on the truck, unloading duration, lairage duration, transport + lairage duration, slaughter score) showed no appreciable relation with the cluster classification. Other parameters (i.e., irregular behaviors at loading, average vehicle speed, waiting time at the slaughterhouse, pigs unloaded per hours, total irregular behaviors, groups stability, farm score, transport score, and TSWI) seemed to show an overall negative relationship with the meat quality clusters (as the value of the variables increased, shipments were more likely to be classified in the LQ clusters). However, as previously described, these variables failed to reach statistically significant differences between clusters. Similarly, a positive correlation (leading also in this case to no statistically significant differences between clusters) was observed only for the variable 'waiting time at the farm' (as the waiting time increased, the shipments were more likely to be classified in the HQ cluster). This may indicate that a short waiting time at the farm, especially if the weather is mild, may give to the animals the possibility to adapt (at least partially) to the truck environment before the beginning of the journey.

According to our statistical model, in fact, a 14-min waiting time increased the probability of having HQ meat (specificity 0.70, sensibility 0.59).

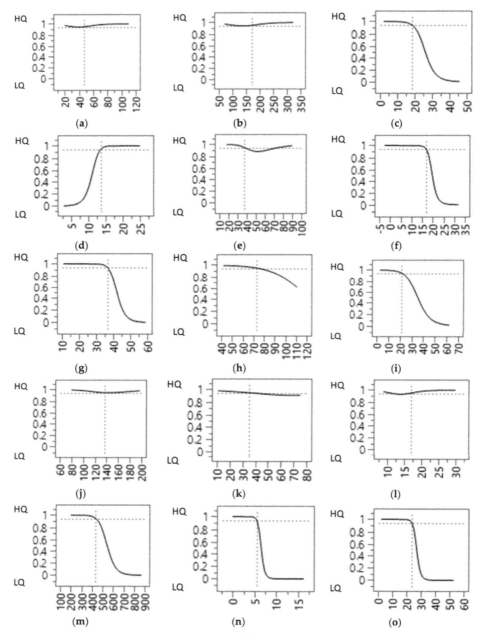

Figure 2. *Cont.*

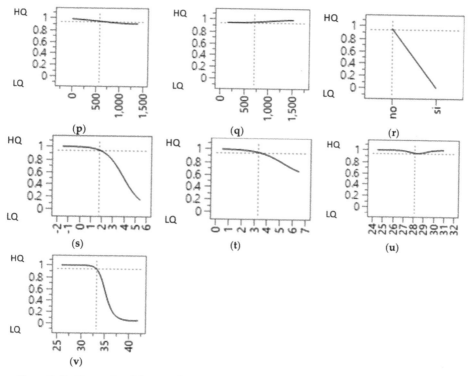

Figure 2. Profile graphs of the neural network model for all the pre-slaughter variables presented in Table 2. For each graph, the name of the variable plotted on the *x*-axis is indicated below the figure. (HQ = High quality cluster; LQ = Low quality cluster). Variable names highlighted in bold character indicate statistically significant differences (*p* < 0.05) between clusters, as presented in Table 2. (**a**) Loading duration, min. (**b**) Pigs loaded per hour, n. (**c**) Irregular behaviors at loading, %. (**d**) Waiting time at the farm, min. (**e**) **Journey duration, min.** (**f**) **Ambient temperature, °C.** (**g**) **Distance traveled, km.** (**h**) Average vehicle speed, km/h. (**i**) Waiting time at slaughterhouse, min. (**j**) Total journey duration, min. (**k**) Total waiting time on the truck, min. (**l**) Unloading duration, min. (**m**) Pigs unloaded per hour, n. (**n**) **Irregular behaviors at unloading, %.** (**o**) Total irregular behaviors. (**p**) Lairage duration, min. (**q**) Transport + lairage duration, min. (**r**) Stable (unmixed) groups, odds ratio. (**s**) On-departure (at farm) score, pts. (**t**) Transport score, pts. (**t**) Slaughter score, pts. (**u**) TSWI, pts.

Among the variables which, as described in Section 3.3, statistically differed between the two clusters (journey duration, ambient temperature, distance traveled, irregular behavior at unloading), three (namely ambient temperature, distance traveled, irregular behaviors at unloading) showed a negative correlation with the cluster classification. More specifically, for ambient temperature, the observed cut-off value (as assessed using the ROC curve) was at 22 °C (sensitivity 0.88; specificity 0.60); and transports carried out above this temperature had a greater probability of resulting in lower meat quality. Previous studies on Italian heavy pigs found an increase in transport losses during the summer [12], and in particular when the THI (temperature humidity index) exceeded 78.5 (corresponding, for example, to combinations of temperature and relative humidity of about 35° and 20%, or 30°C and 50%, or 27 °C and 80%) [13]. Our results, therefore, indicate that adverse effects on meat quality can be already observed at lower ambient temperatures. Interestingly, even lower temperatures were indicated in studies on the mortality of market-weight pigs, in which in-transit losses have been reported to increase beyond ambient temperatures of 16–17 °C [45,46]. It is also worth pointing out that, in terms of thermal comfort, a more accurate evaluation of the heat stress level experienced by the animals could be carried out by implementing more complex measurements, such as continuous monitoring of the pigs' internal temperature [47], monitoring the microclimate inside the tuck (e.g., by assessing times derivatives of temperature or enthalpy [48]) or including a quantification of the heat and moisture generated by animals during transportation [49]. Such complex evaluations, however, fall outside the scope of the present paper, in which the evaluation of pre-slaughter variables was carried out only using a checklist system and no sensors were installed on the truck or placed on/inside the animals' body.

As concerns irregular behaviors at unloading, the observed threshold was at 5.9% (sensitivity 0.74; specificity 0.90), implying that transports in which more than this percentage of animals showed slipping, falling, or and overlapping at unloading were more likely to belong to the LQ cluster.

As concerns distance traveled, the cut-off value was 26 km (sensitivity 0.80; specificity 0.79), with animals transported for 26 km or above having lower meat quality. Journey duration showed a bimodal trend, in which transports lasting between 38 min (sensitivity 0.80; specificity 0.73) and 66 min (sensitivity 0.30; specificity 0.94) were associated with worse meat quality. This seems to indicate that shorter transports do not consistently affect meat quality. As concerns longer journeys, it has previously been observed that, provided that conditions on the means of transportation guarantee adequate comfort, animals may (at least partially) recover from the stress and muscular fatigue experienced during loading [38].

These threshold values could be used as indicators (or risk factors) to identify which shipments of heavy pigs deserve particular attention. Guaranteeing better transportation conditions during these shipments (e.g., by installing cooling systems on the trucks, reducing stocking densities, providing adequate bedding, etc.) can help to improve meat quality, together with animal welfare. However, given the relatively limited variability of some of the examined parameters (e.g., distance traveled, transportation scores, journey duration), these results should be validated under more variable transport conditions. Additionally, it should also be observed that the calculated welfare indexes (on-departure score, transport score, slaughter score, and TSWI) showed no appreciable correlation with meat quality, probably because all the transports monitored in this study fell in the moderate-to-high animal welfare level, reducing the variability in the calculated indexes [14]. For all the above reasons, further validation of these results under more variable pre-slaughter welfare conditions is warranted.

4. Conclusions and Future Work

This study aimed at identifying the pre-slaughter parameters which cause the largest variation in the meat quality of Italian heavy pigs. A wide range of pre-slaughter variables was assessed, alongside with some previously-described indexes and scores (on-departure score, transport score, slaughter score, and TSWI). Our results identified some pre-slaughter conditions (ambient temperatures above 22 °C, distance traveled 26 km or above, travel duration between 38 and 66 min, more than 5.9% of animals showing irregular behaviors at unloading) which increased the risk of worse meat quality in Italian heavy pigs. While some of the described effects have previously been observed (despite at different thresholds) also in lighter pigs, to the best of our knowledge, no study addressed the relationship between irregular behaviors during unloading and meat quality. Notwithstanding the need for further validation of our results, these parameters offer a first guide for the identification of those shipments that may require additional attention in terms of animal welfare in order to obtain meat suitable for high-quality productions. Lastly, additional ethical consideration should be drawn to the fact that, despite transports were carried out under overall moderate-to-high welfare conditions, as much as 25% of the loins analyzed in the present study were classified as 'lower quality'. This aspect urges a wider reflection on possible strategies to be adopted in order to improve animal welfare and product quality.

Author Contributions: Conceptualization, L.S., E.N., and D.C.; methodology, A.G. (Alessandro Gastaldo), M.B., A.B., V.M., and A.G. (Anna Garavaldi), software, A.G. (Alessandro Gastaldo) and M.B.; validation, L.S., A.G. (Alessandro Gastaldo), M.B., A.B., V.M., and A.G. (Anna Garavaldi); formal analysis, L.S., E.N. and D.C.; investigation, A.G. (Alessandro Gastaldo), M.B., A.B., V.M. and A.G. (Anna Garavaldi); Resources, L.S., G.M., and E.N.; data curation, L.S. and D.C.; writing—original draft preparation, E.N.; writing—review and editing, E.N., L.S., V.M. and G.M.; visualization, E.N., L.S. and D.C.; supervision, A.G. (Alessandro Gastaldo), M.B., A.B. and E.N.; project administration, A.G. (Alessandro Gastaldo), M.B., A.B. and L.S.; funding acquisition, A.G. (Alessandro Gastaldo) and L.S. All authors have read and agreed to the published version of the manuscript.

Funding: This research was funded by Regione Emilia-Romagna (Emilia Romagna region)—Misura 124 del Programma di Sviluppo Rurale 2007–2013 (Measure 124 of the Regional Rural Development Program 2007–2013), project title: "Benessere dei suini nelle fasi di trasporto e macellazione e qualità percepita della carne" (Pig welfare during transport and slaughter and perceived meat quality).

Acknowledgments: The authors would like to acknowledge the support given by the slaughterhouse O.P.A.S. (Carpi, Italy) and all the farms involved in the trial. The authors would also like to thank Carlo Bianco for his thoughtful comments on the form and content of the manuscript.

Conflicts of Interest: The authors declare no conflict of interest.

References

1. Chulayo, A.Y.; Tada, O.; Muchenje, V. Research on pre-slaughter stress and meat quality: A review of challenges faced under practical conditions. *Appl. Anim. Husb. Rural Dev.* **2012**, *5*, 1–6.

2. Rioja-Lang, F.C.; Brown, J.A.; Brockhoff, E.J.; Faucitano, L. A Review of Swine Transportation Research on Priority Welfare Issues: A Canadian Perspective. *Front. Vet. Sci.* **2019**, *6*, 36. [CrossRef] [PubMed]

3. Consortium for Parma Ham. Prosciutto di Parma (Parma Ham) Protected Designation of Origin. 1992. Available online: https://www.prosciuttodiparma.com/wp-content/uploads/2019/07/Parma_Ham_Specifications_Disciplinare_Consolidato_Nov_13.pdf (accessed on 10 December 2020).

4. Wu, F.; Vierck, K.R.; DeRouchey, J.M.; O'Quinn, T.G.; Tokach, M.D.; Goodband, R.D.; Dritz, S.S.; Woodworth, J.C. A review of heavy weight market pigs: Status of knowledge and future needs assessment. *Transl. Anim. Sci.* **2017**, *1*, 1–15. [CrossRef] [PubMed]

5. Bertol, T.M.; Oliveira, E.A.; Coldebella, A.; Kawski, V.L.; Scandolera, A.J.; Warpechowski, M.B. Meat quality and cut yield of pigs slaughtered over 100 kg live weight. *Arquivo Brasileiro de Medicina Veterinária e Zootecnia* **2015**, *67*, 1166–1174. [CrossRef]

6. Barducci, R.S.; Zhou, Z.Y.; Wormsbecher, L.; Roehrig, C.; Tulpan, D.; Bohrer, B.M. The relationship of pork carcass weight and leanness parameters in the Ontario commercial pork industry. *Transl. Anim. Sci.* **2020**, *4*, 331–338. [CrossRef]

7. Price, H.E.; Lerner, A.B.; Rice, E.A.; Lowell, J.E.; Harsh, B.N.; Barkley, K.E.; Honegger, L.T.; Richardson, E.; Woodworth, J.C.; Tokach, M.D. Characterizing ham and loin quality as hot carcass weight increases to an average of 119 kilograms. *Meat Muscle Biol.* **2019**, *3*. [CrossRef]

8. Latorre, M.A.; García-Belenguer, E.; Ariño, L. The effects of sex and slaughter weight on growth performance and carcass traits of pigs intended for dry-cured ham from Teruel (Spain)1. *J. Anim. Sci.* **2008**, *86*, 1933–1942. [CrossRef]

9. Latorre, M.A.; Lázaro, R.; Valencia, D.G.; Medel, P.; Mateos, G.G. The effects of gender and slaughter weight on the growth performance, carcass traits, and meat quality characteristics of heavy pigs1. *J. Anim. Sci.* **2004**, *82*, 526–533. [CrossRef]

10. Gallo, L.; Dalla Bona, M.; Cecchinato, A.; Schiavon, S. Effect of growth rate on live performance, carcass and green thigh traits of finishing Italian heavy pigs. *Ital. J. Anim. Sci.* **2017**, *16*, 652–658. [CrossRef]

11. Čandek-Potokar, M.; Škrlep, M. Factors in pig production that impact the quality of dry-cured ham: A review. *Animal* **2012**, *6*, 327–338. [CrossRef]

12. Nannoni, E.; Liuzzo, G.; Serraino, A.; Giacometti, F.; Martelli, G.; Sardi, L.; Vitali, M.; Romagnoli, L.; Moscardini, E.; Ostanello, F. Evaluation of pre-slaughter losses of Italian heavy pigs. *Anim. Prod. Sci.* **2017**, *57*, 2072–2081. [CrossRef]

13. Vitali, A.; Lana, E.; Amadori, M.; Bernabucci, U.; Nardone, A.; Lacetera, N. Analysis of factors associated with mortality of heavy slaughter pigs during transport and lairage1. *J. Anim. Sci.* **2014**, *92*, 5134–5141. [CrossRef] [PubMed]

14. Sardi, L.; Gastaldo, A.; Borciani, M.; Bertolini, A.; Musi, V.; Martelli, G.; Cavallini, D.; Rubini, G.; Nannoni, E. Identification of possible pre-slaughter indicators to predict stress and meat quality: A study on heavy pigs. *Animals* **2020**, *10*, 945. [CrossRef] [PubMed]

15. EU Directive 2010/63/EU of the European Parliament and of the Council of 22 September 2010 on the protection of animals used for scientific purposes. *Off. J. Eur. Union* **2010**, *L276*, 33–79.

16. EC Council Directive 2008/120/EC of 18 December 2008 laying down minimum standards for the protection of pigs. *Off. J. Eur. Union* **2008**, *L47*, 5–13.

17. EC Council Regulation (EC) No 1/2005 of 22 December 2004 on the protection of animals during transport and related operations and amending Directives 64/432/EEC and 93/119/EC and Regulation (EC) No 1255/97. *Off. J. Eur. Union* **2005**, *L3*, 1–44.

18. EC Council Regulation (EC) No 1099/2009 of 24 September 2009 on the protection of animals at the time of killing. *Off. J. Eur. Union* **2009**, *L303*, 1–30.

19. Barbari, M.; Gastaldo, A.; Rossi, P. Farm Welfare Index for assessment of wellbeing in swine farms. In Proceedings of the International Conference: "Innovation Technology to Empower Safety, Health and Welfare in Agriculture and Agro-food Systems", Ragusa, Italy, 15–17 September 2008; pp. 1–7.

20. Siegel, P.B.; Honaker, C.F. General principles of stress and well-being. In *Livestock Handling and Transport*, 4th ed.; Grandin, T., Ed.; CABI: Wallingford, UK, 2014; pp. 14–22. ISBN 9781780643212.

21. Broom, D.M. Welfare of transported animals: Factors influencing welfare and welfare assessment. In *Livestock Handling and Transport*, 4th ed.; Grandin, T., Ed.; CABI: Wallingford, UK, 2014; pp. 23–38. ISBN 9781780643212.

22. Anderson, D.B. Relationship of blood lactate and meat quality in market hogs. In Proceedings of the Reciprocal Meat Conference, Lubbock, TX, USA, 17–20 June 2010.

23. Adenkola, A.Y.; Ayo, J.O. Physiological and behavioural responses of livestock to road transportation stress: A review. *Afr. J. Biotechnol.* **2010**, *9*, 4845–4856.

24. Kanda, K.; Sugama, K.; Sakuma, J.; Kawakami, Y.; Suzuki, K. Evaluation of serum leaking enzymes and investigation into new biomarkers for exercise-induced muscle damage. *Exerc. Immunol. Rev.* **2014**, *20*, 39–54.

25. Addis, P.B.; Nelson, D.A.; Ma, R.T.-I.; Burroughs, J.R. Blood Enzymes in Relation to Porcine Muscle Properties. *J. Anim. Sci.* **1974**, *38*, 279–286. [CrossRef]

26. Bacci, M.L.; Nannoni, E.; Govoni, N.; Scorrano, F.; Zannoni, A.; Forni, M.; Martelli, G.; Sardi, L. Hair cortisol determination in sows in two consecutive reproductive cycles. *Reprod. Biol.* **2014**, *14*, 218–223. [CrossRef] [PubMed]

27. CIE (Commission Internationale de l'Eclairage). *Colorimetry*; Pubbl. n. 15; CIE: Wien, Austria, 1976; p. 78.

28. Honikel, K.O. Reference methods for the assessment of physical characteristics of meat. *Meat Sci.* **1998**, *49*, 447–457. [CrossRef]

29. Della Casa, G.; Bochicchio, D.; Faeti, V.; Marchetto, G.; Poletti, E.; Rossi, A.; Garavaldi, A.; Panciroli, A.; Brogna, N. Use of pure glycerol in fattening heavy pigs. *Meat Sci.* **2009**, *81*, 238–244. [CrossRef] [PubMed]

30. Fischer, K. Drip loss in pork: Influencing factors and relation to further meat quality traits. *J. Anim. Breed. Genet.* **2007**, *124*, 12–18. [CrossRef] [PubMed]

31. Feiner, G. (Ed.) 4—Definitions of terms used in meat science and technology. In *Woodhead Publishing Series in Food Science, Technology and Nutrition*; Woodhead Publishing: Cambridge, UK, 2006; pp. 46–71. ISBN 978-1-84569-050-2.

32. Kim, Y.H.B.; Warner, R.D.; Rosenvold, K. Influence of high pre-rigor temperature and fast pH fall on muscle proteins and meat quality: A review. *Anim. Prod. Sci.* **2014**, *54*, 375–395. [CrossRef]

33. Tornberg, E. Biophysical aspects of meat tenderness. *Meat Sci.* **1996**, *43*, 175–191. [CrossRef]

34. Čobanović, N.; Stajković, S.; Blagojević, B.; Betić, N.; Dimitrijević, M.; Vasilev, D.; Karabasil, N. The effects of season on health, welfare, and carcass and meat quality of slaughter pigs. *Int. J. Biometeorol.* **2020**. [CrossRef]

35. Warner, R.D.; Kauffman, R.G.; Greaser, M.L. Muscle protein changes post mortem in relation to pork quality traits. *Meat Sci.* **1997**, *45*, 339–352. [CrossRef]

36. Virgili, R.; Degni, M.; Schivazappa, C.; Faeti, V.; Poletti, E.; Marchetto, G.; Pacchioli, M.T.; Mordenti, A. Effect of age at slaughter on carcass traits and meat quality of Italian heavy pigs. *J. Anim. Sci.* **2003**, *81*, 2448–2456. [CrossRef]

37. Warriss, P.D.; Brown, S.N.; Bevis, E.A.; Kestin, S.C. The influence of pre-slaughter transport and lairage on meat quality in pigs of two genotypes. *Anim. Sci.* **1990**, *50*, 165–172. [CrossRef]

38. Pérez, M.P.; Palacio, J.; Santolaria, M.P.; Aceña, M.C.; Chacón, G.; Gascón, M.; Calvo, J.H.; Zaragoza, P.; Beltran, J.A.; García-Belenguer, S. Effect of transport time on welfare and meat quality in pigs. *Meat Sci.* **2002**, *61*, 425–433. [CrossRef]

39. Gonzalez-Rivas, P.A.; Chauhan, S.S.; Ha, M.; Fegan, N.; Dunshea, F.R.; Warner, R.D. Effects of heat stress on animal physiology, metabolism, and meat quality: A review. *Meat Sci.* **2020**, *162*, 108025. [CrossRef] [PubMed]

40. Dalla Costa, O.A.; Faucitano, L.; Coldebella, A.; Ludke, J.V.; Peloso, J.V.; dalla Roza, D.; Paranhos da Costa, M.J.R. Effects of the season of the year, truck type and location on truck on skin bruises and meat quality in pigs. *Livest. Sci.* **2007**, *107*, 29–36. [CrossRef]

41. Correa, J.A.; Torrey, S.; Devillers, N.; Laforest, J.P.; Gonyou, H.W.; Faucitano, L. Effects of different moving devices at loading on stress response and meat quality in pigs. *J. Anim. Sci.* **2010**, *88*, 4086–4093. [CrossRef]

42. Goumon, S.; Faucitano, L. Influence of loading handling and facilities on the subsequent response to pre-slaughter stress in pigs. *Livest. Sci.* **2017**, *200*, 6–13. [CrossRef]

43. Sommavilla, R.; Faucitano, L.; Gonyou, H.; Seddon, Y.; Bergeron, R.; Widowski, T.; Crowe, T.; Connor, L.; Scheeren, B.M.; Goumon, S.; et al. Season, Transport Duration and Trailer Compartment Effects on Blood Stress Indicators in Pigs: Relationship to Environmental, Behavioral and Other Physiological Factors, and Pork Quality Traits. *Animals* **2017**, *7*, 8. [CrossRef]

44. Rocha, L.M.; Dionne, A.; Saucier, L.; Nannoni, E.; Faucitano, L. Hand-held lactate analyzer as a tool for the real-time measurement of physical fatigue before slaughter and pork quality prediction. *Animal* **2015**, *9*, 707–714. [CrossRef]

45. Haley, C.; Dewey, C.E.; Widowski, T.; Friendship, R. Relationship between estimated finishing-pig space allowance and in-transit loss in a retrospective survey of 3 packing plants in Ontario in 2003. *Can. J. Vet. Res.* **2010**, *74*, 178–184.

46. Warriss, P.D.; Brown, S.N. A survey of mortality in slaughter pigs during transport and lairage. *Vet. Rec.* **1994**, *134*, 513. [CrossRef]

47. Mitchell, M.A.; Kettlewell, P.J.; Villarroell, M.; Farish, M.; Harper, E. Assessing potential thermal stress in pigs during transport in hot weather—Continuous physiological monitoring. *J. Vet. Behav.* **2010**, *5*, 61–62. [CrossRef]

48. Villarroel, M.; Barreiro, P.; Kettlewell, P.; Farish, M.; Mitchell, M. Time derivatives in air temperature and enthalpy as non-invasive welfare indicators during long distance animal transport. *Biosyst. Eng.* **2011**, *110*, 253–260. [CrossRef]

49. Mitchell, M.A.; Kettlewell, P.J. Engineering and design of vehicles for long distance road transport of livestock (ruminants, pigs and poultry). *Vet. Ital.* **2008**, *44*, 201–213. [PubMed]

Publisher's Note: MDPI stays neutral with regard to jurisdictional claims in published maps and institutional affiliations.

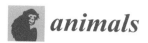

Article

Characterization of Subcutaneous Fat of Toscano Dry-Cured Ham and Identification of Processing Stage by Multivariate Analysis Approach Based on Volatile Profile

Francesco Sirtori [1,*], Chiara Aquilani [1], Corrado Dimauro [2], Riccardo Bozzi [1], Oreste Franci [1], Luca Calamai [1], Antonio Pezzati [1] and Carolina Pugliese [1]

[1] Dipartimento di Scienze e Tecnologie Agrarie, Alimentari, Ambientali e Forestali, Università di Firenze, Scuola di Agraria, Via delle Cascine 5, 50144 Florence, Italy; chiara.aquilani@unifi.it (C.A.); riccardo.bozzi@unifi.it (R.B.); oreste.franci@unifi.it (O.F.); luca.calamai@unifi.it (L.C.); antonio.pezzati@unifi.it (A.P.); carolina.pugliese@unifi.it (C.P.)

[2] Dipartimento di Agraria, Università Degli Studi di Sassari, Viale Italia 39, 07100 Sassari, Italy; dimauro@uniss.it

* Correspondence: francesco.sirtori@unifi.it

Simple Summary: Dry-cured ham has a characteristic flavor that originates from biochemical reactions during processing and seasoning of hams. In the case of Toscano dry-cured ham, the Protected Designation of Origin (PDO) states the minimum seasoning length in 12 months, but seasoning can be extended achieving favorable outcomes on sensory characteristics, and above all on aroma. The present study focused on subcutaneous fat of ham. Color of seasoned ham and fat composition of green and seasoned hams were studied. Special attention was paid on the study of volatile compounds, the main substances perceived by smell, present in fat. These compounds are present in large numbers, and they can be used as markers of a specific seasoning stage. For this purpose, they were analyzed by different statistical techniques to select the ones which are the most characteristic of each specific processing (0, 1, 3, 6 months) and seasoning (12, 14, 16, or 18 months) classes.

Abstract: During ham processing the action of endogenous proteolytic and lipolytic enzymes leads to the development of volatile compounds (VOCs) responsible of typical aromas. Protected Designation of Origin (PDO) of Toscano ham requires at least 12 months of ripening but extended seasoning might improve flavor and economic value. This study aimed at assessing the evolution of color, fatty acids, and VOCs profile in subcutaneous fat, and, among VOCs, at identifying possible markers characterizing different seasoning length. For this purpose, a reduced pool of VOCs was selected by 3 multivariate statistical techniques (stepwise discriminant analysis, canonical discriminant analysis and discriminant analysis) to classify hams according to ripening (<12 months) or seasoning (≥12 months) periods and also to seasoning length (S12, S14, S16, or S18 months). The main VOCs chemical families steadily increased along ripening. Aldehydes and hydrocarbons reached their peaks at S16, acids and ketones remained constant from R6 to S16, whereas esters started decreasing after 12 months of seasoning. Stepwise analysis selected 5 compounds able to discriminate between ripening and seasoning periods, with 1,1-diethoxyhexane and dodecanoic acid being the most powerful descriptors for ripening and seasoning period, respectively. Instead, 12 compounds were needed to correctly classify hams within seasoning. Among them, undecanoic acid methyl ester, formic acid ethyl ester, 2,4,4-trimethylhexane, and 6-methoxy-2-hexanone had a central role in differentiating the seasoning length.

Keywords: pork; solid-phase microextraction; mass spectrometry; aroma; meat

Citation: Sirtori, F.; Aquilani, C.; Dimauro, C.; Bozzi, R.; Franci, O.; Calamai, L.; Pezzati, A.; Pugliese, C. Characterization of Subcutaneous Fat of Toscano Dry-Cured Ham and Identification of Processing Stage by Multivariate Analysis Approach Based on Volatile Profile. *Animals* **2021**, *11*, 13. https://doi.org/10.3390/ani11010013

Received: 4 December 2020
Accepted: 18 December 2020
Published: 23 December 2020

Publisher's Note: MDPI stays neutral with regard to jurisdictional claims in published maps and institutional affiliations.

1. Introduction

Fat content is one of the main factors characterizing the quality of the meat. Its quantitative and qualitative characteristics affect many aspects linked both to the general quality of products and to consumer acceptability [1–3]. In the last years consumers have put increasing pressure on the manufacturers to produce healthier products but also with certain quality characteristics that distinguish the production process. In fact, it is important for producers to develop new lines of products or to change already existing ones in order to meet different consumer requests [3]. In the last years, Protected Designation of Origin (PDO) productions have been affected by changes in the dry-cured process due to market demands. In addition to the reduction of fat, salt, and preserving agents, there was also a request to extend the seasoning period, especially for hams. The recipe reformulation is likely to have impact on the sensory qualities and on the development of the aroma [4]. Aroma is produced by an interaction of factors including the manufacture process [5]. PDO Toscano dry-cured ham production lasts for at least 12 months. During the process numerous changes linked to water loss, salt intake, lipolysis, and proteolysis take place [6]. Sensory characteristics of the hams are mainly linked to physical and biochemical reactions caused by endogenous proteolytic and lipolytic enzymes during the drying and ripening/maturation phases [7]. The standardization of the seasoning process has meant that the qualitative variations of the products are mainly due to the intrinsic characteristics of the fresh hams [8]. With the modification of the seasoning time, chemical and sensory changes strongly depend on the duration of the ripening process [9]. An elongation of the process is generally considered a sign of high quality due to enzymatic processes which lead to an improvement of the texture and flavor of this product. Furthermore, this extension is generally linked to higher end-user prices [10]. The Canonical Discriminant Analysis (CDA) is a multivariate statistical technique which identifies a set of variables that maximizes the groups separation, whereas the Discriminant Analysis (DA) was applied to classify the samples in the different groups [11] Considering the number of variables involved, the CDA and the DA, were preferred to Principal Component Analysis (PCA) to analyze data.

The aim of this work was to study the evolution of color, fatty acids, and volatile compounds (VOCs) profile in subcutaneous fat, and, among VOCs, to identify possible markers characterizing different seasoning length.

2. Materials and Methods

2.1. Samples

In an industrial plant, thirty hams weighing 15.60 ± 1.06 kg were randomly selected and underwent the same manufacturing "Toscano" PDO Consortium manufacturing protocol, consisting of the following stages: salting (15–18 days), pre-resting (15 days), resting (60–70 days), drying (10 days), and ripening (~240 days). At the end of the ripening, hams were randomly allotted into 3 groups of 10 hams each. The first group (S14) was seasoned until 14 months, the second group (S16) until 16 months, and the third group (S18) up to 18 months. At the end of each established seasoning time, hams were dissected, and the external fat was trimmed and analyzed. Hams reached the average final weight of 10.73 ± 0.88 kg, in accordance with the PDO protocol.

Moreover, the external fat of hams belonging to group S18 was sampled along the whole processing and ripening periods to assess VOCs profile. Specifically, samples were taken at 0, 1, 3, 6, 12, 14, 16, and 18 months as described below, in paragraph 2.3 "Volatile compounds analysis".

2.2. Physical and Chemical Parameters

Results on chemical composition of sliced hams, comprehensive of lean and fat, were reported in a previous research [11]. At the end of each seasoning time (14, 16, or 18 months) the trimmed fat of each sample was analyzed to assess instrumental color. As regards moisture, fat, and fatty acids profile, analysis was performed at time 0 and at the end of the seasoning time. Moisture was determined by lyophilizing to constant weight 40 g of sample, according to AOAC methods [12]. Instrumental color was assessed immediately after trimming by a Minolta Chromameter CR200 with illuminant C (Konica Minolta,

Tokyo, Japan) according to CIELab coordinate system, where L* indicates lightness (or darkness), a* is the color's position on the red-green axis and b* on the yellow-blue axis. Fatty acids were determined using a Varian GC-430 apparatus equipped with a flame ionization detector (FID) (AgilentManufacturer, Santa Clara, CA, USA) as reported by Sirtori et al. [13]. The individual methyl esters were identified by their retention time using an analytical standard (F.A.M.E. Mix, C8-C22 Supelco 18,9201AMP). Response factors based on the internal standard (C19:0) were used for quantification and results were expressed as g/100g of sample.

2.3. Volatile Compound Analysis

Analysis on VOCs profile were carried out by repeated sampling on each ham of group S18 ($n = 10$). Sampling took place at time 0 (R0, green ham) and after 1 (R1), 3 (R3), 6 (R6) months of ripening and at 12 (S12), 14 (S14), 16 (S16), and 18 (S18) months of seasoning. Fat was sampled using a 5-mm punch corer positioned approximately in the same location every sampling time. After each sampling, the hole was filled with a mixture of lard, salt, and pepper to prevent oxidation reactions and microbial contaminations. Subsequently, 1g of homogenized fat was grounded by liquid nitrogen and then transferred to 10 mL screw cap headspace vials adding for each sample 1 mL of distilled water and approximately 1 g of NaCl. The vials were supplemented with 40 µL of internal standard mix (ethylacetate-d8; toluene-d8; ethyl hexanoate d11; hexanoic acid d11; 3,4-dimethylphenol), either isotopologues, i.e., deuterated analogues of compounds present in the samples, added to the samples immediately before the analyses [14]. The volatile compound profile was obtained by Solid Phase Microextraction Gas Chromatography-Mass Spectrometry (SPME–GC–MS) technique. An Agilent 7890 Chromatograph (Agilent, Santa Clara, CA, USA) equipped with a 5975A MSD with EI ionisation was used for analysis. A three-phase DVB/Carboxen/PDMS 75-µm SPME fibre (Supelco, Bellafonte, PA, USA) was exposed in the head space of the vials at 60 °C for 30 min for volatile compound sampling after a 5-min equilibration time. A Gerstel MPS2 XL autosampler (GERSTEL GmbH & Co.KG, Mülheim an der Ruhr, Germany) equipped with a magnetic transportation adapter and a temperature-controlled agitator (250 rpm with on/cycles of 10 s) was used for ensuring consistent SPME extraction conditions. Chromatographic conditions were column J&W Innovax (Agilent, Santa Clara, CA, USA) 30 m, 0.25 mm, ID 0.5 µm DF; injection temperature 250 °C, splitless mode, oven program 40° for 1 min then 2 °C/min to 60 °C, then 3 °C/min to 150 °C, then 10 °C/min to 200 °C, and then 25 °C/min to 260 °C for 6.6 min. Mass spectra were acquired within the 29–350 M/Z interval with an Agilent 5975C MSD spectrometer (Agilent, Santa Clara, CA, USA) at a scan speed in order to obtain three scans/s. The identification of volatile compounds was obtained by matching the peak spectra with library spectral database and by matching of the calculated Kovats index (KI) with the KI retrieved from literature. Data are expressed as normalized area ratios with the appropriate internal standard (IS) [15].

2.4. Statistical Analysis

Color data were analyzed using SAS Software [16] according to the following linear model:

$$y_{ijl} = \mu + RT_i + \varepsilon_{ijl} \qquad (1)$$

where y is the investigated variable; µ the overall mean; RT the fixed effect of processing stage; ε the random residual error. Tukey's test with a *p*-value threshold lower than 0.05 was used to compare means.

Fat, moisture, fatty acids, and VOCs data were analyzed using SAS Software [16] according to the following linear model:

$$y_{ijl} = \mu + RT_i + H_j + \varepsilon_{ijl} \qquad (2)$$

where y is the investigated variable; μ the overall mean; RT the fixed effect of processing stage (2 levels for fat, moisture, and fatty acids; 8 levels for VOCs); H the random effect of ham (with repeated measures in time); ε the random residual error. Tukey's test with a *p*-value threshold lower than 0.05 was used to compare means.

VOCs trend during ripening and seasoning was also analyzed by SAS software (SAS Institute, Inc., Charlotte, NC, USA) applying 3 multivariate statistical techniques: stepwise discriminant analysis (SDA), CDA, and DA. The aim of multivariate analysis was to assess if there were groups of VOCs able to characterize the different ripening and seasoning times studied. Furthermore, multivariate approach was also used to outline the contribution of the identified VOCs in properly classifying hams according to their seasoning time only.

Groups separation was tested by Hotelling's T-square test [17]. However, this test can be developed only if the pooled (co)variance matrix of data is not singular. In our research, the number of hams (rows in the matrix of data) is lower than the number of volatile compounds (columns). In this condition, any multivariate technique becomes meaningless because the (co)variance matrix does not have a full rank [18]. Therefore, a reduction of the space-variables was required. For this reason, before CDA and DA, the SDA was applied to the data to select a restricted subset of linearly independent variables, the VOCs, able to discriminate groups [19]. The obtained compounds were used in the CDA and the DA.

The CDA derives a set of new variables, called canonical functions (CAN), that are linear combination of the original compounds. For k-groups involved in the CDA, k-1 CANs are extracted. The structure of a CAN is:

$$CAN = c_1 X_1 + c_2 X_2 + \ldots \ldots + c_n X_n \tag{3}$$

where c_n are the canonical coefficients (CCs) and Xi are the scores of original variables. CCs indicate the partial contribution of each variable in composing the CAN. The greater the CC, the more the variable contributes to compose the CAN.

The distance between groups was evaluated by using the Mahalanobis' distance, whereas the effective groups' separation was tested with the corresponding Hotelling's T-square test (De Maesschalck et al., 2000). Finally, the DA was performed to classify ham samples into seasoning groups.

The above-mentioned statistical approaches were successively applied to volatile compounds data according to the following two scenarios. In the first scenario, VOCs data were arranged in two major seasoning classes: the low maturing class (LMC) with samples belonging to 0, 1, 3, and 6 months; the high maturing class (HMC) with samples belonging to 12, 14, 16, and 18 months of seasoning. In the second scenario, only samples belonging to HMC were considered.

The discriminant procedures were applied to detect the most discriminant compounds able to correctly separate groups involved in the two scenarios. To validate the results, considering the reduced number of involved hams, the leave-one-out cross-validation technique was adopted. In practice, in each scenario, SDA, CDA, and DA were applied 10 times (being 10 the hams involved in the study) by using, at each run, one ham as validation sample. At the end, ten datasets of variables were obtained. Since compounds selected at each round could be different, the ten groups of variables were joined. The resulting compounds were used to develop the final run of CDA and DA.

3. Results and Discussion

3.1. Physical and Chemical Parameters

Subcutaneous fat is an important component of the final product, indeed, even when ham is sold in slices, fat is commonly left on. However, few studies have investigated its characteristics separately from the other section of the slice. Instrumental color parameters are shown in Table 1. According to CIELAB color values, L* and a* were affected by different seasoning times, whereas b* did not change significantly. Since b* variable is linked to yellowness and the formation of yellow-colored polymers has been associated to oxidative deterioration [20], it seems that the oxidative status of subcutaneous fat was not affected by the tested seasoning lengths. On the contrary, L* reached the greatest values as seasoning time increased, while a* showed the highest score in S16 hams and the lowest in S18 hams with S14 samples being similar to both. Analogous L* scores were reported by Tomažin et al. [21] studying the effect of sex and salting time on dry-cured ham characteristics. L* has been positively correlated to fat saturation [22], which is in accordance with the slightly higher content of saturated fatty acids (SFA) of S18 hams, as shown in Table 2. Compared to our results, higher values of a* and b* and lower of L* were observed in Iberian and Iberian × Duroc dry-cured hams reared according to two different systems [22].

Table 1. Instrumental color of subcutaneous fat trimmed from Toscano dry-cured ham.

	Seasoning			RMSE [1]	*p*
	S14 (*n* = 10)	S16 (*n* = 10)	S18 (*n* = 10)		
Instrumental color					
L*	76.125 [b]	77.948 [a,b]	79.068 [a]	1.923	0.0178
a*	2.804 [a,b]	3.763 [a]	2.238 [b]	1.086	0.0302
B*	3.964	3.192	4.158	0.912	0.0869

[1] Root mean square error. Different letters (a,b) within the same chemical family indicate significant differences (*p* < 0.05) among maturing times.

Table 2. Moisture and fatty acids profile of raw and seasoned (S14, S16, S18) subcutaneous fat of Toscano dry-cured ham.

		Seasoning			RMSE [1]	*p*
	R0 (*n* = 30)	S14 (*n* = 10)	S16 (*n* = 10)	S18 (*n* = 10)		
Moisture (%)	16.955 [a]	2.941 [b]	3.161 [b]	2.744 [b]	7.288	<0.0001
Total lipids	68.423 [b]	76.718 [a]	76.246 [a]	78.091 [a]	4.774	<0.0001
C12:0	0.051	0.0386	0.025	0.027	0.029	0.0343
C14:0	0.420 [a,b]	0.434 [a,b]	0.409 [b]	0.459 [a]	0.040	0.0366
C14:1-n5	0.005 [a,b]	0.005 [a,b]	0.004 [b]	0.005 [a]	0.001	0.0055
C15:0	0.011	0.011	0.010	0.013	0.002	0.1094
C16:0	5.599 [b]	6.103 [a]	5.942 [a,b]	6.460 [a]	0.462	<0.0001
C16:1	0.893	0.928	0.902	0.990	0.102	0.0992
C17:0	0.064	0.066	0.068	0.078	0.014	0.1070
C17:1	0.067	0.067	0.067	0.079	0.015	0.1955
C18:0	2.326 [b]	2.628 [a]	2.624 [a]	2.745 [a]	0.235	<0.0001
C18:1	11.289 [b]	12.578 [a]	12.253 [a]	12.959 [a]	0.041	<0.0001
C18:2-n6cis	2.962	3.210	3.167	2.966	0.404	0.2549
C18:3-n3	0.203	0.217	0.215	0.206	0.022	0.2212
C20:0	0.047	0.051	0.0471	0.052	0.007	0.1340
C20:1	0.270	0.296	0.276	0.295	0.036	0.2295
C20:2-n6	0.157 [b]	0.187 [a]	0.181 [a,b]	0.164 [a,b]	0.028	0.0126
C20:3-n6	0.027	0.025	0.023	0.022	0.006	0.0697
C20:4-n6	0.062 [a]	0.059 [a,b]	0.058 [a,b]	0.050 [b]	0.010273	0.0235
C20:3-n3	0.090 [b]	0.104 [a]	0.102 [a,b]	0.103 [a,b]	0.014215	0.0111
C22:4-n6	0.087	0.105	0.106	0.103	0.022764	0.0714
C22:5-n3	0.081	0.097	0.097	0.096	0.020967	0.0624
C20:5-n3	0.000	0.009	0.000	0.009	0.015231	0.2337
SFA	8.521 [b]	9.333 [a]	9.126 [a,b]	9.834 [a]	0.694	<0.0001
MUFA	12.524 [b]	13.873 [a]	13.503 [a]	14.329 [a]	0.994	<0.0001
PUFA	3.671	4.013	3.945	3.720	0.479	0.1671
PUFA-n6	3.297	3.587	3.531	3.305	0.439	0.2058
PUFA-n3	0.320	0.355	0.340	0.340	0.039	0.0725

[1] Root mean square error. Different letters (a,b) within the same chemical family indicate significant differences (*p* < 0.05) among maturing times.

Total lipids (Table 2) significantly increased moving from raw to seasoned hams, but not among different seasoning classes. The most abundant fatty acid was the oleic (C18:1), followed by palmitic (C16:0), linoleic (C18:2), and stearic (C18:0) acids, in agreement with several studies [14,23,24]. Myristic and myristoleic acids showed the highest content in S18 hams and lowest in S16 ones, with R0 and S14 hams showing intermediate amounts.

Palmitic, stearic, and oleic acids showed lower content in R0 hams than in dry-cured ones, with no differences among seasoning classes. Monounsaturated fatty acids (MUFA) content was greater in seasoned than in raw hams, in accordance with oleic acid content, which is the major contributor to MUFA group in pork. This evolution was also observed by Narvàez-Rivas et al. [25] studying the changes in the fatty acid profile of subcutaneous fat of Iberian ham during dry-curing process. However, they also reported a decrease in the most important polyunsaturated fatty acids, which was not observed in the present study except for arachidonic fatty acid. Significant differences were observed only for eicosadienoic and eicosatrienoic fatty acids, but their amounts were at the lowest level in R0 samples, whereas polyunsaturated fatty acids (PUFA) showed similar amounts regardless seasoning length. Eventually, saturated fatty acids (SFA) were affected by seasoning with the lowest content in R0 hams and the highest in S12 and S18 hams, while S14 samples were similar to both. SFA are generally considered stable along processing and seasoning [25] phases, but an increase in this group was already reported in intramuscular fat of Iberian ham during the dry-curing process [26]. Probably, the decrease of moisture during processing leads to changes in sample composition and stable compounds, as SFA are detected in greater concentration.

3.2. Evolution of Volatile Compounds from Raw to Cured Ham

Volatile compounds develop over the ripening process, leading to the typical aroma of dry-cured products. Among the several compounds normally generated by the enzymatic and oxidative processes taking place in the tissues, aldehydes play a prominent role in characterizing dry-cured products' aroma. Aldehydes are considered important contributors to overall aroma both for being strongly present in finished products and for their low thresholds making them easily detectable by assessors and consumers [27]. Twenty-nine aldehydes were identified in Toscano ham samples (Table 3), most of them characterized by low concentrations in green hams, whereas their presence in the cured product was considerable. The most abundant compounds in raw hams were 2-methylundecanal, 2,6-dimethyl-benzaldehyde, 2,4-dimethyl-benzaldehyde; during post-salting also pentanal and hexanal increased significantly. These two latter compounds were typical of dry-cured hams. Hexanal was reported to be the most abundant aldehyde in subcutaneous fat of Iberian ham [19,23,28], arising from linoleic acid oxidation, which is widely available in this tissue. Hexanal is also considered an important indicator of lipid oxidation; in fact, even if it contributes to the ham overall aroma with grassy and fresh notes, its excessive presence easily leads to unpleasant rancid notes and flavors [28]. Besides hexanal, also the others observed linear aldehydes originated from unsaturated fatty acids: i.e., pentanal, heptanal, octanal, and nonanal were all oxidation products of one or both oleic and linoleic acids [29]. Among linear saturated aldehydes displayed in Table 1, hexanal resulted the most abundant compound between 12 and 16 months, followed by pentanal and nonanal. These compounds reached the highest values at 16 months and drop dramatically in the last two months of ripening. This is consistent with the results reported by Andrès et al. [30], who also observed a minor peak in saturated aldehydes during the drying phase, a slight decrease at the beginning of the cellar period, probably due to further reactions with other components, and a huge increase during cellar period, that authors associated to a reduction in the activity of antioxidative systems or to a development of an intense lipolysis. Pentanal and nonanal contribute to the overall aroma with slightly fruity, nut-like notes and fatty, citrus-like notes, respectively [31]. As regard unsaturated aldehydes, 2-heptenal was the most abundant just as 2,4-heptadienal was for polyunsaturated ones. They were both characterized by green and fatty notes [31,32]. Additionally, in these groups there was an increase up to 16 months of seasoning followed by a sharp drop in the S18 hams. Probably, the cause of this decrease is to be found in the progressive disappearance of the fatty acid precursors of these aromatic compounds [33]. In fact, unsaturated aldehydes have their origin in the autoxidation of unsaturated fatty acids, in particular linoleic and linolenic acid that, in this study, although not significantly, showed a positive trend up to 14 months and then they slowly decreased.

Table 3. Effect of ripening and seasoning times on volatile compounds of subcutaneous fat Toscano dry-cured ham (*n* = 10).

Volatile Compound	KI [1]	ID [2]	RMSE [3]	Time								p
				R0	R1	R3	R6	S12	S14	S16	S18	
Aldehydes												
2-methylbutanal	880	MS/KI	0.05	0.02 c	0.01 c	0.03 c	0.11 b	0.16 a,b	0.13 a,b	0.19 a	0.11 b	<0.0001
3-methylbutanal	884	MS/KI	0.05	0.01 e	0.02 e	0.05 d,e	0.12 b,c,d	0.19 a,b	0.14 a,b,c	0.21 a	0.09 c,d,e	<0.0001
Pentanal	974	MS/KI	2.28	0.15 c	1.40 b,c	2.12 b,c	1.42 b,c	8.27 a	2.50 b,c	3.78 b	1.07 b,c	<0.0001
Hexanal	1081	MS/KI	3.23	0.17 c	1.90 c	3.05 b,c	4.03 b,c	8.59 a	7.42 a,b	11.72 a	2.24 c	<0.0001
Heptanal	1183	MS/KI	0.26	0.01 d	0.18 d	0.30 d	0.28 d	1.04 a,b	0.70 b,c	1.22 a	0.31 c,d	<0.0001
Octanal	1287	MS/KI	0.73	0.04 b	0.08 b	0.13 b	0.22 b	0.53 b	2.22 a	2.00 a	0.08 b	<0.0001
2-Heptenal	1318	MS/KI	2.92	0.07 c	0.33 c	1.37 c	3.94 b,c	7.32 a,b	8.06 a,b	10.80a	3.70 b,c	<0.0001
Nonanal	1392	MS/KI	0.54	0.05 c	0.18 c	0.34 c	0.72 b,c	1.29 b	1.38 a,b	2.11 a	0.41 c	<0.0001
2,4 hexadienal	1402	MS/KI	0.69	0.04c	0.01 c	0.18 c	0.69 b,c	1.26 a,b	1.61 a,b	2.11 a	0.59 b,c	<0.0001
2-octenal	1442	MS/KI	0.70	0.02 c	0.05 c	0.27 c	1.53 a,b	1.39 b	1.46 a,b	2.45 a	0.59 b,c	<0.0001
2,4 heptadienal	1493	MS/KI	2.38	0.16 d	0.24 d	0.28 c,d	1.29 c,d	3.41 b,c	5.82 a,b	8.22 a	1.82 c,d	<0.0001
Decanal	1498	MS/KI	0.13	0.01 b	0.02 b	0.02 b	0.09 a,b	0.04 b	0.03 b	0.23 a	0.03 b	0.008
2,4-Heptadienal (E,E)-	1501	MS/KI	2.80	0.15 c	0.11 c	0.58 c	2.19 b,c	5.54 b	6.25 b	10.70 a	2.43 b,c	<0.0001
Benzaldehyde	1515	MS/KI	0.68	0.01 c	0.14 c,d	0.28 c,d	0.85 b,c,d	1.03 b,c	6.25 b	10.70 a	2.43 b,c	<0.0001
2-nonenal	1532	MS/KI	0.97	0.00 c	0.06 c	0.30 b,c	1.36 b,c	1.38 b,c	1.56 d	2.82 a	0.66 b,c,d	<0.0001
2-methylundecanal	1644	MS/KI	18.86	11.68 b	15.30 b	13.64 b	23.42 b	29.19 a,b	1.62 b	3.43 a	0.70 b,c	<0.0001
2-Dodecenal	1844	MS/KI	0.93	0.03 d	0.00 c,d	0.22 c,d	0.90 b,c,d	1.72 b	32.14 a,b	51.96a	9.25 b	<0.0001
Benzeneacetaldehyde	1646	MS/KI	1.72	0.01 d	0.07 d	0.20 d	1.95 b,c,d	1.44 c,d	1.39 b,c	3.51 a	0.62 b,c,d	<0.0001
trans, trans-nona-2,4-dienal	1704	MS/KI	2.52	0.12 c	0.04 c	0.51 c	2.74 b,c	4.05 b	4.02 a,b	6.07 a	3.85 a,b,c	<0.0001
2-undecenal	1717	MS/KI	1.00	0.04 c	0.04 c	0.18 c	0.74 b,c	1.72 b	4.80 b	9.13 a	1.36 b,c	<0.0001
2,4 decadienal	1797	MS/KI	3.49	0.17 b	0.23 b	0.24 b	1.48 b	2.21 b	1.40 a	3.73 b,c	0.51 b,c	<0.0001
2,6-dimethylbenzaldehyde	1640	MS/KI	4.20	2.98 d	5.55 b,c,d	4.46 c,d	10.29 a,b,c	11.81 a,b	4.67 b	10.50 a	0.93 b	<0.0001
									8.13 a,b,c,d	13.59 a	2.39 d	<0.0001

[1] Kovat's index (KI), [2] Identification (ID) was carried out by comparing each mass spectrum in NIST 05 or Wiley 7 databases (MS); matching with reported Kovat's indices (KI), [3] Root mean square error, Different letters (a,b,c,d,e) within the same chemical family indicate significant differences (*p* < 0.05) among maturing times.

Three branched aldehydes were observed. Two-methylbutanal and 3-methylbutanal were observed in low concentrations, but they are both considered important contributors to dry-cured ham's aroma. Two-methyl butanal is associated with nutty, cheesy, and salty notes, while 3-methyl butanal is characterized by fruity, acorn-like, cheesy notes [31,32]. They displayed the same trend commonly described for dry-cured ham. Indeed, they showed a moderate increase in post-salting period and a deep increase during drying and cellar periods [33]. Branched aldehydes of ham were originated mainly by amino acids degradation, but there is not accordance about the pathway. Some authors postulated a microbial formation, since microorganisms are able to metabolize L-isoleucine to 2-methylbutanal and L-leucine to 3-methybutanal [33,34]; on the contrary other authors rejected this hypothesis due to the ham low microbial count, especially in the inner parts such as muscles, and postulated a non-enzymatic process via Strecker reaction [35,36], adducing the long dry-curing period as a possible alternative to high temperature in promote this kind of reaction [37]. In fat tissue, amino acids are low represented, and likely, they were quickly decomposed leading to a low concentration of branched aldehydes if compared to those usually found in muscle tissues [38,39]. Among the identified branched aldehydes, the 2-methylundecanal resulted also the most abundant volatile compound found in all samples. This compound has not been reported in dry-cured ham. It is found naturally in kumquat peel oil [31], and it is commonly used as odorant for soaps, detergents, and perfumes [40] thanks to its herbaceous, orange, fatty, and ambergris-like smell. It has also been reported in rabbit meat, but it was not classified among key odorants [41]. A recent study on interactions between protozoa and foodborne pathogenic bacteria has listed 2-methylundecanal among the VOCs originated from Listeria spp. [42], whereas European Food Safety Authority (EFSA) has defined 2-methylundecanal, among the flavoring compounds approved for addition in animal feed [43]. However, in the present study, the presence of 2-methylundecanal cannot be certainly attributed to feed rather than to microbiological metabolism or contaminant. Eventually, four aromatic aldehydes were found: benzaldehyde, benzeneacetaldehyde, 2,6-dimethylbenzaldehyde, and 2,4-dimethylbenzaldehyde. They are generally linked to amino acid degradation [44].

During the drying and the cellar periods they quickly increased until the 16th month, when together represented the 14% of the total aldehydes, then, as for the other compounds, their quantity dramatically drops. Benzaldehyde and benzeneacetaldehyde were largely reported in dry-cured ham and described as unpleasant bitter almond flower, solvent-like, fruity notes [45].

Another important chemical family in dry-cured products is the esters. These compounds were generally associated to the microorganism esterase activity, but, due to the low bacterial count in ham, an alternative pathway was hypothesized. Flores et al. [46] proposed that esters could also be formed from the interaction of free fatty acids and alcohols generated by lipid oxidation in intramuscular tissues. In our study twenty esters were observed, which is a quite high number if compared with results reported by several authors [38,47]. It is worth noting that most of the studies on ham employed samples of *Biceps femoris* or *Semimembranosus* muscles, in which the fat content was very low compared to our samples. So, being the esters produced by the interaction of two lipid oxidation products, the free fatty acids and the alcohols, the greatest number of esters identified in the present work could be well explained by the matrix used. Additionally, a microbial contribution cannot be excluded being the sampling carried out on subcutaneous fat not covered by skin, where moulds and yeasts develop during the ripening and tissues are easily accessible for microbial esterase enzymes. Eventually, subcutaneous fat is also in close contact with salt used for the manufacturing, in which a considerable number of microbial communities belonging to *Micrococcaceae* was found [48]. These microorganisms were previously found in ham and associated with a significant lipolytic activity [35]. Esters developed during the ripening process, resulting thus significantly higher in finished products respect to green hams [47]. Accordingly, in the present study, the highest concentration of these compounds was observed at the end of ripening, in S12 samples (Figure 1).

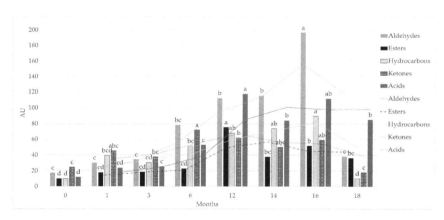

Figure 1. Total amounts of aldehydes, ketones, esters and hydrocarbons from R0 to S18 Toscano dry-cured hams. AU = Abundance units. Different letters (a,b,c,d) within the same chemical family indicate significant differences (*p* < 0.05) among maturing times.

Thirteen hydrocarbons were identified from R0 to S18. Hydrocarbons generally followed the trend showed by aldehydes, with an overall gradual increase until S16 and a final drop at S18. Four n-alkanes (hexane, decane, tridecane and pentadecane) were detected; they are likely products derived from lipid oxidation, as reported by several authors [49,50]. The other hydrocarbons detected are mainly branched alkanes, but two branched alkene and one branched alkyne were also identified. This chemical family is widely known in dry-cured ham, both in fat and lean matrix [39,45], but to the best of our knowledge, except for n-alkanes, none of the other compounds detected in the present study has been previously reported in literature. The identification of these compounds is likely challenging without a specific SPME fiber [51]. Despite their strong presence in dry-cured ham, most of them usually have high odor thresholds and are considered not important contributors to the aroma of dry-cured products [49]. In this study, only one aromatic hydrocarbon was found. Styrene was already reported in ham fat [39,50], its origin was alternatively reported as contaminant of plastic bags [39] or as product of degradation of phenylalanine [52], moreover styrene was associated with a penetrating odor and sweet smell [53].

Twelve ketones were found in subcutaneous fat. Three of them were aliphatic ketones (2-decanone, 2-undecanone, 2-pentadecanone). Aliphatic ketones are characteristics of dry-cured ham, being already reported by several authors both in lean and fat tissues [14,33,44,54]. 2-decanone and 2-undecanone reached their peak at S6, whereas 2-pentadecanone was related to the early ripening stages and then significantly decreased. Their aromatic notes have been described as fruity, spicy, and sometimes cheesy notes [55]. Three unsaturated ketones (1-octen-3-one, 4-hexen-2-one, 3-octen-2-one), five among polyunsaturated and methyl branched ketones (4-methyl-2-hexanone, 2,3-octanedione, 6-methyl-5-hepten-2-one, 6-methoxy 2-hexanone, 3,5-octadien-2-one), and one aromatic ketone (acetophenone) were also identified. Four-hexen-2-one is the most abundant compound for this family, it reached its maximum at 6 months of ripening then considerably declined until S18. However, at the best of our knowledge, it is the first time that this compound is reported in ham, while it was already found in pork loin and belly [56], but odor description was not reported. Concerning unsaturated and polyunsaturated ketones, 1-octen-3-one, 3-octen-2-one, 2,3-octanedione, 6-methyl-5-hepten-2-one and 3,5-octadien-2-one were already observed in fat of dry-cured ham [23,33,39]. Moreover, 1-octen-3-one was also identified as odor-active compound in ham, and described as spicy, mushroom, dirty [32]. Among the other compounds, 3-octen-2-one and 6-methyl-5-hepten-2-one have been reported as aroma active compounds in fermented meat. They were reported to have mushroom, metal and resin, pine, herbal, synthetic notes [5]. Different pathways are related to the formation of unsaturated and polyunsaturated ketones, with lipid autoxidation and microbial metabolism (β-oxidation) being the main ones [46]. Even though the microbial pathway has often been discarded for dry-cured ham due to its small internal microbial population [28], in the case of subcutaneous fat, this pathway is likely concurrent to autoox-idation considering the greater exposure of sampled fat to the external environment during processing, ripening and seasoning. For instance, Andrade et al. [57], working on Iberian dry-cured ham, assumed that 2-butanone was produced by yeasts population. Accordingly, ketones resulted in being the most abundant family in early ripening phases, declining from S12 when aldehydes became the most represented group of VOCs (Figure 1).

Alcohols detected in subcutaneous fat consisted of 12 compounds. Most of them were also observed in fat [47], whole slice [30], and lean tissue [58] of Iberian ham [45] and Toscano ham [11,59]. Alcohols showed a very regular trend constantly increasing from R0 to S16 when the greatest amount for almost every compound was observed. The great increase of this family from green to seasoned fat of dry-cured ham is in accordance with results reported by Narváez-Rivas et al. [47]. After the 16th month of seasoning, they dropped at lower values. Linear and branched alcohols are known as products of lipid oxidation, whereas methyl branched ones were also linked to Strecker degradation [38]. Previous studies reported that 1-hexanol originates from palmitoleic and oleic fatty acids oxidation, while 1-octanol seems to be formed from oleic acid oxidation [60]. The most abundant alcohol observed resulted 2-octen-1-ol, followed by 1-octen-3-ol. As for many straight-chain unsaturated alcohols, they have low odor thresholds. 2-octen-1-ol is described as oily, slightly nutty and fatty waxy [31]; 1-octen-3-ol is often associated to mushroom-like, earth, fatty, and sometimes rancid notes in dry-cured products [54,61].

Carboxylic acids showed an increasing trend from green to seasoned hams. Most of the identified compounds reached the highest concentration between 12 and 16 months of seasoning and they generally decreased at S18. This is in accordance with their origin being products from hydrolysis of triglycerides and phospholipids, or from the oxidation of unsaturated fatty acids [62]. Twelve acids were identified in seasoned fat of Cinta Senese [14], however, concerning only the subcutaneous fat, few studies reported the presence of carboxylic acids. Specifically, butanoic and hexanoic acids were observed in French and Spanish dry-cured ham [19,28,39], but not in the present study. Most of the literature references about carboxylic acids in dry-cured ham refer to volatile profile of lean tissue. Nevertheless, even in this matrix, a great variability in type and number of identified compounds was observed [30,44,63,64].

Three last compounds were identified, one nitrogenous compound, one furanone, and one furan. Both furan and furanone reached their peak during the early stage of seasoning. Two-pentylfurane was detected in subcutaneous fat of Teruel white hams, Iberian hams, Spanish white hams, and French white hams [19,39]. Its trend was consistent with its origin connected to lipid oxidation [30] and in accordance with results reported for Toscano ham [11,65] and Iberian ham [58], even if these studies refer to lean matrix. Due to its quite low odor threshold, it might contribute to overall aroma by vegetable aromatic note [37]. 2(3H)dihydro-5-penthylfuranone is a lactone, it was observed only by Ruiz et al. [66] in dry-cured ham. Nevertheless, lactones have been widely reported in ham and dry-cured products with γ-butyrolactone, γ-octalactone, and γ-nonalactone being the most frequently detected in Iberian ham [45]. Similarly to 2-pentylfuran, also 2(3H)dihydro-5-penthylfuranone was likely a product of lipid oxidation of fatty acids or unsaturated aldehydes. Indeed this is considered the main origin of lactones, even if also Maillard reaction was also proposed as a possible pathway [37].

3.3. Prediction of the Maturing Time by a Multivariate Approach

Several authors proposed a multivariate approach to classify dry-cured ham relying on VOCs profile. The main approach used was PCA [28,33], but also other approaches were tested, including Linear Discriminant Analysis (LDA) [33], Partial Least Square-Discriminant Analysis regression [67], and stepwise linear discriminant analysis [19,28]. In the present study three multivariate approaches were applied together to tentatively discriminate between ripening and seasoning (first scenario) and, within seasoning, to classify hams according to seasoning length (second scenario). In the first scenario, 5 compounds were selected by SDA (Table 4), Then, using the selected variables, the CDA was able to significantly ($p < 0.001$) split hams belonging to LMC (R0, R1, R3, R6) from hams belonging to HMC (S12, S14, S16, S18) (Figure 2). In details, the presence of 1,1-diethoxy-hexane was characteristics of LMC hams, whereas the other 4 compounds were related to HMC samples. Especially dodecanoic acid, with a canonical coefficient (CC) of 2.42, resulted the most characterizing compound of Toscano ham's fat during late seasoning. Lastly, the DA correctly assigned all samples to their group of origin. Dodecanoic acid contribution in describing high maturing classes of Toscano dry-cured ham was previously observed also in *Semimembranosus* muscle (CC = 4.20) [11]. In subcutaneous fat it displayed a very clear ascending trend during ripening and reached consistent amounts in seasoning. However, it has a very high perception threshold [31], so despite being an important descriptor from the chemical point of view, it is likely not perceivable by sensorial assessment. On the contrary, to the best of our knowledge, 1,1-diethoxyhexane was not previously reported in subcutaneous fat of dry-cured products.

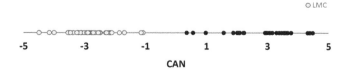

Figure 2. Separation of subcutaneous fat volatile compounds (VOCs) selected by SDA relatively to their capability of correctly differentiating Toscano dry-cured ham samples between low maturing classes (<12 months) and high maturing classes (≥12 months).

Table 4. Volatile compounds of subcutaneous fat of Toscano dry-cured ham selected by stepwise discriminant analysis. Canonical discriminant analysis scores (Can1) were used to separate low maturing classes (LMC) and high maturing classes (HMC).

Subcutaneous Fat Samples			
	Chemical Family	Can1	Sensory Descriptors [a]
1,1-diethoxyhexane	Hydrocarbon	−0.82	Cognac, pear, floral, hyacinth, apple, fruity [1]
3-methyl-ethyl ester butanoic acid	Ester	0.03	Strong, fruity, vinous, apple-like
2,4-dimethylbenzaldehyde	Aldehyde	0.13	Mild, sweet, bitter-almond
Butanoic acid, ethyl ester	Ester	0.45	Fruity odor with pineapple undertone and sweet
Dodecanoic acid	Acid	2.42	Fatty, creamy, cheese-like, waxy

[a] As reported in Burdock, G.A, 2010 [31], except for: [1] Based on online databases www.thegoodscentscompany.com.

In the second scenario, 12 VOCs were identified by SDA to discriminate samples into seasoning classes (Table 5) and then used to correctly assign samples to each group. The first and second canonical functions accounted for the 87% of the total variance and they were able to highlight differences among groups (Figure 3a). Can1 separated S12, S14, and S18 groups from S16. Among the compounds that weighed the most in Can1 there were 3 ketones (2,3-octanedione, 4-methyl-2-hexanone, and 6-methoxy-2-hexanone) and 1 aldehyde (decanal) (Figure 3b). Can2 separated samples belonging to S12 from the other groups. In this case, the most important compounds were 2 esters (formic acid ethyl ester and undecanoic acid, methyl ester), 1 hydrocarbon (2,4,4-trimethylhexane), and 1 ketone (6-methoxy-2-hexanone). 2,3-octanedione, 4-methyl-2-hexanone and decanal resulted in the highest CCs of Can1. Among them, special importance in overall aroma of dry-cured ham is attributed to 2,3-octanedione, which has a "warmed-over" flavor [31]. Moreover, decanal, which originates from autoxidation of oleic fatty acid, was already identified among the main descriptors to characterize samples from different dry-curing periods by LDA [33]. According to Figure 3a,b, this compound, together with 4-methyl-2-hexanone, were mainly involved in the discrimination of S16 from S12, S14, and S18. Focusing on Can2, 4 compounds had CCs higher than 1. These compounds were: undecanoic acid methyl ester (−1.22), formic acid ethyl ester (+1.18), 2,4,4-trimethylhexane (−1.13) and 6-methoxy-2-hexanone (+1.03). According to Figure 3a, formic acid ethyl ester and 6-methoxy-2-hexanone were linked to S12 hams, whereas undecanoic acid methyl ester and 2,4,4-trimethylhexane resulted to be good descriptors of hams seasoned for more than 12 months. In comparison with the previous study on VOCs of *Semimembranosus* muscle [11], a lower number of VOCs were needed to correctly classify samples according to their actual ripening and seasoning stage. This suggests that, in subcutaneous fat, there are compounds that could be powerful markers for assessing processing stages of hams.

Table 5. Volatile compounds of subcutaneous fat of Toscano dry-cured ham selected by stepwise discriminant analysis. Canonical discriminant analysis scores (Can1, Can2, and Can3) were used to separate hams belonging to different seasoning lengths (S12, S14, S16, S18).

Subcutaneous Fat Samples	Chemical Family	Can1	Can2	Can3	Sensory Descriptors [a]
1,1-diethoxyhexane	Hydrocarbon	−0.75	−0.44	−0.03	Cognac, pear, floral, hyacinth, apple, fruity [1]
Pentanoic acid, ethyl ester	Ester	0.48	0.12	0.74	Fruity, apple-like
4-methyl-2-hexanone	Ketone	2.17	0.93	0.64	Fruity [2]
2,4,4-trimethylhexane	Hydrocarbon	0.37	−1.13	0.69	-
2,3-octanedione	Ketone	−3.26	0.20	0.55	Green, spicy, cilantro, fatty, leafy, cortex, herbal, warmed-over
Formic Acid, ethyl ester	Ester	−0.10	1.18	−0.88	Pungent, rum-like, pineapple
6-methoxy-2-hexanone	Ketone	−0.76	1.03	0.63	Fruity e spicy [3]
Decanal	Aldehyde	1.07	−0.06	−0.30	Sweet, waxy, floral, citrus, fatty
Acetic acid, ethenyl ester	Ester	0.88	0.04	−0.50	Wine, fruity [4]
dihydro-5-penthyl-2(3H) furanone	Furanone	0.00	0.85	0.57	Coconut and fatty
Hexadecanoic acid, ethyl ester	Ester	0.81	0.45	0.02	Mild, waxy sweet
Undecanoic acid, methyl ester	Ester	−0.07	−1.22	0.02	Fatty, waxy fruity [1]
Proportion of explained variation		0.56	0.31	0.13	

[a] As reported in Burdock, G.A, 2010 [31], except for: [1] Based on online databases www.thegoodscentscompany.com; [2] Reale et el., 2019 [68]; [3] Luna et al., 2006 [19]; [4] Lin et al., 2014 [69].

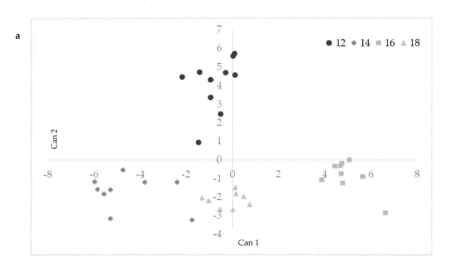

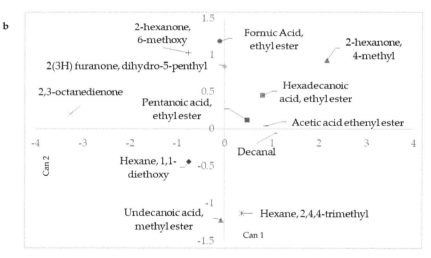

Figure 3. Scores (**a**) of canonical discriminant analysis within high maturing class (HMC) samples: S12, S14, S16, and S18 months of seasoning. (**b**) Loadings of canonical discriminant analysis within HMC.

4. Conclusions

In conclusion, instrumental color of subcutaneous fat was affected by time, especially L* score was higher for longer seasoning time, partially in agreement with the greater degree of saturation observed in the higher maturing classes. Oleic acid, the main contributor to MUFA amount, showed no difference among seasoning groups. According to VOCs profile, almost every identified compound was affected by ripening and seasoning times. Regardless of single compounds, the main chemical families steadily increased until R6, then different trends were observed. Aldehydes and hydrocarbons reached their peaks at S16, ketones and acids instead showed the highest total content at R6 and R12, respectively. Lastly, esters started to decrease after 12 months of seasoning. Moreover, at S18 most of the main compounds involved in dry-cured ham overall aroma already declined to value similar to ripening phases. In the future, it would be interesting to thoroughly investigated also the enzymatic activity taking place during the different processing stages. The multivariate approach adopted highlighted the importance of 5 compounds present in subcutaneous fat to discriminate between ripening and seasoning stages (1,1-diethoxyhexane, 3-methyl-ethyl ester butanoic acid, 2,4-dimethyl-benzaldehyde, butanoic acid ethyl ester, dodecanoic acid). Instead, 12 compounds were selected to classify hams according to seasoning length. Among them, 4 VOCs with CCs > 1 (undecanoic acid methyl ester, formic acid ethyl ester, 2,4,4-trimethylhexane, and 6-methoxy-2-hexanone) had a central role in differentiating the clusters.

Author Contributions: Conceptualization, C.P. and O.F.; methodology, F.S. and L.C.; software F.S. and C.D.; formal analysis, F.S. and A.P.; data curation, C.A. and F.S.; writing—original draft preparation, C.A. and F.S.; writing—review and editing, R.B. and C.D.; supervision, C.P.; project administration, C.P.; funding acquisition, O.F. All authors have read and agreed to the published version of the manuscript.

Funding: This research was funded by Regione Toscana and Consorzio del Prosciutto Toscano.

Data Availability Statement: The data presented in this study are available on request from the corresponding author.

Acknowledgments: The authors would like to thank Aldo Neri and the staff of Valdinievole salumi srl.

Conflicts of Interest: The authors declare no conflict of interest. The funders had no role in the design of the study; in the collection, analyses, or interpretation of data; in the writing of the manuscript, or in the decision to publish the results.

References

1. Fernandez, X.; Monin, G.; Talmant, A.; Mourot, J.; Lebret, B. Influence of intramuscular fat content on the quality of pig meat-2. Consumer acceptability of m. longissimus lumborum. *Meat Sci.* **1999**, *53*, 67–72. [CrossRef]
2. Aquilani, C.; Sirtori, F.; Franci, O.; Acciaioli, A.; Bozzi, R.; Pezzati, A.; Pugliese, C. Effects of Protein Restriction on Performances and Meat Quality of Cinta Senese Pig Reared in an Organic System. *Animals* **2019**, *9*, 310. [CrossRef]
3. Cardona, M.; Gorriz, A.; Barat, J.M.; Fernández-Segovia, I. Perception of fat and other quality parameters in minced and burger meat from Spanish consumer studies. *Meat Sci.* **2020**, *166*, 108138. [CrossRef]
4. Flores, M. Understanding the implications of current health trends on the aroma of wet and dry cured meat products. *Meat Sci.* **2018**, *144*, 53–61. [CrossRef]
5. Flores, M.; Olivares, A. Flavor. In *Handbook of Fermented Meat and Poultry*, 2nd ed.; Wiley: Hoboken, NJ, USA, 2014; pp. 217–225. ISBN 9781118522653.
6. Čandek-Potokar, M.; Škrlep, M. Factors in pig production that impact the quality of dry-cured ham: A review. *Animal* **2012**, *6*, 327–338. [CrossRef]
7. Dall'Olio, S.; Aboagye, G.; Nanni Costa, L.; Gallo, M.; Fontanesi, L. Effects of 17 performance, carcass and raw ham quality parameters on ham weight loss at first salting in heavy pigs, a meat quality indicator for the production of high quality dry-cured hams. *Meat Sci.* **2020**, *162*, 108012. [CrossRef]
8. Bosi, P.; Russo, V. The production of the heavy pig for high quality processed products. *Ital. J. Anim. Sci.* **2004**, *3*, 309–321. [CrossRef]
9. Prevolnik, M.; Andronikov, D.; Žlender, B.; Font-i-Furnols, M.; Novič, M.; Škorjanc, D.; Čandek-Potokar, M. Classification of dry-cured hams according to the maturation time using near infrared spectra and artificial neural networks. *Meat Sci.* **2014**, *96*, 14–20. [CrossRef]
10. Hersleth, M.; Lengard, V.; Verbeke, W.; Guerrero, L.; Næs, T. Consumers' acceptance of innovations in dry-cured ham: Impact of reduced salt content, prolonged aging time and new origin. *Food Qual. Prefer.* **2011**, *22*, 31–41. [CrossRef]
11. Sirtori, F.; Dimauro, C.; Bozzi, R.; Aquilani, C.; Franci, O.; Calamai, L.; Pezzati, A.; Pugliese, C. Evolution of volatile compounds and physical, chemical and sensory characteristics of Toscano PDO ham from fresh to dry-cured product. *Eur. Food Res. Technol.* **2020**, *246*, 409–424. [CrossRef]
12. Association of Officia Analytical Chemist. *Official Methods of Analysis (AOAC)*, 19th ed.; Association of Officia Analytical Chemist: Gaithersburg, MD, USA, 2012.
13. Sirtori, F.; Crovetti, A.; Acciaioli, A.; Bonelli, A.; Pugliese, C.; Bozzi, R.; Campodoni, G.; Franci, O. Effect of replacing a soy diet with Vicia faba and Pisum sativum on performance, meat and fat traits of Cinta Senese pigs. *Ital. J. Anim. Sci.* **2015**, *14*, 99–104. [CrossRef]

14. Pugliese, B.C.; Sirtori, F.; Ruiz, J.; Martin, D.; Franci, O. Effect of pasture on chestnut or acorn on fatty acid composition and aromatic profile of fat of Cinta Senese dry-cured ham. *Grasas Aceites* **2009**, *60*, 271–276. [CrossRef]

15. McNaught, A.D.; Wilkinson, A. *Compendium of Chemical Terminology, The Gold Book*, 2nd ed.; Wiley: Blackwell, UK, 1997; ISBN 0865426848.

16. SAS Institute Inc. *SAS/STAT®9.3 User's Guide*; SAS Institute Inc.: Cary, NC, USA, 2011.

17. De Maesschalck, R.; Jouan-Rimbaud, D.; Massart, D.L.L. The Mahalanobis distance. *Chemom. Intell. Lab. Syst.* **2000**, *50*, 1–18. [CrossRef]

18. Dimauro, C.; Cellesi, M.; Pintus, M.A.; MacCiotta, N.P.P. The impact of the rank of marker variance-covariance matrix in principal component evaluation for genomic selection applications. *J. Anim. Breed. Genet.* **2011**, *128*, 440–445. [CrossRef] [PubMed]

19. Luna, G.; Aparicio, R.; García-González, D.L. A tentative characterization of white dry-cured hams from Teruel (Spain) by SPME-GC. *Food Chem.* **2006**, *97*, 621–630. [CrossRef]

20. Ruiz, J.; García, C.; Muriel, E.; Andrés, A.I.; Ventanas, J. Influence of sensory characteristics on the acceptability of dry-cured ham. *Meat Sci.* **2002**, *61*, 347–354. [CrossRef]

21. Tomažin, U.; Škrlep, M.; Prevolnik Povše, M.; Batorek Lukač, N.; Karolyi, D.; Červek, M.; Čandek-Potokar, M. The effect of salting time and sex on chemical and textural properties of dry cured ham. *Meat Sci.* **2020**, *161*, 107990. [CrossRef]

22. Carrapiso, A.I.; García, C. Instrumental colour of Iberian ham subcutaneous fat and lean (biceps femoris): Influence of crossbreeding and rearing system. *Meat Sci.* **2005**, *71*, 284–290. [CrossRef]

23. Timón, M.L.; Ventanas, J.; Carrapiso, A.I.; Jurado, A.; García, C. Subcutaneous and intermuscular fat characterisation of dry-cured Iberian hams. *Meat Sci.* **2001**, *58*, 85–91. [CrossRef]

24. Larrea, V.; Pérez-Munuera, I.; Hernando, I.; Quiles, A.; Lluch, M.A. Chemical and structural changes in lipids during the ripening of Teruel dry-cured ham. *Food Chem.* **2007**, *102*, 494–503. [CrossRef]

25. Narváez-Rivas, M.; Vicario, I.M.; Constante, E.G.; León-Camacho, M. Changes in the fatty acid and triacylglycerol profiles in the subcutaneous fat of Iberian ham during the dry-curing process. *J. Agric. Food Chem.* **2008**, *56*, 7131–7137. [CrossRef] [PubMed]

26. Martín, L.; Córdoba, J.J.; Ventanas, J.; Antequera, T. Changes in intramuscular lipids during ripening of Iberian dry-cured ham. *Meat Sci.* **1999**, *51*, 129–134. [CrossRef]

27. Gandemer, G. Lipids in muscles and adipose tissues, changes during processing and sensory properties of meat products. *Meat Sci.* **2002**, *62*, 309–321. [CrossRef]

28. Sánchez-Peña, C.M.; Luna, G.; García-González, D.L.; Aparicio, R. Characterization of French and Spanish dry-cured hams: Influence of the volatiles from the muscles and the subcutaneous fat quantified by SPME-GC. *Meat Sci.* **2005**, *69*, 635–645. [CrossRef] [PubMed]

29. Belitz, H.; Grosch, W.; Schieberle, P. *Aroma Compounds BT—Food Chemistry*; Belitz, H.D., Grosch, W., Schieberle, P., Eds.; Springer: Berlin/Heidelberg, Germany, 2004; pp. 342–408. ISBN 978-3-662-07279-0.

30. Andrés, A.I.; Cava, R.; Ruiz, J. Monitoring volatile compounds during dry-cured ham ripening by solid-phase microextraction coupled to a new direct-extraction device. *J. Chromatogr. A* **2002**, *963*, 83–88. [CrossRef]

31. Burdock, G.A. *Fenaroli's Handbook of Flavor Ingredients*; CRC Press, Taylor & Francis Group: Boca Raton, FL, USA, 2010; ISBN 9781420090772.

32. García-González, D.L.; Tena, N.; Aparicio, R. Contributing to interpret sensory attributes qualifying Iberian hams from the volatile profile. *Grasas Aceites* **2009**, *60*, 277–283. [CrossRef]

33. Narváez-Rivas, M.; Gallardo, E.; León-Camacho, M. Chemical changes in volatile aldehydes and ketones from subcutaneous fat during ripening of Iberian dry-cured ham. Prediction of the curing time. *Food Res. Int.* **2014**, *55*, 381–390. [CrossRef]

34. Hinrichsen, L.L.; Andersen, H.J. Volatile Compounds and Chemical Changes in Cured Pork: Role of Three Halotolerant Bacteria. *J. Agric. Food Chem.* **1994**, *42*, 1537–1542. [CrossRef]

35. Ventans, J.; Córdoba, J.J.; Antequera, T.; Garcia, C.; López-Bote, C.; Asensio, M.A. Hydrolysis and Maillard Reactions During Ripening of Iberian Ham. *J. Food Sci.* **1992**, *57*, 813–815. [CrossRef]

36. Smit, B.A.; Engels, W.J.M.; Smit, G. Branched chain aldehydes: Production and breakdown pathways and relevance for flavour in foods. *Appl. Microbiol. Biotechnol.* **2009**, *81*, 987–999. [CrossRef]

37. Andres, A.I.; Cava, R.; Ventanas, S.; Muriel, E.; Ruiz, J. Effect of salt content and processing conditions on volatile compounds formation throughout the ripening of Iberian ham. *Eur. Food Res. Technol.* **2007**, *225*, 677–684. [CrossRef]

38. García-González, D.L.; Aparicio, R.; Aparicio-Ruiz, R. Volatile and amino acid profiling of dry cured hams from different swine breeds and processing methods. *Molecules* **2013**, *18*, 3927–3947. [CrossRef] [PubMed]

39. Narváez-Rivas, M.; Gallardo, E.; Ríos, J.J.; León-Camacho, M. A tentative characterization of volatile compounds from Iberian dry-cured ham according to different anatomical locations. A detailed study. *Grasas Aceites* **2010**, *61*, 369–377.

40. Gibka, J.; Gliński, M. Synthesis and olfactory properties of 2-alkylalkanals, analogues of 2-methylundecanal. *Flavour Fragr. J.* **2006**, *21*, 480–483. [CrossRef]

41. Xie, Y.J.; He, Z.F.; Zhang, E.; Li, H.J. Technical note: Characterization of key volatile odorants in rabbit meat using gas chromatography mass spectrometry with simultaneous distillation extraction. *World Rabbit Sci.* **2016**, *24*, 313–320. [CrossRef]

42. Gaines, A.; Ludovice, M.; Xu, J.; Zanghi, M.; Meinersmann, R.J.; Berrang, M.; Daley, W.; Britton, D. The dialogue between protozoa and bacteria in a microfluidic device. *PLoS ONE* **2019**, *14*, e0222484. [CrossRef]

43. EFSA Panel on Additives and Products or Substances used in Animal Feed (FEEDAP). Scientific Opinion on the safety and efficacy of branched-chain primary aliphatic alcohols/aldehydes/acids, acetals and esters with esters containing branched-chain alcohols and acetals containing branched-chain aldehydes (chemical group 2) when used as flavourings for all animal species. *EFSA J.* **2012**, *10*, 2927.

44. Petričević, S.; Marušić Radovčić, N.; Lukić, K.; Listeš, E.; Medić, H. Differentiation of dry-cured hams from different processing methods by means of volatile compounds, physico-chemical and sensory analysis. *Meat Sci.* **2018**, *137*, 217–227. [CrossRef]

45. Narváez-Rivas, M.; Gallardo, E.; León-Camacho, M. Analysis of volatile compounds from Iberian hams: A review. *Grasas Aceites* **2012**, *63*, 432–454.

46. Flores, M.; Grimm, C.C.; Toldrá, F.; Spanier, A.M. Correlations of Sensory and Volatile Compounds of Spanish "Serrano" Dry-Cured Ham as a Function of Two Processing Times. *J. Agric. Food Chem.* **1997**, *45*, 2178–2186. [CrossRef]

47. Narváez-Rivas, M.; Narváez-Rivas, M.; Gallardo, E.; León-Camacho, M. Study of volatile alcohols and esters from the subcutaneous fat during ripening of Iberian dry-cured ham. A tool for predicting the dry-curing time. *Grasas Aceites* **2016**, *67*, e166. [CrossRef]

48. Cordero, M.R.; Zumalacárregui, J.M. Characterization of Micrococcaceae isolated from salt used for Spanish dry-cured ham. *Lett. Appl. Microbiol.* **2000**, *31*, 303–306. [CrossRef] [PubMed]

49. Ramírez, R.; Cava, R. Volatile profiles of dry-cured meat products from three different Iberian x Duroc genotypes. *J. Agric. Food Chem.* **2007**, *55*, 1923–1931. [CrossRef] [PubMed]

50. Narváez-Rivas, M.; Gallardo, E.; León-Camacho, M. Evolution of volatile hydrocarbons from subcutaneous fat during ripening of Iberian dry-cured ham. A tool to differentiate between ripening periods of the process. *Food Res. Int.* **2015**, *67*, 299–307. [CrossRef]

51. Petrón, M.J.; Tejeda, J.F.; Muriel, E.; Ventanas, J.; Antequera, T. Study of the branched hydrocarbon fraction of intramuscular lipids from Iberian dry-cured ham. *Meat Sci.* **2005**, *69*, 129–134. [CrossRef] [PubMed]

52. Hidalgo, F.J.; Zamora, R. Conversion of phenylalanine into styrene by 2,4-decadienal in model systems. *J. Agric. Food Chem.* **2007**, *55*, 4902–4906. [CrossRef]

53. Calkins, C.R.; Hodgen, J.M. A fresh look at meat flavor. *Meat Sci.* **2007**, *77*, 63–80. [CrossRef]

54. Pugliese, C.; Sirtori, F.; Škrlep, M.; Piasentier, E.; Calamai, L.; Franci, O.; Čandek-Potokar, M. The effect of ripening time on the chemical, textural, volatile and sensorial traits of Bicep femoris and Semimembranosus muscles of the Slovenian dry-cured ham Kraški pršut. *Meat Sci.* **2015**, *100*, 58–68. [CrossRef]

55. García-González, D.L.; Tena, N.; Aparicio-Ruiz, R.; Morales, M.T. Relationship between sensory attributes and volatile compounds qualifying dry-cured hams. *Meat Sci.* **2008**, *80*, 315–325. [CrossRef]

56. Park, S.Y.; Yoo, S.S.; Uh, J.H.; Eun, J.B.; Lee, H.C.; Kim, Y.J.; Chin, K.B. Evaluation of Lipid Oxidation and Oxidative Products as Affected by Pork Meat Cut, Packaging Method, and Storage Time during Frozen Storage. *J. Food Sci.* **2007**, *72*, C114–C119. [CrossRef]

57. Jesús Andrade, M.; Córdoba, J.J.; Sánchez, B.; Casado, E.M.; Rodríguez, M. Evaluation and selection of yeasts isolated from dry-cured Iberian ham by their volatile compound production. *Food Chem.* **2009**, *113*, 457–463. [CrossRef]

58. Jurado, Á.; Carrapiso, A.I.; Ventanasa, J.; García, C. Changes in SPME-extracted volatile compounds from Iberian ham during ripening. *Grasas Aceites* **2009**, *60*, 262–270. [CrossRef]

59. Barbieri, G.; Bolzoni, L.; Parolari, G.; Virgili, R.; Buttini, R.; Careri, M.; Mangia, A. Flavor compounds of dry-cured ham. *J. Agric. Food Chem.* **1992**, *40*, 2389–2394. [CrossRef]

60. Flores, J. Mediterranean vs northern European meat products. Processing technologies and main differences. *Food Chem.* **1997**, *59*, 505–510. [CrossRef]

61. Théron, L.; Tournayre, P.; Kondjoyan, N.; Abouelkaram, S.; Santé-Lhoutellier, V.; Berdagué, J.L. Analysis of the volatile profile and identification of odour-active compounds in Bayonne ham. *Meat Sci.* **2010**, *85*, 453–460. [CrossRef] [PubMed]

62. Pérez-Palacios, T.; Ruiz, J.; Martín, D.; Grau, R.; Antequera, T. Influence of pre-cure freezing on the profile of volatile compounds during the processing of Iberian hams. *J. Sci. Food Agric.* **2010**, *90*, 882–890. [CrossRef]

63. Martínez-Onandi, N.; Rivas-Cañedo, A.; Ávila, M.; Garde, S.; Nuñez, M.; Picon, A. Influence of physicochemical characteristics and high pressure processing on the volatile fraction of Iberian dry-cured ham. *Meat Sci.* **2017**, *131*, 40–47. [CrossRef]

64. Carrapiso, A.I.; Noseda, B.; García, C.; Reina, R.; Sánchez del Pulgar, J.; Devlieghere, F. SIFT-MS analysis of Iberian hams from pigs reared under different conditions. *Meat Sci.* **2015**, *104*, 8–13. [CrossRef]

65. Pugliese, C.; Sirtori, F.; Calamai, L.; Franci, O. The evolution of volatile compounds profile of "Toscano" dry-cured ham during ripening as revealed by SPME-GC-MS approach. *J. Mass Spectrom.* **2010**, *45*, 1056–1064. [CrossRef]

66. Ruiz, J.; Cava, R.; Ventanas, J.; Jensen, M.T. Headspace Solid Phase Microextraction for the Analysis of Volatiles in a Meat Product: Dry-Cured Iberian Ham. *J. Agric. Food Chem.* **1998**, *46*, 4688–4694. [CrossRef]

67. Shi, Y.; Li, X.; Huang, A. Multivariate analysis approach for assessing coated dry-cured ham flavor quality during long-term storage. *J. Food Sci. Technol.* **2020**. [CrossRef]

68. Reale, A.; Di Renzo, T.; Boscaino, F.; Nazzaro, F.; Fratianni, F.; Aponte, M. Lactic acid bacteria biota and aroma profile of Italian traditional sourdoughs from the irpinian area in Italy. *Front. Microbiol.* **2019**, *10*, 1621. [CrossRef] [PubMed]

69. Lin, M.; Liu, X.; Xu, Q.; Song, H.; Li, P.; Yao, J. Aroma-active components of yeast extract pastes with a basic and characteristic meaty flavour. *J. Sci. Food Agric.* **2014**, *94*, 882–889. [CrossRef] [PubMed]

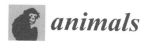

animals

Article

Investigating the Features of PDO Green Hams during Salting: Insights for New Markers and Genomic Regions in Commercial Hybrid Pigs

Martina Zappaterra [1,*], Paolo Zambonelli [1], Cristina Schivazappa [2], Nicoletta Simoncini [2], Roberta Virgili [2], Bruno Stefanon [3] and Roberta Davoli [1,*]

[1] Department of Agricultural and Food Sciences (DISTAL), University of Bologna, Viale Fanin 46, I-40127 Bologna, Italy; paolo.zambonelli@unibo.it
[2] Stazione Sperimentale per l'Industria delle Conserve Alimentari (SSICA), Viale Faustino Tanara 31/A, I-43121 Parma, Italy; cristina.schivazappa@ssica.it (C.S.); nicoletta.simoncini@ssica.it (N.S.); roberta.virgili@ssica.it (R.V.)
[3] Department of Agrifood, Environmental and Animal Science, University of Udine, Via delle Scienze 208, I-33100 Udine, Italy; bruno.stefanon@uniud.it
[*] Correspondence: martina.zappaterra2@unibo.it (M.Z.); roberta.davoli@unibo.it (R.D.)

Simple Summary: In recent years, the meat industry is looking with increased interest at the implementation of non-invasive new tools for predicting the final quality of dry-cured hams and monitoring ham aging. The selection of raw meat and the control of the salting procedure to predict the quality of dry-cured hams are of primary importance for meat processors. The identification of genetic markers associated with ham traits and related to different aptitudes of the thighs towards salting phases and weight losses is a primary goal for the Italian pig production chain. This paper addresses the need for investigating the associations between genomic markers and ham traits obtained through the application of non-invasive technologies for monitoring hams before and during the salting process. To our knowledge, this is the first study investigating the markers and genes associated with ham traits obtained through the use of Ham Inspector™ apparatus.

Citation: Zappaterra, M.; Zambonelli, P.; Schivazappa, C.; Simoncini, N.; Virgili, R.; Stefanon, B.; Davoli, R. Investigating the Features of PDO Green Hams during Salting: Insights for New Markers and Genomic Regions in Commercial Hybrid Pigs. *Animals* 2021, *11*, 68. https://doi.org/10.3390/ani11010068

Received: 15 December 2020
Accepted: 28 December 2020
Published: 1 January 2021

Abstract: Protected Designation of Origin (PDO) dry-cured hams production is greatly dependent on raw meat quality. This study was performed to identify genetic markers associated with the quality of dry-cured ham. Carcass traits of 229 heavy pigs belonging to three commercial genetic lines were registered (weight, EUROP classification). Phenotypic traits (*Semimembranosus* muscle ultimate pH, ham weight and lean meat content, adsorbed salt) of the corresponding thighs, undergone PDO ham process in three different plants, were measured, using a fast and non-invasive technology. Green ham weight and lean meat percentage influenced the estimated salt content and the weight loss during salting, even if the processing plant greatly affected the variability of the measured ham traits. The genomic data were obtained with the GeneSeek Genomic Profiler (GGP) 70k HD Porcine Array, using the slaughter day and the sex of the animals in the statistical analyses. The phenotypic traits were associated with the genotypes through GenAbel software. The results showed that 18 SNPs located on nine porcine chromosomes were found to be associated with nine phenotypic traits, mainly related to ham weight loss during salting. New associations were found between markers in the genes *Neural Precursor Cell Expressed Developmentally Down-Regulated 9* (*NEDD9*, SSC7), *T-Cell Lymphoma Invasion and Metastasis 2* (*TIAM2*, SSC1), and the ham quality traits. After validation, these SNPs may be useful to improve the quality of thighs for the production of PDO dry-cured hams.

Keywords: swine; genetic marker; ham processing; ham quality

1. Introduction

The production of Protected Designation of Origin (PDO) Parma and San Daniele hams plays an economic role of primary importance in the Italian pig production chain [1]

and represents a point of excellence for the Italian pork chain. The quality of the raw meat and the carcass composition greatly influence both the suitability of the thighs to obtain high-quality PDO dry-cured hams such as Parma and San Daniele [2,3]. The fresh thighs used for the production of PDO Parma hams are obtained from heavy pigs slaughtered at a live weight of at least 140 to160 kg, with an age of at least nine months, and belonging to specific selected breeds defined by Parma ham Consortium [4]. These requirements are essential for obtaining hind legs with features suitable for long curing periods; additional required parameters of the thighs are the presence of subcutaneous fat of 15 to 30 mm of thickness to minimize processing losses [2]. These features affect both the aptitude of meat to adsorb salt during the ham salting periods and the weight loss of the ham after salting during the long maturation, which may last from 12 to 24 or more months [5]. However, over time, extensive analytical surveys were carried out to determine the contribution of this food to sodium intake, and medical and public health organizations recommended to reduce sodium dietary intake to prevent hypertension and other diseases [5,6]. On the other hand, an excessive reduction in the amount of adsorbed salt can worsen the technological performances, causing an increase in proteolysis, higher softness, and the production of off-flavors due to the release of free amino acids and peptides during ripening [5,6]. The research on environmental and genetic factors involved in salt adsorption and in the sodium amount of dry-cured ham has attracted great interest based on these contrasting nutritional and technological requirements behind the issue of sodium reduction. Several factors contribute to influencing the final salt amount in dry-cured hams; among them, a crucial role is represented by the know-how of the different ham processors [5]. The ham weight and size, the inter- and intramuscular fat content, the thickness of subcutaneous fat, and the lean meat content of the hind leg represent the main factors that can influence also the aptitude of the ham to adsorb salt [7–10]. The study and identification of genes and genetic markers associated with these traits could provide new and important tools for the ham industry for improving ham yield during processing. Also the physico-chemical modifications of thigh muscles post-mortem, such as pH decline, water activity, proteolytic and lipolytic reactions, produce changes in color, taste, flavor, texture [11], and salt absorption in the hams [5]. These traits are affected, at least in part, by the animal genetic background as reported by studies indicating genetic markers associated with *Semimembranosus* muscle (SM) pH and drip loss [12,13], and with enzymes activity in San Daniele hams [14]. Most of these association studies have been performed on the purebred pig lines used in the two-way or three-way crossbreeding schemes [12,15], but few association studies exist between genetic markers and ham ripening related traits measured directly in heavy pigs used for dry-cured ham production. Moreover, the genetic improvement of quality traits of dry-cured hams is difficult because these characteristics cannot be easily measured in live animals and are cost-effective phenotypes.

In recent years, different non-invasive technologies based on X-rays or near-infrared (NIR) spectroscopy were investigated as quality control techniques in the ham industry [16]. Magnetic induction technology is among the most promising to estimate lean content in green hams [17] and the salt absorbed by processed hams [18]. These new non-invasive technologies allow for the collecting of a huge number of phenotypic data. Thus, the identification of genetic markers and new tools to assess and help to predict these traits may be of primary importance for pig production chain and ham processors [10,14,19].

This work aims to investigate the variability of green ham traits in a sample of 229 commercial hybrid heavy pigs during salting and the genomic regions associated with the measured phenotypes. These regions will be singled out through a Genome-Wide Association Study (GWAS), which will allow identifying DNA markers and candidate genes associated with phenotypic characteristics of the fresh hams measured during the first stages of the ham processing. The identified SNPs might be of interest to improve ham yield after salting and the quality of the finished product. The identification of genetic markers associated with the quality of the thighs for PDO dry-cured hams can offer new helpful tools for the highly innovative pig production chain.

2. Materials and Methods

2.1. Animal Data Availability

The samples and hams used in the present study were obtained from the slaughtering of commercial heavy pigs intended for human consumption, and thus the present research did not need approval from a research ethics committee. The heavy pig hybrids were slaughtered in commercial abattoirs in four slaughter days between March and July 2018. The animals were slaughtered in compliance with the European rules [20,21] on the protection of animals during transport and related operations and slaughtering. All slaughter procedures were monitored by the veterinary team appointed by the Italian Ministry of Health. The carcasses came from crossbred pigs reared in three different farms and were obtained from the crossbreeding of the three main breeds reared in Italy for heavy pig production, namely Large White, Landrace, and Duroc. These commercial hybrids were kept in collective pens until they reached the slaughter weight. The pigs were fed diets complying with the dietary inclusion limits established by the Parma Ham Consortium [4] and were slaughtered at an average live weight of 160 kg. Each farm sent their heavy pigs to a specific abattoir, and the thighs were then processed by a specific processing plant. Thus, the farm of farrowing, abattoir, and ham processing plants are collinear variables. Similarly, also the slaughter days match with the farms, abattoirs, and plants, with the thighs coming from the same slaughter day for the hams of plant 1, from two slaughter days for hams processed in plant 2, and from one day of slaughtering for ham processed in plant 3.

2.2. Carcass and Ham Traits

A total of 229 fresh hams were collected from carcasses classified as "U", "R", and "O" in compliance with Commission Implementing Decision, 2014/38/EU [22]. Pig carcasses were graded according to the European EUROP carcass grading system [22] which considers the lean meat content estimated for the whole carcass. In particular, carcasses classified as "U" are characterized by a lean meat content between 50% and 55%, carcasses "R" are characterized by a lean meat content between 45% and 50%, and carcasses "O" are characterized by a lean meat content between 40% and 45%. Fresh hams were elaborated at three different dry-cured ham processing plants operating in accordance with tutelary regulations of Parma ham manufacturing [23,24]. A sample of SM was collected for the genomic analyses, and frozen at −20 °C until processed for DNA extraction.

The pH of fresh hams was measured in SM with a Hamilton glass electrode probe attached to a portable pH meter (WTW pH3110, Weilheim, Germany). Homogeneous sets of hams in terms of muscle pH at 24 h post-mortem (pHu) ranged between 5.50 and 5.90 were used for each plant.

Then, all fresh hams underwent traditional salting for Italian dry-cured ham, based on a two-step addition of salt [25], following the standard procedure of each plant.

2.3. Non-Invasive Magnetic Induction (MI) System Analysis

The lean amount of green hams and the salt content of the salted ones were determined by the Ham Inspector™ apparatus (Lenz, Barcelona, Spain). The system based on electromagnetic induction (MI) technology generates a signal with an amplitude depending on the ham lean amount and salt content, estimated using a proper calibration [17,18].

Two hundred and twenty-nine fresh hams were scanned with the MI system set in the "RAW" mode, installed at each plant. The lean amount expressed as a percentage of ham weight was estimated by using previously developed predictive models reported in Simoncini et al. [17]. This model was improved, including a greater number of dissected and analyzed hams, and estimating the new prediction accuracy (RMSE = 1.34%). After the first salting and at the end of the salting steps, the unabsorbed salt was brushed away, and the same salted hams were scanned with the MI system set in the "salted" mode. The salt content of the lean part, expressed as a percentage on a wet basis, was estimated by using a previously developed predictive model, in accordance with Schivazappa et al. [18].

Prediction accuracy of the model including a greater number of dissected and analyzed salted hams was estimated (RMSE = 0.14%).

All scanned hams were tempered at 3 ± 0.5 °C and temperature tested with the thermometer Ebro TFX 410 Pt1000 (Xylem Inc, Rye Brook, NY, USA) inserted into SM muscle (5 cm depth) to avoid possible drifts of MI signal, associated with variations in sample temperature.

The weight of the fresh hams as well as their weights during the salting process (after the first salting and at the end of the salting period) was recorded by the MI apparatus in order to calculate the corresponding weight losses, expressed as percentage loss of fresh ham weight.

2.4. Statistical Analyses of Ham Traits

All statistics of phenotypic traits were obtained by SPSS version 22.0 software platform (SPSS Inc., Chicago, IL, USA); normal distribution of data was investigated before statistical analyses. The boxplot procedure was applied to present the distribution of measured lean percentage of hams, differently labeled according to the EUROP grid (lean carcass grading). Data of ham traits were analyzed using Generalized Linear Model (GLM) procedure; the models included the processing plant and the sex of the pigs respectively, as fixed factors. These factors were included in the model since they are known to affect ham quality [3]. The Least Significant Difference (LSD) posthoc test was applied to compare the Estimated Marginal Means (EMMs). Finally, the Pearson's correlation analysis was performed to investigate the relationships between all quality and technological traits of hams in each processing plant.

2.5. Genotyping and Association Study

The collected SM samples were used for the genomic analyses. DNA extractions were carried out using a standard protocol by an outsource laboratory (Agrotis S.r.L.-LGS, Cremona, Italy, http://www.lgscr.it/ENG/index.html) where the genotype analyses were also performed. For the genotyping, the GeneSeek® Genomic Profiler-GGP-70k HD Porcine chip (Illumina, San Diego, CA, USA; https://emea.illumina.com/products/by-type/microarray-kits/ggp-porcine.html) containing 68516 SNPs was used using the procedures indicated by the company. The SNPs were mapped using *Sus scrofa* Genome Assembly Build 11.1 (NCBI: https://www.ncbi.nlm.nih.gov/assembly/GCF_000003025.6; ENSEMBL: https://www.ensembl.org/Sus_scrofa/Info/Index). The sex of the animals (females, castrated males) was obtained on the basis of the genotypes for the sex chromosomes. The genotypic data were filtered using gPLINK (version 2.050, based on PLINK version 1.07) [26] and GenAbel (version 1.8-0, run on R version 3.4.4) [27] discarding the markers or samples not passing these thresholds: all the markers with call rate < 90%, with minor allele frequency < 5%, which are not in Hardy-Weinberg equilibrium [28] (p-value < 0.001); all the individuals with more than 10% missing genotypes and with Identity by State (IBS) > 90%. After filtering, 54,569 SNPs and 169 individuals were retained. The large number of excluded animals (n = 60) was because their IBS was above the threshold set at 90%. The association analyses were carried out using *polygenic_hglm* and *qtscore* functions implemented on the GenAbel package according to the procedure described in Nicolazzi et al. [29]. The statistical model included the day of slaughter and the sex as predictive variables, together with the effect of the SNP and the genomic kinship matrix. The genomic kinship matrix was obtained with GenAbel and was used to estimate the relatedness between the animals. Pedigree data were not available for these animals since commercial hybrids are obtained from heterospermic artificial insemination. Also, the information concerning litters and dams was not available. These data can be available in fully controlled experimental studies, but they are difficult to obtain in commercial farm conditions, where cross-fostering is a common practice. The p-values of the associations between ham traits and SNPs were corrected for the "deflation" factor, as reported by GenAbel. Markers were considered significant with corrected p-values below the chromosome-wide significant threshold (Table S1), and the trend towards the significance threshold was set at 5.00×10^{-5} [30]. The markers with corrected *p*-values below these thresholds were further considered for the estimation of the genotypic effects. Their genotypes were extracted from the PED file generated through the gPLINK tool using in-house implemented scripts in the R environment [31]. Linear mixed models were performed to obtain the Estimated Least Squares Means (LSM) for the genotypes of the significant markers. The associated traits were used as dependent variables; the genotype of each marker taken individually was modeled as a predictive variable together with the fixed effects of sex and slaughter day. The linear regression model did not include the random effect of the genomic kinship matrix. For each marker found with the GWAS, the additive and dominance genetic effects were also estimated. The additive effect was estimated as half of the difference between the two homozygous groups: a = 1/2(BB − AA), with A and B that indicate the first and the second allele of the analyzed markers, respectively. The dominance effect was estimated as the difference between the heterozygous group and the average of the two homozygous groups in each locus: d = AB − 1/2(AA + BB). These analyses were performed using functions in the packages *nlme* [32], *lsmeans* [33], *lme4* [34], and *car* [35] in the R environment [31]. The genes located in the region flanking the identified markers (±500 kilobases from the associated marker) were further considered for the identification of candidate genes for the traits. The list of the flanking genes was obtained using the BioMart tool [36] and was submitted to David Bioinformatics Resources version 6.8 on-line tool (https://david.ncifcrf.gov/). Candidate genes were identified on the basis of their location (the nearest gene to the significant marker) and biological role. In order to find possible splice sites or motifs with biological relevance, the sequences flanking the intronic variants found associated with ham traits were submitted to the Tomtom tool in MEME Suite version 5.3.0 [37] (http://meme-suite.org/). The found motifs are ranked based on their Bonferroni significance (*q*-value) for the found match between the query sequence (or its complementary) and the motif in JASPAR CORE 2014 database.

3. Results

3.1. Ham Quality and Technological Traits

The variability noticed for ham lean % is reported in Figure 1. The boxplot displays the distribution of the lean % of hams estimated by Ham Inspector[TM], in relation to the lean % of the corresponding carcasses according to EUROP classification [22]. The EUROP classification of the original carcass is printed on the skin of each fresh ham supplied to dry-cured ham producers, to provide information on the lean % expected in fresh ham.

The class R, corresponding to an estimated lean % of the carcass in the range 45 to 50% is the most abundant (n = 110) compared to classes O (lean % = 40 to 45%, n = 36) and U (lean %= 50 to 55%, n = 62). In the current study, the lean % of the hams scanned by Ham Inspector[TM] shows higher values (R = 62.3 ± 2.7, U = 63.0 ± 2.0, O = 61.6 ± 2.2) than those estimated from the EUROP classification of the corresponding whole carcass.

All fresh hams were processed in three different manufacturing plants in accordance with tutelary regulations of Parma ham [23,24].

The results of GLM analysis including "processing plant" and "sex" as fixed effects and their interaction are summarized in Table 1. For each trait, the EMMs (Estimated Marginal Means), the standard error, and the corresponding significance level are reported.

Differences in the measured ham traits between processing plants (*p* < 0.001) were detected. In particular, processing plant 1 handles the heaviest hams between the tested plants (15.1 kg), and hams leaner (62.7%) than plant 3 (60.6%). This condition affects salting weight losses, yielding higher values at the end of salting for plant 1 compared to other plants. The salt % predicted in ham lean content after both salting steps differed significantly between processing plants (*p* < 0.001), reporting greater values for plant 3 and 2, respectively (Table 1).

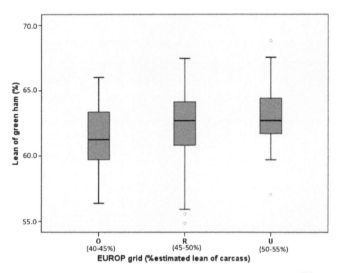

Figure 1. Boxplots of the lean content (%) estimated by Ham Inspector™ for the green hams grouped according to the EUROP classes (U, R, and O) of the corresponding carcasses. For each EUROP class, the range of % estimated lean carcass is reported. Blank circles represent outliers.

The sex of the pigs generated differences for the lean % of green hams ($p < 0.001$) and their weight loss after the first ($p < 0.05$) and at the end of the salting ($p < 0.01$; Table 1), and the predicted salt contents ($p < 0.01$). The higher lean % of green hams from females caused higher weight losses during salting, and higher values of salt content at the end of salting (2.60%) if compared to barrows (2.53%). As for the salt content at the end of salting, the interaction between processing plant and sex was significant ($p < 0.05$): the three plants differed regardless of the sex of the animal, but in the case of females the salt values were higher than in barrows.

The results of the Pearson's correlation analysis performed between ham traits measured in each processing plant are reported in Tables S2–S4. The strongest and most significant correlations were found in plant 2 (Table S3): pH was negatively correlated with salt content measured at the first salting step (r = −0.241, $p < 0.01$) and the weight loss at the end of salting (r = −0.388, $p < 0.001$). The weight of green hams was negatively correlated with salt content after the first salting in all tested processing plants (Tables S2–S4), whereas, only for plant 2, the negative correlation coefficient with salt content at the end of the salting process was significant (r = −0.486, $p < 0.001$; Table S3). For all processing plants (Tables S2–S4), the lean % of green hams was positively related to ham weight losses and to the salt contents predicted after the first and at the end of the salting steps. In each processing plant, the highest positive correlation coefficients have been found between green ham weight and ham weight after the first salting (plant 1: r = 0.999, $p < 0.001$; plant 2 r = 0.999, $p < 0.001$; plant 3 r = 0.998, $p < 0.001$), green ham weight and ham weight at the end of salting (plant 1: r = 0.997, $p < 0.001$; plant 2 r = 0.999, $p < 0.001$; plant 3 r = 0.996, $p < 0.001$), and between ham weight after first and at the end of salting (plant 1: r = 0.997, $p < 0.001$; plant 2 r = 0.999, $p < 0.001$; plant 3 r = 0.999, $p < 0.001$).

3.2. Association Study Results

The performed GWAS allowed the identification of eight markers displaying a Bonferroni corrected *p*-value significant at the chromosome-wide level, reported in bold in Table 2. The most significant association was found for pHu, which is linked to WU_10.2_18_17949287 marker. This SNP is an intergenic variant located at 17 Mb on *Sus scrofa* chromosome 18 (SSC18). Green ham lean % showed an association with a region on SSC4 at 2 Mb, where the marker ASGA0016987 is located. This SNP is an exon variant of a non-coding transcript (ENSSSCT00000066959.1), and most of the genes comprised in the flanking region are non-coding genes. Green ham weight, ham weight after first salting, and ham weight at the end of the salting showed an association with the same two markers, namely CASI0010463 and WU_10.2_14_144250775. The first is located on SSC15 at 12 Mb, in an intron of the gene *Neurexophilin 2* (*NXPH2*). WU_10.2_14_144250775 is an intergenic variant in a region characterized by high gene density, on SSC14 at 132 Mb. Two SNPs were significant for ham weight loss after first salting: ASGA0031014, an intron variant of the gene *Neural Precursor Cell Expressed, Developmentally Down-Regulated 9* (*NEDD9*), and WU_10.2_10_74620421, a variant in a non-coding transcript on SSC10. Salt content at the end of salting showed two markers displaying a chromosome-wide significant association. The first (INRA0000796) is located on SSC1 at 13 Mb, and is an intron variant of the gene *Regulator of G Protein Signaling 17* (*RGS17*); the second (ASGA0102337) is an intron variant of the gene *GRAM Domain Containing 1B* (*GRAMD1B*), located on SSC9 at 50 Mb. Eleven markers showed less significant associations with the ham traits, with adjusted p-values comprised between the chromosome-wide significance level and the threshold of 5.00×10^{-5} (Table 2). The complete lists of the top 20 markers most associated with the measured traits are reported in File S1. Table S5 reports the complete list of all the genes located in the regions flanking the markers reported in Table 2. The results of the functional association obtained for the genes in Table S5 are reported in Table S6. No significant terms were identified, and none of them seemed to indicate a direct involvement of the candidate genes in muscle or fat development. Thus, further discussion of the obtained associations was based on the review of the scientific literature.

For each of the found markers, the LSM of the genotypes were estimated and reported in Table 3. For pHu, both markers showed genotype distributions quite unbalanced, with GG genotype poorly represented (WU_10.2_18_17949287) or not represented at all (WU_10.2_4_91195648) in our sample. Other identified markers showed a genotypic class poorly represented ($n < 10$ animals, i.e., ASGA0016987, ALGA0002237, CASI0010463, WU_10.2_7_118557013) or completely lacking (ALGA0044906, INRA0000796). The weights of fresh thighs and hams after first and at the end of salting were associated with the same markers, namely CASI0010463 and WU_10.2_14_144250775. Furthermore, the marker ASGA0026341 showed an additive genetic effect on both ham weights after first salting and at the end of salting. In fact, the AA animals for this marker showed lower ham weights than GG pigs (Table 3). Additive genetic effects were also found for H3GA0000815, WU_10.2_7_118557013, WU_10.2_14_36295226, and ASGA0031014 (Table 3). In particular, the AA animals for the H3GA0000815 SNP were associated with a lower lean % in green hams; the A allele of WU_10.2_7_118557013 was related to higher weights at the end of salting; the G allele of ASGA0031014 showed lower weight losses, and the GG animals for the WU_10.2_14_36295226 SNP presented a higher % of salt adsorbed at first salting. Concerning the ASGA0031014 marker, the three genotypic classes were well represented, following the 1:2:1 ratio.

The results obtained with MEME Suite indicated that none of the identified intronic variants were located in splice sites, but the marker ASGA0031014 fell into an intronic region of the gene *Neural Precursor Cell Expressed, Developmentally Down-Regulated 9* (*NEDD9*) harboring several binding sites recognized by *Forkhead box O* (*FOXO*) transcription factors (Table S7). The in-silico analysis indicated that the mutation ASGA0031014 changed the sequence recognized by *FOXO3* (q-value = 0.050; Figure S1a), *FOXO1* (q-value = 0.074; Figure S1b), and *FOXO4* (q-value = 0.074; Figure S1c). The sequences recognized by these transcription factors are the reverse complement of the region flanking ASGA0031014, since the *NEDD9* gene is located on the reverse strand (strand −1 in Table S5). For this reason, ASGA0031014 has T/C as alternate alleles in Figure S1.

Table 1. Effect of the processing plant (PP) and sex (S) of the animals on the traits (Estimated Marginal Means ± standard error) of hams (green and after salting steps).

Ham Traits	Processing Plant (PP)				Sex (S)			PPxS
	1	2	3	p-Value	Barrow	Female	p-Value	p-Value
	n. 60	n.120	n.50		n. 105	n. 125		
pH$_u$	5.63^c ± 0.02	5.69^b ± 0.01	5.79^a ± 0.02	<0.001	5.71 ± 0.01	5.70 ± 0.01	n.s.	n.s.
Weight $_{GH}$, kg [1]	15.10^a ± 0.10	13.90^b ± 0.10	12.60^c ± 0.20	<0.001	13.90 ± 0.11	13.80 ± 0.10	n.s.	n.s.
Lean $_{GH}$, % [2]	62.70^a ± 0.30	62.90^a ± 0.20	60.60^b ± 0.30	<0.001	61.10 ± 0.20	62.90 ± 0.20	<0.001	n.s.
Weight $_{1S}$, kg [3]	14.90^a ± 0.10	13.70^b ± 0.10	12.50^c ± 0.20	<0.001	13.70 ± 0.10	13.60 ± 0.10	n.s.	n.s.
Weight Loss $_{1S}$, % [4]	1.31 ± 0.03	1.26 ± 0.02	1.36 ± 0.04	n.s.	1.28 ± 0.03	1.35 ± 0.02	<0.05	n.s.
Salt $_{1S}$, % [5]	1.06^c ± 0.01	1.21^b ± 0.01	1.46^a ± 0.02	<0.001	1.22 ± 0.01	1.27 ± 0.01	<0.001	n.s.
Weight $_{ES}$, kg [6]	14.60^a ± 0.10	13.50^b ± 0.10	12.20^c ± 0.20	<0.001	13.70 ± 0.10	13.40 ± 0.10	n.s.	n.s.
Weight Loss $_{ES}$, % [7]	3.13^a ± 0.06	2.64^b ± 0.04	2.72^b ± 0.07	<0.001	2.73 ± 0.05	2.93 ± 0.04	<0.01	n.s.
Salt $_{ES}$, % [8]	2.37^c ± 0.02	2.80^a ± 0.02	2.52^b ± 0.03	<0.001	2.53 ± 0.02	2.60 ± 0.02	<0.01	<0.05
Salt $_{1S}$ /Salt $_{ES}$, % [9]	44.70^b ± 0.30	43.00^c ± 0.20	57.50^a ± 0.40	<0.001	48.50 ± 0.30	48.30 ± 0.20	n.s.	n.s.

Estimated Marginal Means with different letters along rows are significantly different (LSD posthoc test); n.s: not significant. [1] Weight of green hams measured with Ham Inspector^{TM} and expressed in kg. [2] Lean content of green hams estimated by Ham Inspector^{TM} and expressed as a percentage of green ham weight (%). [3] Weight of hams measured with Ham Inspector^{TM} and expressed in kg. [4] Weight loss measured after 1st salting and expressed as percentage loss of green ham weight (%). [5] Salt (as NaCl) content of the lean part of salted hams at 1st salting, estimated by Ham Inspector^{TM} and expressed as a percentage of wet weight (%). [6] Weight of hams measured at the end of salting with Ham Inspector^{TM} and expressed in kg. [7] Weight loss measured at the end of salting and expressed as percentage loss of green ham weight (%). [8] Salt (as NaCl) content of the lean part of salted hams at the end of salting, estimated by Ham Inspector^{TM} and expressed as a percentage of wet weight (%). [9] Ratio between salt at 1st salting step and salt content at the end of salting, expressed as percentage (%).

Table 2. The list of the significant markers, with the associated traits, the marker position, the type of variant, and the list of the candidate genes in the regions flanking the significant markers. Chromosome-wide significant markers are in bold.

Trait	Marker	Marker Rs Code	Position[1]	MAF[2]	Pc1df[3]	Type of Variant	Candidate Genes in the Region[4]
pH$_u$	WU_10.2_18_17949287	rs321317414	18:17,103,785	0.22	2.54×10^{-6}	intergenic variant	PLXNA4, MKLN1
	WU_10.2_4_91195648	rs342976952	4:83,519,869	0.13	3.94×10^{-5}	intron variant of the gene CD247	DCAF6, MPC2, ADCY10, MPZL1, RCSD1, CREG1, CD247, POU2F1, DUSP27, GPA33, MAEL
Lean $_{GH}$, %[5]	ASGA0016987	rs80994554	4:2,020,990	0.25	1.42×10^{-5}	exon variant of a non-coding transcript	ADGRB1, MROH5, PTP4A3, GPR20, SLC45A4
	ALGA0002237	rs80883186	1:30,193,313	0.16	3.07×10^{-5}	intergenic variant	SGK1, SLC2A12, TBPL1, TCF21, EYA4
	H3GA0000815	rs80848905	1:11,662,820	0.35	4.72×10^{-5}	intron variant of the gene TIAM2	NOX3, TFB1M, TIAM2, SCAF8
	ASGA0001055	rs80923830	1:11,684,450	0.33	4.72×10^{-5}	intron variant of the gene TIAM2	NOX3, TFB1M, TIAM2, SCAF8
Weight $_{GH}$, kg[6]	CASI0010463	rs335635913	15:12,997,362	0.13	5.48×10^{-6}	intron variant of the gene NXPH2	NXPH2, SPOPL
	WU_10.2_14_144250775	rs343048625	14:132,664,262	0.40	1.33×10^{-5}	intergenic variant	AWN, PSP-II, SPMI, PSTK, IKZF5, ACADSB, HMX2, HMX3, BUB3
Weight $_{1S}$, kg[7]	CASI0010463	rs335635913	15:12,997,362	0.13	4.13×10^{-6}	intron variant of the gene NXPH2	NXPH2, SPOPL
	WU_10.2_14_144250775	rs343048625	14:132,664,262	0.40	1.26×10^{-5}	intergenic variant	AWN, PSP-II, SPMI, PSTK, IKZF5, ACADSB, HMX2, HMX3, BUB3
	ASGA0026341	rs80859829	5:74,704,457	0.33	4.57×10^{-5}	intergenic variant	ADAMTS20, PUS7L, IRAK4, TWF1, U6, TMEM117
Weight $_{ES}$, kg[8]	CASI0010463	rs335635913	15:12,997,362	0.13	2.15×10^{-6}	intron variant of the gene NXPH2	NXPH2, SPOPL
	WU_10.2_14_144250775	rs343048625	14:132,664,262	0.40	4.27×10^{-6}	intergenic variant	AWN, PSP-II, SPMI, PSTK, IKZF5, ACADSB, HMX2, HMX3, BUB3
	ASGA0026341	rs80859829	5:74,704,457	0.33	2.23×10^{-5}	intergenic variant	ADAMTS20, PUS7L, IRAK4, TWF1, U6, TMEM117
	WU_10.2_7_118557013	rs325887861	7:111,991,773	0.12	4.25×10^{-5}	intergenic variant	EFCAB11, TDP1, KCNK13, PSMC1, NRDE2, CALM1
	ALGA0004906	rs80886909	7:112,364,405	0.08	4.66×10^{-5}	intron variant of the gene TTC7B	PSMC1, NRDE2, CALM1, TTC7B, RPS6K, A5TTC7B

183

Table 2. *Cont.*

Trait	Marker	Marker Rs Code	Position[1]	MAF[2]	Pc1df[3]	Type of Variant	Candidate Genes in the Region[4]
Weight Loss[1S], %[9]	ASGA0031014	rs80963318	7:8,081,734	0.47	1.00×10^{-5}	intron variant of the gene *NEDD9*	*GCM2, ELOVL2, SMIM13, NEDD9, TMEM170B, ADTRP, HIVEP1*
	WU_10.2_10_74620421	-	10:67,919,711	0.25	1.57×10^{-5}	sequence variant of a non-coding gene	*ADARB2*
Weight Loss[ES], %[10]	ALGA0022599	rs80917191	4:6,665,856	0.27	2.90×10^{-5}	intergenic variant	*KHDRBS3*
Salt[1S], %[11]	WU_10.2_14_3629226	rs323879154	14:34,218,184	0.44	1.71×10^{-5}	intron variant of the genes *SUDS3* and *SRRM4*	*SUDS3, TAOK3, VSIG10, WSB2, RFC5, KSR2SUDS3, SRRM4*
	ASGA0000817	rs80921216	1:8,287,008	0.42	2.22×10^{-5}	intergenic variant	*FNDC1, TAGAP, RSPH3, EZR, SYTL3, DYNLT1, TMEM181*
Salt[ES], %[12]	INRA0000796	rs332490862	1:13,370,639	0.08	4.36×10^{-6}	intron variant of the gene *RGS17*	*RGS17, MTRFL1, FBXO5, VIP, MYCT1*
	ASGA0102337	rs81323631	9:50,457,899	0.35	1.46×10^{-5}	intron variant of the gene *GRAMD1B*	*HSPA8, CLMP, GRAMD1B, SCN3B, ZNF202, OR6X1, OR6M1, OR4D5, OR6T1,*

[1] The marker position in *Sus scrofa* Genome Assembly Build 11.1 is reported as *Sus scrofa* chromosome: nucleotide position in base pairs. [2] Minor Allele Frequency. [3] Significance estimates obtained with GenABEL with the correction for inflation factor (stratification effects). Bold values indicate markers significant at the chromosome-wide level. [4] The flanking region is the genomic region located between the marker position ± 500,000 nucleotides. [5] Lean content of green hams estimated by Ham Inspector™ and expressed as a percentage of green ham weight (%). [6] Weight of green hams measured with Ham Inspector™ and expressed in kg. [7] Weight of hams at 1st salting measured with Ham Inspector™ and expressed in kg. [8] Weight of hams at the end of salting measured with Ham Inspector™ and expressed in kg. [9] Weight loss measured after 1st salting and expressed as percentage loss of green ham weight (%). [10] Weight loss measured at the end of salting and expressed as percentage loss of green ham weight (%). [11] Salt (as NaCl) content of the lean part of salted hams at 1st salting, estimated by Ham Inspector™ and expressed as percentage of wet weight (%). [12] Salt (as NaCl) content of the lean part of salted hams at the end of salting, estimated by Ham Inspector™ and expressed as a percentage of wet weight (%).

Table 3. Estimated Least Squares Means (LSM) ± standard errors (S.E.), additive and dominance genetic effects of the markers associated with ham traits. Between brackets are reported the numbers of the observations used for each genotype.

Trait	Marker	Allele		LSM ± S.E (N)			Additive Effect	Dominance Effect
		1	2	11	12	22		
pH_u	WU_10.2_18_17949287	G	A	5.71 a ± 0.04 (10)	5.73 a ± 0.02 (55)	5.70 a ± 0.01 (104)	n.s.	n.s.
	WU_10.2_4_91195648	G	A	- (0)	5.69 a ± 0.02 (43)	5.72 a ± 0.01 (126)	-	-
Lean $_{GH}$, %[1]	ASGA0016987	G	A	63.91 a ± 0.81 (8)	61.91 b ± 0.27 (64)	62.61 ab ± 0.23 (93)	n.s.	0.042
	ALGA0002237	C	A	62.15 a ± 0.21 (115)	63.04 a ± 0.33 (46)	62.47 a ± 1.10 (4)	n.s.	n.s.
	H3GA0000815	G	A	63.57 a ± 0.48 (20)	62.71 a ± 0.25 (75)	61.75 b ± 0.26 (70)	0.0005	n.s.
	ASGA0001055	G	A	61.72 a ± 0.51 (19)	62.61 a ± 0.26 (70)	62.40 a ± 0.25 (76)	n.s.	n.s.
Weight $_{GH}$, kg[2]	CASI0010463	C	A	13.58 ab ± 0.68 (2)	14.05 a ± 0.16 (38)	13.66 b ± 0.09 (125)	n.s.	n.s.
	WU_10.2_14_144250775	G	A	13.93 ab ± 0.20 (24)	13.88 a ± 0.10 (85)	13.48 b ± 0.13 (56)	n.s.	n.s.
Weight $_{IS}$, kg[3]	CASI0010463	C	A	13.42 ab ± 0.69 (2)	13.85 a ± 0.16 (37)	13.48 b ± 0.09 (123)	n.s.	n.s.
	WU_10.2_14_144250775	G	A	13.74 ab ± 0.20 (24)	13.69 a ± 0.11 (83)	13.29 b ± 0.13 (55)	n.s.	n.s.
Weight $_{ES}$, kg[4]	ASGA0026341	G	A	14.01 a ± 0.24 (16)	13.71 a ± 0.11 (78)	13.29 b ± 0.12 (68)	0.009	n.s.
	CASI0010463	C	A	13.12 ab ± 0.69 (2)	13.63 a ± 0.17 (37)	13.24 b ± 0.09 (116)	n.s.	n.s.

185

Table 3. *Cont.*

Trait	Marker	Allele		LSM ± S.E (N)			Additive Effect	Dominance Effect
		1	2	11	12	22		
	WU_10.2_14_144250775	G	A	13.48 ab ± 0.21 (23)	13.48 a ± 0.11 (79)	13.04 b ± 0.13 (52)	n.s.	n.s.
	ASGA0026341	G	A	13.70 a ± 0.25 (16)	13.50 a ± 0.11 (78)	13.05 b ± 0.12 (68)	0.022	n.s.
	WU_10.2_7_118557013	G	A	13.18 c ± 0.09 (120)	13.74 b ± 0.17 (33)	15.19 a ± 0.67 (2)	0.003	n.s.
	ALGA0044906	G	A	13.24 b ± 0.08 (131)	13.81 a ± 0.20 (24)	- (0)	-	-
Weight Loss $_{1S}$, % [5]	ASGA0031014	G	A	1.24 b ± 0.02 (91)	1.37 a ± 0.03 (61)	1.35 ab ± 0.08 (10)	1.23 b ± 0.04 (42)	n.s.
	WU_10.2_10_74620421	G	A	1.24 b ± 0.02 (91)	1.37 a ± 0.03 (61)	1.35 ab ± 0.08 (10)	n.s.	n.s.
Weight Loss $_{ES}$, % [6]	ALGA0022599	G	A	2.82 a ± 0.04 (86)	2.81 a ± 0.05 (57)	2.90 a ± 0.11 (12)	n.s.	n.s.
Salt $_{1S}$, % [7]	WU_10.2_14_36295226	G	A	1.26 a ± 0.02 (28)	1.25 ab ± 0.01 (85)	1.21 b ± 0.01 (49)	0.036	n.s.
	ASGA0000817	G	A	1.25 a ± 0.01 (51)	1.23 a ± 0.01 (87)	1.24 a ± 0.02 (24)	n.s.	n.s.
Salt $_{ES}$, % [8]	INRA0000796	C	A	- (0)	2.62 a ± 0.03 (21)	2.63 a ± 0.01 (134)	-	-
	ASGA0102337	G	A	2.62 a ± 0.04 (17)	2.62 a ± 0.02 (73)	2.64 a ± 0.02 (65)	n.s.	n.s.

LSM with different letters along rows are significantly different for *p* < 0.10 adjusted with the Tukey test. "." means that additive and dominance effect cannot be estimated for that marker as two genotypes were found in the samples. n.s. stands for not significant. [1] Lean content of green hams estimated by Ham Inspector[TM] and expressed as a percentage of green ham weight (%). [2] Weight of green hams measured with Ham Inspector[TM] and expressed in kg. [3] Weight of hams at 1st salting measured with Ham Inspector[TM] and expressed in kg. [4] Weight of hams at the end of salting measured with Ham Inspector[TM] and expressed in kg. [5] Weight loss measured after 1st salting and expressed as percentage loss of green ham weight (%). [6] Weight loss measured at the end of salting and expressed as percentage loss of green ham weight (%). [7] Salt (as NaCl) content of the lean part of salted hams at 1st salting, estimated by Ham Inspector[TM] and expressed as a percentage of wet weight (%). [8] Salt (as NaCl) content of the lean part of salted hams at the end of salting, estimated by Ham Inspector[TM] and expressed as a percentage of wet weight (%).

4. Discussion

The development of new technologies enabling a fast and non-invasive measure of green ham potential to be processed into typical dry-cured ham is a goal for pig production chain and PDO ham producers. In the last decade, technologies such as those based on X-rays have been studied [16], with the aim of monitoring and gathering information in a non-invasive way on green hams intended for dry curing, focusing on their qualitative traits and the amount of salt absorbed during processing. The Ham Inspector™ system permits an on-line and non-invasive inspection of the hams, a classification of thighs based on the lean content (calculated as a percentage of green ham weight), and an estimation of salt amount adsorbed in the lean part during the salting stages. The use of Ham Inspector™ in three processing plants qualified for the production of PDO Parma ham provided the phenotypic data and information to perform the GWAS. At present, green hams allowed to be processed into PDO Parma hams are those labeled as U, R, and O according to the EUROP grid, with a few specific exceptions [38]. In the current study, a high variability in ham lean % within U, R, and O classes was detected. In particular, the thigh lean % estimated from Ham Inspector™ was higher than the lean % of the corresponding carcasses estimated from EUROP grading. Thus, the thigh lean % given by Ham Inspector™ and the carcass lean % obtained from EUROP grading provide different information. This is anyway expected, because ham is a lean cut, with a higher lean % than that of the corresponding EUROP carcass class. The measures estimated by Ham Inspector™ about the lean-to-fat ratio of each thigh proved to be crucial to homogenously group hams during processing [6]. Processing plants showed differences for all the measured phenotypes, except for ham weight loss after the first salting. This result must be carefully evaluated as the on-field conditions of the present study did not permit to distinguish the specific effect of the processing plant, which included also the effects of the pig genetic type, farm management, and abattoir. Thus, the effect of the processing plant may be overestimated in the present study. The effect of the lean amount of green hams on the processing weight losses is underlined by the positive and significant correlation coefficients displayed in the three plants. This is in line with previous findings: weight losses are indeed known to be greater in hams obtained from animals with greater lean %, whereas the presence of inter, intramuscular and covering fat, containing less water than muscular tissue, is associated with a reduction of weight losses [2]. As can be expected, the lean % of green hams was strongly related to salt content after the first salting period and at the end of salting: this behavior is related to the higher salt and water diffusion coefficients of Fick's law in lean hams than in the fat ones [39]. Currently, the variability detected in the phenotypic traits of processed ham as a consequence of the differences in raw matter and in the production plants remains in full compliance with the tutelary guidelines of Parma hams [23].

With the aim of finding genomic regions and candidate genes associated with the green ham weight, lean %, salting losses, and contents of adsorbed salt, we used sex and slaughter day (and thus also the ham processing plant) as fixed effects in the GWAS model. GWAS indicated eight markers significant at the chromosome-wide level, and eleven with a Pc1df below the threshold of 5.00×10^{-5}. The most significant association was found between pHu and the WU_10.2_18_17949287 marker, which is located in an intergenic region of SSC18, harboring the genes *Plexin A4* (*PLXNA4*), and *Muskelin 1* (*MKLN1*). This association signal with the *PLXNA4* region could support the findings reported by Bordbar et al. [40] in Simmental beef cattle. These authors found that the bovine *PLXNA4* gene harbored 18 SNPs significantly associated with muscle development in the Simmental breed. Despite this strong association, no clear biologic evidence supporting the *PLXNA4* role in bovine muscle development was found [40]. The pHu variability was also found associated with the WU_10.2_4_91195648 marker, on SSC4. Anyway, both WU_10.2_18_17949287 and WU_10.2_4_91195648 markers showed unbalanced genotype distributions, which may have biased the association results, causing an overestimation of the marker effects.

Thigh lean % was associated with the marker H3GA0000815 located in an intronic region of the gene *T-Cell Lymphoma Invasion And Metastasis 2* (*TIAM2*). Among the identified associations, the H3GA0000815 marker showed the clearest additive effect, with the GG animals showing a higher lean % than those with the AA genotype. The lower frequency observed for the GG genotype in our samples suggests that the favorable allele G may be used in selection schemes to increase lean mass deposition in the pig breeds used for the production of PDO hams. Interestingly, the *TIAM2* gene was found in a previous study to be located in a region displaying a selective signature in a Duroc pig population [41]. This gene encodes a guanine nucleotide exchange factor with a role in intracellular signal transduction and in the regulation of cell migration and cell focal adhesions [42]. Cell migration and focal adhesions are essential steps in organogenesis, and also muscle development is known to involve a series of morphogenetic events including cell fusion, migration, and epidermal attachment [43]. Despite the fact that this result seems to agree with a previous study [41], to date, it is not possible to draw a clear hypothesis linking this gene with thigh lean % as the knowledge of the *TIAM2* gene and its roles in pig muscle development is still mostly unknown.

The variability of green ham weight, and ham weight after first salting and at the end of the salting period showed to be associated with the same markers, indicating a pleiotropic effect of these mutations. The LSM estimated for these markers were concordant among the measured traits, with the same genotypic class displaying higher estimated LSM for the weights of the fresh thigh and the ham after first salting and at the end of salting. This pattern was expected given the degree of shared variability between these three traits, as demonstrated by their high and positive phenotypic correlations, indicating that the higher the weight of the fresh thigh, the heavier are the same hams after first salting and at the end of salting period. Ham weights at the first salting and at the end of salting were significantly associated with the two markers ASGA0026341 and WU_10.2_7_118557013. An additive effect was found for both these markers, which are located in intergenic regions on SSC5 and SSC7, respectively. This is not surprising, since the literature indicates that the majority of GWAS peaks are located in non-coding or intergenic regions [44], and may therefore be a signal indicating that the found association may be due to causal mutations in closely located genes or to mutations in a still unknown gene. Among the genes located near WU_10.2_7_118557013 is *Calmodulin 1* (*CALM1*), which encodes for one of three calcium-binding calmodulin proteins. *CALM1* mediates the control of a large number of enzymes, ion channels, aquaporins, and other proteins through calcium-binding, and controls also the transport of glucose and other sugars in hepatic cells [45]. Its gene expression was also found to be downregulated in the *Longissimus* muscle of pigs with a high deposition of intramuscular fat [46], suggesting that this gene may have a role also in the metabolic pathways influencing pig meat quality.

The ham weight loss after first salting was found to be associated with ASGA0031014, on SSC7. The alleles for this marker show a significant additive effect and balanced genotype distributions in the considered sample. The most favorable genotype for this locus was GG, which displayed the lowest weight losses during processing. This mutation is an intron variant of the gene *NEDD9*, which codes for a focal adhesion protein that acts as a scaffold to regulate signaling complexes important in cell attachment, migration, and invasion [47], as well as apoptosis and the cell cycle [48]. Some studies of different authors reported that *NEDD9* is essential for the Transforming Growth Factor β (TGF-β) signaling pathway [49,50]. Moreover, members of the TGF-β superfamily can profoundly regulate mesenchymal stem cell differentiation, as well as adipogenesis and myogenesis [51,52]. Due to the involvement of *NEDD9* in TGF-β signaling, it is, therefore, possible that changes in its gene sequence may affect also TGF-β signaling and the differentiation of mesenchymal stem cells during muscle development. Furthermore, *NEDD9* is known to take part in the inhibition of primary cilia formation during embryogenesis [53]. Primary cilia are non-motile organelles that have been shown to play an important role as antennae to extracellular stimuli during embryogenesis [53], adipogenesis, and myofibrogenesis [54]. In our previous study, we found several genes related to primary cilia associated with intramuscular fat deposition [55], and *NEDD9* may take part in this complex signaling pathway related to muscle and adipose tissue development in embryogenesis. Interestingly, the marker ASGA0031014 fell into an intronic region harboring several sequences recognized by FOXO transcriptional regulators. In particular, this intronic variant is located in a site matching the motifs recognized by *FOXO1, FOXO3,* and *FOXO4* transcription regulators, suggesting that changes in this sequence may also affect the ability of those transcription regulators to recognize this binding site. This hypothesis seems to be supported in the literature, which indicated that *NEDD9* gene expression was found to be regulated by another forkhead box member (*FOXC1*) [56] and that *FOXO1* has a major role in the regulation of skeletal muscle differentiation and fiber type specification in mammals [57]. Taken together, these results suggest that ASGA0031014 may be a useful marker for the improvement of ham yield during processing. Our hypothesis needs anyway a validation with further specific studies.

In addition to these markers, other mutations were associated with the ham traits, even though they did not present significant additive effects. Among the markers associated with the ham weights at the first and at the end of the salting steps is CASI0010463, an intron variant of the *Neurexophilin 2* (*NXPH2*) gene. A Run of Homozygosity (ROH) region was found in the *NXPH2* gene in Valdostana Black Pied and Valdostana Chestnut bovine breeds [58]. This evidence seems to suggest a possible role of *NXPH2* in livestock traits related to muscle development and production efficiency. However, this gene has never been studied before in pigs and the limited knowledge of the *NXPH2* gene does not permit to reach a complete interpretation of the associations found for this gene in the present study. Another marker associated with green ham weight, ham weight after first salting, and ham weight at the end of salting is WU_10.2_14_144250775. This marker results to be unmapped in the latest release of the Ensembl database [59], while it was located at 132,664,262 bp on SSC14 in Illumina 11.1 mapping. Following the latter mapping, WU_10.2_14_144250775 is an intergenic variant. The closest genes to this marker are *Acyl-CoA Dehydrogenase Short/Branched Chain* (*ACADSB*), *H6 Family Homeobox 2* (*HMX2*), *H6 Family Homeobox 3* (*HMX3*), and *BUB3 Mitotic Checkpoint Protein* (*BUB3*). The sequence comprising *ACADSB, HMX2, HMX3,* and *BUB3* is highly conserved between mammals [60], suggesting that this region could be of primary biological importance. Anyway, no clear association exists between muscle development and deposition, and these genes. Further investigation should be dedicated to testing the role of these genes located in this SSC14 region on production traits and porcine muscle development. Also of interest is the marker ASGA0102337, an intron variant of the *GRAM Domain Containing 1B* (*GRAMD1B*) gene. This gene codes for a cholesterol transporter that mediates non-vesicular transport of cholesterol from the plasma membrane to the endoplasmic reticulum [61,62]. *GRAMD1B* gene expression in muscle was found associated with obesity in the mouse model [63], and mutations in its sequence were associated with feed efficiency in a beef cattle population with individuals from various breeds [64]. As fat deposition is important in determining salting losses and salt uptake of the green hams, mutations in the *GRAMD1B* sequence may also influence salting and maturation traits. However, the possible effect of this gene on ham quality traits needs confirmation with studies in larger samples.

5. Conclusions

To our knowledge, this is the first study describing significant associations between porcine candidate genes and ham traits, measured in a non-invasive way using a Magnetic Induction System. This on-line and non-invasive technology allows the estimation of green ham lean % and the salt content in the salted ones, on a great number of hams during processing. The GWAS identified several markers associated with the measured traits, and SNPs in candidate genes related to the neuromuscular junction, and muscle development during embryonic stages were found associated with lean % and ham weights. Among the markers associated with ham traits, the marker located in *NEDD9* could be of particular interest for further studies and for implementing selection schemes aimed at improving ham yields after the salting steps. Further studies including a greater number of hams and different processing conditions are needed to strengthen the investigated associations.

Supplementary Materials: The following are available online at https://www.mdpi.com/2076-2615/11/1/68/s1, Table S1: The Chromosome-wide thresholds for significance calculated for each chromosome; Table S2: Pearson's correlation coefficients (above the diagonal) and corresponding *p*-values (below the diagonal) between processing and analytical traits of hams (green and after 1st and at the end of salting steps) in Plant 1; Table S3: Pearson's correlation coefficients (above the diagonal) and corresponding *p*-values (below the diagonal) between processing and analytical traits of hams (green and after 1st and at the end of salting steps) in Plant 2; Table S4: Pearson's correlation coefficients (above the diagonal) and corresponding *p*-values (below the diagonal) between processing and analytical traits of hams (green and after 1st and at the end of salting steps) in Plant 3; Table S5: List of the genes in the regions flanking the markers associated with ham traits; Table S6: Results of the functional enrichment analysis performed on the list of the genes located in the regions flanking the markers associated with ham traits; Table S7: Results of the Tomtom tool with the binding sites recognized by different transcription regulators on the sequence flanking the marker ASGA0031014; Figure S1: The sequence flanking the marker ASGA0031014 (position 17) is recognized by the transcription factors (**a**) *Forkhead box O 3* (*FOXO3*; upper sequence), with the alternate allele C (or G if we consider the complementary DNA sequence) possibly changing the binding site recognized by *FOXO3* (*q*-value = 0.050); (**b**) *Forkhead box O 1* (*FOXO1*; upper sequence), with the alternate allele C (or G if we consider the complementary DNA sequence) possibly changing the binding site recognized by *FOXO1* (*q*-value = 0.074); (**c**) *Forkhead box O 4* (*FOXO4*; upper sequence), with the alternate allele C (or G if we consider the complementary DNA sequence) possibly changing the binding site recognized by *FOXO4* (*q*-value = 0.074); File S1: Tables with the top 20 markers associated with each ham trait and their complete output information obtained with GenAbel package.

Author Contributions: Conceptualization, M.Z. and R.D.; methodology, M.Z., N.S., and R.V.; formal analysis, P.Z., M.Z., N.S., and C.S.; investigation, M.Z., P.Z., N.S., B.S., C.S., R.V., and R.D.; resources, C.S., N.S., and M.Z.; data curation, P.Z., N.S., C.S., and R.D.; writing—original draft preparation, M.Z., N.S., R.D., and R.V.; writing—review and editing, M.Z., P.Z., N.S., R.D., and R.V.; supervision, R.D. and B.S.; project administration, R.V., R.D., and M.Z.; funding acquisition, R.D. and R.V. All authors have read and agreed to the published version of the manuscript.

Funding: This research was funded by the AGER CARIPLO Italian foundation, grant number 2017–2022, project "ProSuIT-Tecnologia (T) a favore (Pro) della suinicoltura italiana (Su-I)", and by AGER-Agroalimentare e ricerca: Advanced research in genomics and processing technologies for the Italian heavy pig production-Hepiget project, grant number 2011-0279.

Institutional Review Board Statement: Ethical review and approval were waived for this study, as the samples and hams used in the present study were obtained from commercial heavy pigs intended for human consumption. This study did not involve live animals.

Informed Consent Statement: Not applicable.

Data Availability Statement: The data presented in this study are available on request from the corresponding authors. The data are not publicly available due to confidentiality agreements. Supporting data can be made available to bona fide researchers subject to a non-disclosure agreement.

Acknowledgments: The authors thank Raffaele Mazza from Agrotis-Laboratorio Genetica e Servizi-Associazione Italiana Allevatori (Cremona, Italy) for performing the genotyping and for his support and help. The authors thank Illumina Technical support for providing the updated manifest file with the SNPs annotated with version 11.1 of the porcine genome. The authors thank Tania Toscani from the Consorzio del Prosciutto di Parma for her support and help, and the Consorzio del Prosciutto di Parma for co-financing the trials with Ham Inspector™ in ham processing plants.

Conflicts of Interest: The authors declare no conflict of interest. The funders had no role in the design of the study; in the collection, analyses, or interpretation of data; in the writing of the manuscript, or in the decision to publish the results.

References

1. Carni, I.M. Carne Suina e Salumi. Available online: http://www.ismeamercati.it/carni/carne-suina-salumi (accessed on 22 October 2020).
2. Bosi, P.; Russo, V. The production of the heavy pig for high quality processed products. *Ital. J. Anim. Sci.* **2004**, *3*, 309–321. [CrossRef]
3. Candek-Potokar, M.; Skrlep, M. Factors in pig production that impact the quality of dry-cured ham: A review. *Anim. Int. J. Anim. Biosci.* **2012**, *6*, 327–338. [CrossRef] [PubMed]
4. Prosciutto di Parma (Parma Ham) Protected Designation of Origin (Specifications and Dossier Pursuant to Article 4 of Council Regulation EEC no. 2081/92 Dated 14 July 1992). *Offic. J. L* **1992**, *208*, 9–14.
5. Schivazappa, C.; Virgili, R. Impact of salt levels on the sensory profile and consumer acceptance of Italian dry-cured ham. *J. Sci. Food Agric.* **2020**, *100*, 3370–3377. [CrossRef] [PubMed]
6. Pinna, A.; Saccani, G.; Schivazappa, C.; Simoncini, N.; Virgili, R. Revision of the cold processing phases to obtain a targeted salt reduction in typical Italian dry-cured ham. *Meat Sci.* **2020**, *161*, 107994. [CrossRef]
7. Fernández, A.; de Pedro, E.; Núñez, N.; Silió, L.; García-Casco, J.; Rodríguez, C. Genetic parameters for meat and fat quality and carcass composition traits in Iberian pigs. *Meat Sci.* **2003**, *64*, 405–410. [CrossRef]
8. Davoli, R.; Catillo, G.; Serra, A.; Zappaterra, M.; Zambonelli, P.; Zilio, D.M.; Steri, R.; Mele, M.; Buttazzoni, L.; Russo, V. Genetic parameters of backfat fatty acids and carcass traits in Large White pigs. *Anim. Int. J. Anim. Biosci.* **2019**, *13*, 924–932. [CrossRef]
9. Davoli, R.; Luise, D.; Mingazzini, V.; Zambonelli, P.; Braglia, S.; Serra, A.; Russo, V. Genome-wide study on intramuscular fat in Italian Large White pig breed using the PorcineSNP60 BeadChip. *J. Anim. Breed. Genet.* **2016**, *133*, 277–282. [CrossRef]
10. Davoli, R.; Schivazappa, C.; Zambonelli, P.; Braglia, S.; Rossi, A.; Virgili, R. Association study between single nucleotide polymorphisms in porcine genes and pork quality traits for fresh consumption and processing into Italian dry-cured ham. *Meat Sci.* **2017**, *126*, 73–81. [CrossRef]
11. Toldrá, F.; Flores, M.; Sanz, Y. Dry-cured ham flavour: Enzymatic generation and process influence. *Food Chem.* **1997**, *59*, 523–530. [CrossRef]
12. Davoli, R.; Zappaterra, M.; Zambonelli, P. Genome-wide association study identifies markers associated with meat ultimate pH in Duroc pigs. *Anim. Genet.* **2019**, *50*, 154–156. [CrossRef] [PubMed]
13. Zappaterra, M.; Sami, D.; Davoli, R. Association between the splice mutation g.8283C>A of the PHKG1 gene and meat quality traits in Large White pigs. *Meat Sci.* **2019**, *148*, 38–40. [CrossRef]
14. Renaville, B.; Piasentier, E.; Fan, B.; Vitale, M.; Prandi, A.; Rothschild, M.F. Candidate gene markers involved in San Daniele ham quality. *Meat Sci.* **2010**, *85*, 441–445. [CrossRef] [PubMed]
15. Fontanesi, L.; Schiavo, G.; Gallo, M.; Baiocco, C.; Galimberti, G.; Bovo, S.; Russo, V.; Buttazzoni, L. Genome-wide association study for ham weight loss at first salting in Italian Large White pigs: Towards the genetic dissection of a key trait for dry-cured ham production. *Anim. Genet.* **2017**, *48*, 103–107. [CrossRef] [PubMed]
16. Fulladosa, E.; Muñoz, I.; Serra, X.; Arnau, J.; Gou, P. X-ray absorptiometry for non-destructive monitoring of the salt uptake in bone-in raw hams during salting. *Food Control* **2015**, *47*, 37–42. [CrossRef]
17. Simoncini, N.; Virgili, R.; Schivazappa, C.; Pinna, A.; Rossi, A.; Álvarez, J. Assessment of fat and lean content in Italian heavy green hams by means of on-line non-invasive techniques. In Proceedings of the 58th International Congress of Meat Science and Technology, Montreal, QC, Canada, 12–17 August 2012; p. 4.
18. Schivazappa, C.; Virgili, R.; Simoncini, N.; Tiso, S.; Álvarez, J.; Rodríguez, J.M. Application of the magnetic induction technique for the non-destructive assessment of salt gain after the salting process of Parma ham. *Food Control* **2017**, *80*, 92–98. [CrossRef]
19. Otto, G.; Roehe, R.; Looft, H.; Thoelking, L.; Knap, P.W.; Rothschild, M.F.; Plastow, G.S.; Kalm, E. Associations of DNA markers with meat quality traits in pigs with emphasis on drip loss. *Meat Sci.* **2007**, *75*, 185–195. [CrossRef]
20. EUR-Lex—32009R1099—EN—EUR-Lex. Available online: https://eur-lex.europa.eu/eli/reg/2009/1099/oj (accessed on 28 October 2020).
21. EUR-Lex—32005R0001—EN—EUR-Lex. Available online: https://eur-lex.europa.eu/legal-content/EN/ALL/?uri=celex%3A3 2005R0001 (accessed on 28 October 2020).
22. 2014/38/EU: Commission Implementing Decision of 24 January 2014 Authorising Methods for Grading Pig Carcases in Italy (Notified under Document C(2014) 279). *Offic. J. Eur. Union* **2014**, *23*, 35–40.
23. *Commission Implementing Regulation (EU) No 1208/2013 of 25 November 2013 Approving Minor Amendments to the Specification for a Name Entered in the Register of Protected Designations of Origin and Protected Geographical Indications (Prosciutto di Parma (PDO))*; Publications Office of the European Union: Luxembourg, 2013; Volume 317.
24. Council Regulation (EEC) No 2081/92 of 14 July 1992 on the Protection of Geographical Indications and Designations of Origin for Agricultural Products and Foodstuffs. *Offic. J. L* **1992**, *208*, 1–9.
25. Parolari, G. Review: Achievements, needs and perspectives in dry-cured ham technology: The example of Parma ham/ Revisión: Avances, necesidades y perspectivas de la tecnología del jamón curado: El ejemplo del jamón de Parma. *Food Sci. Technol. Int.* **1996**, *2*, 69–78. [CrossRef]
26. Purcell, S.; Neale, B.; Todd-Brown, K.; Thomas, L.; Ferreira, M.A.R.; Bender, D.; Maller, J.; Sklar, P.; de Bakker, P.I.W.; Daly, M.J.; et al. PLINK: A Tool Set for Whole-Genome Association and Population-Based Linkage Analyses. *Am. J. Hum. Genet.* **2007**, *81*, 559–575. [CrossRef]

27. Aulchenko, Y.S.; Ripke, S.; Isaacs, A.; van Duijn, C.M. GenABEL: An R library for genome-wide association analysis. *Bioinform. Oxf. Engl.* **2007**, *23*, 1294–1296. [CrossRef] [PubMed]
28. Hardy, G.H. Mendelian proportions in a mixed population. *Science* **1908**, *28*, 49–50. [CrossRef] [PubMed]
29. Nicolazzi, E.L.; Biffani, S.; Biscarini, F.; Wengel, P.O.t.; Caprera, A.; Nazzicari, N.; Stella, A. Software solutions for the livestock genomics SNP array revolution. *Anim. Genet.* **2015**, *46*, 343–353. [CrossRef] [PubMed]
30. Burton, P.R.; Clayton, D.G.; Cardon, L.R.; Craddock, N.; Deloukas, P.; Duncanson, A.; Kwiatkowski, D.P.; McCarthy, M.I.; Ouwehand, W.H.; Samani, N.J.; et al. Genome-wide association study of 14,000 cases of seven common diseases and 3,000 shared controls. *Nature* **2007**, *447*, 661–678. [CrossRef]
31. R Core Team. *R: A Language and Environment for Statistical Computing*; R Foundation for Statistical Computing: Vienna, Austria, 2020.
32. Pinheiro, J.; Bates, D.; DebRoy, S.; Sarkar, D.; R Core Team. {nlme}: Linear and Nonlinear Mixed Effects Models; R Package Version 3.1-150. 2020. Available online: https://cran.r-project.org/web/packages/nlme/nlme.pdf (accessed on 28 October 2020).
33. Lenth, R.V. Least-Squares Means: The R Package lsmeans. *J. Stat. Softw.* **2016**, *69*, 1–33. [CrossRef]
34. Bates, D.; Mächler, M.; Bolker, B.; Walker, S. Fitting Linear Mixed-Effects Models Using lme4. *J. Stat. Softw.* **2015**, *67*, 1–48. [CrossRef]
35. Fox, J.; Weisberg, S. *An R Companion to Applied Regression*; SAGE Publications, Inc: Thousand Oaks, CA, USA, 2011; ISBN 978-1-4129-7514-8.
36. Baker, M. Quantitative data: Learning to share. *Nat. Methods* **2012**, *9*, 39–41. [CrossRef]
37. Gupta, S.; Stamatoyannopoulos, J.A.; Bailey, T.L.; Noble, W.S. Quantifying similarity between motifs. *Genome Biol.* **2007**, *8*, R24. [CrossRef]
38. Istituto Parma Qualità. Istituto Nord Est Qualità Impiego delle Nuove Equazioni e Criteri di Accettazione delle Carcasse Suine- Circolare Unificata N. 11/2014; 2014. Available online: http://www.parmaqualita.it/IPQ/datiute/6/112014 CRITERIACCETTABILITACARCASSE.pdf (accessed on 28 October 2020).
39. Harkouss, R.; Chevarin, C.; Daudin, J.-D.; Sicard, J.; Mirade, P.-S. Development of a multi-physical finite element-based model that predicts water and salt transfers, proteolysis and water activity during the salting and post-salting stages of the dry-cured ham process. *J. Food Eng.* **2018**, *218*, 69–79. [CrossRef]
40. Bordbar, F.; Jensen, J.; Zhu, B.; Wang, Z.; Xu, L.; Chang, T.; Xu, L.; Du, M.; Zhang, L.; Gao, H.; et al. Identification of muscle-specific candidate genes in Simmental beef cattle using imputed next generation sequencing. *PLoS ONE* **2019**, *14*, e0223671. [CrossRef] [PubMed]
41. Diao, S.; Luo, Y.; Ma, Y.; Deng, X.; He, Y.; Gao, N.; Zhang, H.; Li, J.; Chen, Z.; Zhang, Z. Genome-wide detection of selective signatures in a Duroc pig population. *J. Integr. Agric.* **2018**, *17*, 2528–2535. [CrossRef]
42. Rooney, C.; White, G.; Nazgiewicz, A.; Woodcock, S.A.; Anderson, K.I.; Ballestrem, C.; Malliri, A. The Rac activator STEF (Tiam2) regulates cell migration by microtubule-mediated focal adhesion disassembly. *EMBO Rep.* **2010**, *11*, 292–298. [CrossRef] [PubMed]
43. Maartens, A.P.; Brown, N.H. The many faces of cell adhesion during Drosophila muscle development. *Dev. Biol.* **2015**, *401*, 62–74. [CrossRef]
44. Watanabe, K.; Taskesen, E.; van Bochoven, A.; Posthuma, D. Functional mapping and annotation of genetic associations with FUMA. *Nat. Commun.* **2017**, *8*, 1826. [CrossRef]
45. Chen, Z.; Ding, L.; Yang, W.; Wang, J.; Chen, L.; Chang, Y.; Geng, B.; Cui, Q.; Guan, Y.; Yang, J. Hepatic Activation of the FAM3C-HSF1-CaM Pathway Attenuates Hyperglycemia of Obese Diabetic Mice. *Diabetes* **2017**, *66*, 1185–1197. [CrossRef]
46. Hamill, R.M.; McBryan, J.; McGee, C.; Mullen, A.M.; Sweeney, T.; Talbot, A.; Cairns, M.T.; Davey, G.C. Functional analysis of muscle gene expression profiles associated with tenderness and intramuscular fat content in pork. *Meat Sci.* **2012**, *92*, 440–450. [CrossRef]
47. Zhong, J.; Baquiran, J.B.; Bonakdar, N.; Lees, J.; Ching, Y.W.; Pugacheva, E.; Fabry, B.; O'Neill, G.M. NEDD9 Stabilizes Focal Adhesions, Increases Binding to the Extra-Cellular Matrix and Differentially Effects 2D versus 3D Cell Migration. *PLoS ONE* **2012**, *7*, e35058. [CrossRef]
48. Semelakova, M.; Grauzam, S.; Betadthunga, P.; Tiedeken, J.; Coaxum, S.; Neskey, D.M.; Rosenzweig, S.A. Vimentin and Non-Muscle Myosin IIA are Members of the Neural Precursor Cell Expressed Developmentally Down-Regulated 9 (NEDD9) Interactome in Head and Neck Squamous Cell Carcinoma Cells. *Transl. Oncol.* **2018**, *12*, 49–61. [CrossRef]
49. Vogel, T.; Ahrens, S.; Büttner, N.; Krieglstein, K. Transforming Growth Factor β Promotes Neuronal Cell Fate of Mouse Cortical and Hippocampal Progenitors In Vitro and In Vivo: Identification of Nedd9 as an Essential Signaling Component. *Cereb. Cortex* **2010**, *20*, 661–671. [CrossRef]
50. Omata, Y.; Nakamura, J.; Koyama, T.; Yasui, T.; Hirose, J.; Izawa, N.; Matsumoto, T.; Imai, Y.; Seo, S.; Kurokawa, M.; et al. Identification of Nedd9 as a TGF-β-Smad2/3 Target Gene Involved in RANKL-Induced Osteoclastogenesis by Comprehensive Analysis. *PLoS ONE* **2016**, *11*, e0157992. [CrossRef] [PubMed]
51. Ignotz, R.A.; Massagué, J. Type beta transforming growth factor controls the adipogenic differentiation of 3T3 fibroblasts. *Proc. Natl. Acad. Sci. USA* **1985**, *82*, 8530–8534. [CrossRef] [PubMed]
52. Rebbapragada, A.; Benchabane, H.; Wrana, J.L.; Celeste, A.J.; Attisano, L. Myostatin Signals through a Transforming Growth Factor β-Like Signaling Pathway To Block Adipogenesis. *Mol. Cell. Biol.* **2003**, *23*, 7230–7242. [CrossRef] [PubMed]

53. Bangs, F.K.; Schrode, N.; Hadjantonakis, A.-K.; Anderson, K.V. Lineage specificity of primary cilia in the mouse embryo. *Nat. Cell Biol.* **2015**, *17*, 113–122. [CrossRef] [PubMed]

54. Arrighi, N.; Lypovetska, K.; Moratal, C.; Giorgetti-Peraldi, S.; Dechesne, C.A.; Dani, C.; Peraldi, P. The primary cilium is necessary for the differentiation and the maintenance of human adipose progenitors into myofibroblasts. *Sci. Rep.* **2017**, *7*, 15248. [CrossRef] [PubMed]

55. Zappaterra, M.; Gioiosa, S.; Chillemi, G.; Zambonelli, P.; Davoli, R. Muscle transcriptome analysis identifies genes involved in ciliogenesis and the molecular cascade associated with intramuscular fat content in Large White heavy pigs. *PLoS ONE* **2020**, *15*, e0233372. [CrossRef]

56. Shagisultanova, E.; Gaponova, A.V.; Gabbasov, R.; Nicolas, E.; Golemis, E.A. Preclinical and clinical studies of the NEDD9 scaffold protein in cancer and other diseases. *Gene* **2015**, *567*, 1–11. [CrossRef]

57. Xu, M.; Chen, X.; Chen, D.; Yu, B.; Huang, Z. FoxO1: A novel insight into its molecular mechanisms in the regulation of skeletal muscle differentiation and fiber type specification. *Oncotarget* **2016**, *8*, 10662–10674. [CrossRef]

58. Mastrangelo, S.; Jemaa, S.B.; Ciani, E.; Sottile, G.; Moscarelli, A.; Boussaha, M.; Montedoro, M.; Pilla, F.; Cassandro, M. Genome-wide detection of signatures of selection in three Valdostana cattle populations. *J. Anim. Breed. Genet.* **2020**, *137*, 609–621. [CrossRef]

59. rs343048625 (SNP)—Explore This Variant—Sus_scrofa—Ensembl Genome Browser 101. Available online: http://uswest.ensembl.org/Sus_scrofa/Variation/Explore?v=rs343048625;vdb=variation (accessed on 12 October 2020).

60. England, S.J.; Cerda, G.A.; Kowalchuk, A.; Sorice, T.; Grieb, G.; Lewis, K.E. Hmx3a does not require its homeodomain for its essential functions in spinal cord, ear and lateral line development. *bioRxiv* **2020**, *68*. [CrossRef]

61. Sandhu, J.; Li, S.; Fairall, L.; Pfisterer, S.G.; Gurnett, J.E.; Xiao, X.; Weston, T.A.; Vashi, D.; Ferrari, A.; Orozco, J.L.; et al. Aster Proteins Facilitate Nonvesicular Plasma Membrane to ER Cholesterol Transport in Mammalian Cells. *Cell* **2018**, *175*, 514–529.e20. [CrossRef] [PubMed]

62. Kutyavin, V.I.; Chawla, A. Aster: A New Star in Cholesterol Trafficking. *Cell* **2018**, *175*, 307–309. [CrossRef] [PubMed]

63. Farber, C.; Aten, J.; Farber, E.; Vera, V.; Gularte-Mérida, R.; Islas-Trejo, A.; Wen, P.; Horvath, S.; Lucero, M.; Lusis, A.; et al. Genetic dissection of a major mouse obesity QTL (Carfhg2): Integration of gene expression and causality modeling. *Physiol. Genomics* **2009**, *37*, 294–302. [CrossRef]

64. Serão, N.V.; González-Peña, D.; Beever, J.E.; Faulkner, D.B.; Southey, B.R.; Rodriguez-Zas, S.L. Single nucleotide polymorphisms and haplotypes associated with feed efficiency in beef cattle. *BMC Genet.* **2013**, *14*, 94. [CrossRef] [PubMed]

MDPI

St. Alban-Anlage 66

4052 Basel

Switzerland

Tel. +41 61 683 77 34

Fax +41 61 302 89 18

www.mdpi.com

Animals Editorial Office

E-mail: animals@mdpi.com

www.mdpi.com/journal/animals

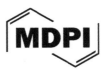

Lightning Source UK Ltd.
Milton Keynes UK
UKHW051330110821
388628UK00003B/177